Business Basics for your Healthcare Practice

Neil Baum • Marc J. Kahn

Business Basics for your Healthcare Practice

Third Edition

Springer

Neil Baum
Urology
Tulane University
New Orleans, LA, USA

Marc J. Kahn
Internal Medicine
University of Nevada, Las Vegas
Las Vegas, NV, USA

ISBN 978-3-032-25240-1 ISBN 978-3-032-25241-8 (eBook)
https://doi.org/10.1007/978-3-032-25241-8

Originally published with the title: The Business of Building and Managing a Healthcare Practice

This Springer imprint is published by the registered company Springer Nature Switzerland AG
The registered company address is: Gewerbestrasse 11, 6330 Cham, Switzerland

The authors dedicate this book to their teachers, patients, and their students.

Preface

Ten Reasons to Read This Book

If you are a medical student, a doctor in training, or a doctor already in practice, you have likely experienced problems that are taking the focus away from patient care and toward potentially mind-numbing administrative tasks and computer data entry. It has been said that the average doctor spends 1–2 hours per day in nonclinical activities, and several hours each evening completing patients' medical records. In spite of these distractions, medicine remains an attractive career choice and the number of applicants to medical schools has not decreased, even though graduating physicians have an average of over $200,000 of debt.

Most physicians have little to no business skills, as standard medical education typically does not equip trainees with this important aspect of the practice of medicine. Physicians are sent out to practice with a strong knowledge of diagnosing and treating medical conditions, but most doctors can't read a profit-and-loss statement for the practice's finances or complete a financial statement for a bank loan. This book is not intended to make you a financial wizard or a number-crunching managing partner of your practice, but the book's purpose is to provide you with basic business principles that will help you to understand the financial landscape of your practice.

Even though there is a trend among young physicians toward employment by a hospital or a large group practice rather than solo or a small practice, physicians will still need to understand certain metrics of business performance and need to know what to do if the numbers are trending in the wrong direction.

These are ten reasons why doctors need to understand basic business practices:

1. Doctors are in an industry where there is a growing demand, a declining supply, and formidable barriers to entry or to join this lofty profession. Every other business or service industry envies this type of economic advantage. If you feel that the healthcare industry is in trouble, imagine working in an industry whose demand is declining, such as selling digital cameras or print newspapers. Can you imagine working in an industry or profession if there is an abundance of competitors who can provide the same services that you do at a much lower cost?

Can you imagine a profession where almost anyone can quickly obtain a license or permission to practice, with minimal or no barriers to entry? The dynamics of our profession assure us that there will always be work and future employment, and if we learn to understand the business side of medical practice, we can enjoy a successful, profitable practice.

2. Physicians have instant status in their community. If you have MD after your name, you have credibility that is immediately accepted by your patients. For example, if a patient comes to a doctor they have never met before, they will divulge the deepest secrets of their past medical history, including menstrual history, bowel habits, and even their sexual history. No other professional can confer instant credibility on new members. We should never take that for granted and always uphold a high standard of confidentiality, ethical behavior, and never flaunt our lofty status with our patients.
3. Physicians are in the top 5% of wage earners in the United States. Many of our nonmedical colleagues are complaining about their incomes. If we compare the average physician's salary with those for all other jobs or professions, our salaries are at the top. Also, most of the other high paying professions do not have the same upside potential that we do. The healthcare profession offers some physicians the opportunity to earn 2–3 times the average physician salary.
4. Physicians are fortunate not to be compelled to retire at a certain age. Since medical practice is less physically demanding than many other occupations, many physicians can work into their 80s if they so desire. A national survey of 1,500 physicians by Wells Fargo found that 25% of respondents will need to work until at least age 80 before having the income in a retirement plan to retire comfortably. Respondents in this survey were between 20 and 70 years old, with incomes ranging from $75,000 to $100,000. Their median retirement savings were only $350,000, which is unlikely to support the standard of living in retirement. Many physicians feel they will need at least $2 million to comfortably retire. Physicians who didn't plan adequately for retirement also have the option of continuing to practice part-time for as long as they choose to work.
5. Doctors, compared to many other professions, have a wonderful lifestyle. The practice of medicine affords most physicians the ability to spend time with their families, take 2–4 weeks of vacation each year, and work 8–10 hour days. Except when physicians are on call, they have reasonable lifestyle choices. Many younger physicians today are opting to work fewer hours per week, even if it means a lower income. Doctors can select their geographic location. Unlike many other occupations that have geographic limitations on where workers can live, or have the possibility of sudden transfer at the whim of a superior, physicians can work nearly anywhere they choose.
6. There are many career opportunities for physicians. Doctors can elect to work for themselves, join a large group practice, or be employed by a hospital or academic healthcare center. While employed physicians must answer to a boss, starting salaries have increased, and these doctors

function relatively independently compared to other career professionals employed by large groups, companies, or organizations.

7. Doctors can carve or sculpt the exact kind of practice that makes them most comfortable. If a doctor is interested in seeing only a certain diagnosis or providing only a limited number of treatment options, they can easily do so. If a doctor wants to see certain kinds of patients, such as geriatric or pediatric patients, this can be easily arranged. If the doctor wishes to see patients who speak only languages other than English, this, too, can easily be achieved. If you want only cash-paying patients, or a concierge practice where a limited number of patients pay an annual fee for 24/7 access to your practice, then this is also within the realm of possibility. There are only a few other professions that afford such choices.
8. For the most part, physicians are told almost daily how terrific they are. There isn't a day that goes by that most physicians don't receive a compliment or accolade about the care they provide. If ego satisfaction and gratification are your drivers, you have selected the right profession. One of us (NHB) has saved complimentary letters from patients and, with the patient's permission, has placed the original letters in a scrapbook that is in the reception area. After nearly 30 years in practice, NHB has 10 leatherbound volumes containing all the letters received from satisfied patients. Also, collecting compliments has become more important than ever, as they can be posted on your website and submitted to online reputation management programs to balance the occasional negative online report from a dissatisfied patient. Certainly, if you have 10–20 positive responses, it will easily dilute the occasional negative note and will not significantly impact your online reputation rating.
9. The practice of medicine provides job security and a future of guaranteed employment. It is a sad commentary that so many graduating lawyers are unable to find a job practicing law. This is not the case with American medical doctors. Everyone who graduates from medical school and a training program can find a job. It may not be a perfect job, but it is nonetheless a profession in demand and will certainly offer job security. Even with artificial intelligence (AI) having a role in both clinical and non-clinical aspects of healthcare, AI will not replace physicians.
10. Even though physicians face the challenge of declining reimbursements and higher overhead costs, such is the case with many careers. These same challenges exist across every industry and profession. These challenges in other industries have led to extinction because competition has created ways to do the same thing either better or more cheaply. Companies, organizations, and practices have done so by becoming more efficient and productive. Ultimately, they have done things better. Healthcare is one of the industries that has focused on increasing efficiency, lowering operating costs, and becoming more productive. This presents an opportunity for improving quality, preserving patient satisfaction, and, yes, improving the bottom line, i.e., increasing productivity.

Despite the hardships and detractors associated with modern healthcare, we have much to be thankful for. Those working in other industries have their lists of complaints, but they are often powerless to make changes. If employees are members of a large organization, there are many layers of bureaucracy to navigate to make changes. Doctors enjoy the opportunity to have significant control and the tools to implement change, and to tweak our practices to improve the services that we provide to our patients. This is especially true if the doctor understands the basic principles of business. If we put our problems and complaints with modern medicine on one side of a balance scale and then compare those issues and concerns to the benefits of being a doctor, we will find that scale tips heavily on the pluses, and we should be thankful that we are physicians and that we can understand and implement basic business concepts to have successful, profitable, and enjoyable practices.

New Orleans, LA, USA Neil Baum
Las Vegas, NV, USA Marc J. Kahn

Contents

1 Why Doctors Need to Consider Medicine a Business 1
Why Do We Become Physicians? 3
The Three Stages of Medical Career 4
Stage 1: Age 20–39—Time and Energy, but No Money 5
Stage 2: Age 40–59—Money and Energy, but No Time 5
Stage 3: Age 60 and Beyond—Money and Time, but No Energy 5
Why Doctors Need to Understand the Basic Principles of Business? 6
Bottom Line 6
References 7

2 Time Value of Money 9
Back to the Case 11
References 12

3 Basic Accounting and Interpretation of Financial Statements ... 13
Basic Accounting 13
Back to the Case 16
Reference 17

4 Contracts and Negotiation 19
Contracts 19
Duration and Geographical Scope 21
Termination and Enforcement 21
Ownership of Patient Files 21
Ownership and Business Transactions 21
Negotiation and Review 22
Negotiation 22
Back to the Case 23

5 Basic Personal Finance and Investing 25
Back to the Case 29
References 30

6 Organized Medicine 31
History of Organized Medicine in the United States 31
What Are the Reasons to Consider Joining Organized Medicine? 32
Back to the Case 35

7 Transitioning from Training to Private Practice 37
Credentialing with Insurance Companies 41
Contracting with Insurance Companies 41
Use of Technology 42
Suggestions for Getting Started 43
Find a Mentor 43
Learn How to Write or Create an Effective Referral Letter 44
Meet the VIPs 44
Meet Other Physicians 44
The Buddy System 44
Contact Nonphysicians 45
Especially for Surgeons 45
Keep in Touch 45
Pharmaceutical Contacts 45
Setting Fees 45
Take a Vacation 46
Back to Neurosurgeon Phil 46
Bottom Line 46
Appendix: Practice Transition List 47
References 52

8 Managing Student Debt 53
Back to Case 55
References 56

9 Obtaining and Maintaining Referrals from Physicians and Other Sources 57
Facts of Life 68
Appendix 70
Exhibit 12–1 Boilerplate "Lazy Person's Referral Letter" 70
Exhibit 12–2 Example of a Birthday Card Sent to Male Colleagues 71
Exhibit 12–3 Sample Letter for Starting a Journal Club Network 73

10 Branding Your Medical Practice: How to Make Your Practice Distinctive and Unique 75
What Is Branding? 76
Benefits of Branding 77
Getting Started to Brand Your Practice 77
Displaying Your Brand 79
Kaila's Story 80
Bottom Line 80

11 Legal Considerations in Hiring and Firing of Healthcare Staff 81
Finding the Match Made in Heaven 81
Screening Applicants 82

The Interview Process 82
Advice on Requesting References 84
Rochelle's Story 85
Bottom Line on Hiring 85
Ready, Aim, Fire! Tactfully Terminating an Employee 85
Case of Terminating Theresa 85
Termination of Employees—Dot Your *I's* and Cross Your *T's* 86
Importance of Documentation 88
Follow Up on the Termination of Theresa 89
Bottom Line on Hiring and Firing 89
Reference 90

12 Malpractice: What You Need to Know to Stay Out of Trouble 91
Types of Malpractice Insurance 91
Finding a Malpractice Carrier 92
To Broker or Not to Broker 93
Bottom Line 93
Reference 94

13 Mid-Level Providers and Use of Scribes to Improve Efficiency and Productivity 95
Who Are the Mid-Level Providers? 95
Where Are MLPs Working? 95
Compensation for MLPs 96
Outcomes and Liability of MLPs 97
Credentialing an MLP 97
Where Do MLPs Come from 97
Do You Need an MLP? 97
Benefits of MLPs 98
How Does the Scribe Work? 99
The Economics of a Scribe 99
Case of Cassandra 101
Bottom Line 101
References 101

14 Team Building for Healthcare Practices 103
Effective Staff Meetings 104
Start Positive 105
Stimulating Staff Involvement 105
The Morning Huddle 106
Practice Retreat [*6*] 107
Practice Retreat Goals and Objectives 107
Retreat Preparation 108
Practice Retreat Facilitation 108
Practice Retreat Objectives 109
Bottom Line 110
References 110

15 Effective and Ethical Marketing of Your Practice 111
Using Social Media 111
Examples of Social Media and Ethical Marketing 112
LinkedIn 112
Facebook 112
X (Previously Twitter) 113
Blogging 113
Getting Started 113
YouTube for Medical Practices 114
Getting Started on YouTube 114
Video Cornerstone of Today's Healthcare Social Strategy 115
TikTok 115
Doximity 116
Instagram 116
QR Codes 116
Sammy's Experience with Social Media 117
References 117

16 One-Page Marketing Plan 119
The Circus and Marketing 119
First Component of the before Phase of the One-Page Marketing Plan 121
Second Component of the Before Phase of the One-Page Marketing Plan 122
Third Component of Phase 1: Reaching Potential Patients Using Social Media 123
Delivering a World-Class Patient Experience 127
Increasing Patient Lifetime Value 128
Orchestrating and Stimulating Referrals 129
Case of Dr. Mendoza 130
References 130

17 Crisis Management 131
Back to Ben and the Hurricane 134
References 134

18 Managing Burnout 135
Definition of Burnout 135
Causes of Burnout 136
Symptoms of Burnout 137
Solutions for Burnout 137
Back to the Case: Lancelot 138
References 139

19 Practice Divorce: Painless Separation from Your Partners 141
References 146

20 Telemedicine 147
Getting Started 147
Selecting a Video Platform 148
Testing It Out and Obtaining Feedback 148

Streaming Online Workflow . . . 149
Influences on Practice Workflow. . . . 149
Telemedicine and the Coronavirus . . . 149
Cost and Complexity. . . . 150
Licensing. . . . 151
Informed Consent . . . 151
Liability Insurance . . . 152
Privacy. . . . 152
Compensation for Telemedicine . . . 152
Virtual Services for Medicare Patients . . . 153
Medicare Telehealth Visits . . . 153
Virtual Check-Ins . . . 153
Using Triangulation . . . 154
Which CPT Codes Should I Use?. . . . 155
Some Final Billing and Coding Advice . . . 156
An Example . . . 156
Using the GT Modifier . . . 156
Modifier 95 . . . 156
Back to the Case . . . 157
References. . . . 157

21 Enhancing Patient Medication Compliance . . . 159
Abner and Drug-Drug Interactions . . . 159
Influencers of Medication Adherence . . . 160
Abner and Compliance . . . 162
References. . . . 163

22 Online Reputation Management . . . 165
Ethically Creating Positive Reviews . . . 166
Managing Negative Reviews. . . . 167
References. . . . 168

23 Surveying Your Practice: Cost-Effective Methods of Identifying the Needs and Wants of Your Patients . . . 169
What to Ask. . . . 170
Whom to Include. . . . 171
Customizing the Survey . . . 171
Implementing the Survey . . . 171
Tabulating the Results. . . . 171
Using the Results . . . 171
Focus Groups . . . 172
Invitations and Reminders . . . 172
Running the Meeting. . . . 174
Follow-Up . . . 174
Suggestion Box . . . 174
Survey Your Peers . . . 175
Asking the Platinum Question . . . 176
Follow-Up on Reginald. . . . 176
References. . . . 177

24 The Use of AI/GPT-4 and Its Implementation into Any Medical Practice . . . 179
What Is GPT-4? . . . 179
History of Innovation and GPT-4 . . . 180
How Does GPT-4 Work? . . . 180
Digitalizing the Doctor-Patient Encounter, Going "Scribe-less" . . . 181
Prior Authorization (PA) Obtained in Minutes, Not Hours . . . 193
Managing Negative Online Reviews . . . 196
How to Write a Job Description for Positions Available in the Office . . . 201
Creating an Informed Consent . . . 201
Provide FAQs for the Common Conditions Seen in the Office . . . 206
Create Blogs for Social Media Sites . . . 210
Creating Patient Education Materials on Tests, Procedures, and Proper Use of Medications . . . 213
Obtain Proper Coding of the Encounter, Procedures, and Tests . . . 216
Request for Summarizing Medical Articles in the Literature . . . 217
Explanation of Benefits (EOB) . . . 218
Use of the Prompt Generator to Enhance the Results of GPT-4 . . . 220
Caveats on GPT-4 . . . 221
Mistakes or Hallucinations . . . 221
Fact-Check AI Content . . . 223
Ethical Concerns of GPT-4 . . . 223
Tanya's Experience with GPT-4 . . . 224
References . . . 225

25 Improving the Health of Populations of Patients . . . 227
Than's Case . . . 229
References . . . 229

26 Concierge Medicine . . . 231
What Is Concierge Medicine? . . . 231
Benefits of Concierge Medicine to Patients . . . 234
What Are the Advantages to Physicians? . . . 234
Getting Started with Concierge Medicine . . . 234
References . . . 236

27 Academic Careers . . . 237
Tenure or Not? . . . 239
Back to the Case . . . 240
References . . . 241

28 The Role of Private Equity . . . 243
Back to the Case . . . 245
References . . . 245

29 Nonclinical Careers . . . 247
MBA . . . 247
MPH . . . 247
MHA . . . 248

MMM ... 248
PhD ... 248
Careers in the Pharmaceutical Industry ... 248
Careers in Consulting ... 249
Careers in Public Health ... 249
Careers in Hospital Administration ... 249
Careers in Academic Administration ... 249
Back to the Case ... 250

30 Five Numbers You Need to Know ... 251
Charges and Receipts ... 251
RVUs ... 252
Accounts Receivable ... 252
Charge Lag ... 253
Denials ... 253
Bottom Line on Business Metrics ... 253

31 Future of Medicine ... 255
Future Changes in Reimbursement ... 257
Future Importance of Medical Quality Assessment ... 258
Future Outcome Metrics ... 259
Back to Case @Rayco ... 259
References ... 259

32 Final Message on the Business of Medicine ... 261
Reference ... 262

Index ... 263

1 Why Doctors Need to Consider Medicine a Business

Case Study: Sally

Sally, a PGY-3 internal medicine resident, spent a rotation with an internist in private practice. She often accompanied him to the doctor's dining room. She heard many doctors complain about decreasing reimbursements, rising overhead, additional government regulations, increasing paperwork, difficulty embracing new technology, increase in nonclinical administrative tasks such as prior authorization, the issue of burnout, and a loss of balance between their professional and personal lives. She seldom heard doctors talk about the joys and benefits of becoming a doctor. She started second-guessing her decision to becoming a physician. This book is not meant to discourage you but to reassure you that you have made an excellent decision to join one of the greatest and most enjoyable professions on this planet. However, to have that enjoyment, it will be necessary to have a modicum of business skills that you probably didn't receive as a medical student.

Physicians who aren't good at business won't survive. —Russel J, *Washington Post*, May 10, 2010.

Let's begin with the topic of becoming a doctor to achieve wealth. Achieving wealth is probably the worst reason to choose medicine as a career. If you compare the incomes of United Parcel Service (UPS) truck drivers and physicians, you will see that achieving wealth is not a viable reason to become a physician. This revealing graph (Fig. 1.1, using a figure from the first edition) shows that a UPS truck driver enters the workforce and begins to earn money at the age of 18. However, a physician usually incurs debt for 8–10 years and enters the workforce around age 30. Therefore, it takes a physician nearly 17 years to equal the accumulated wealth of a UPS truck driver.

Now consider that if the UPS truck driver worked the same hours as a physician—60–70 h a week—and received overtime pay, it would take nearly 24 years for the physician to equal the income of a UPS truck driver.

Any downsides for a doctor? The UPS driver is unlikely to receive a compliment about the delivery they just completed. Whereas the physician is likely to receive multiple warm fuzzies (compliments) every day in practice.

The UPS driver, who drives and delivers packages 6–8 h a day, is probably bored after a few hours in the truck, which may not have air conditioning. However, a physician has a variety of activities, and no day or patient is ever the same. Boredom is never an issue in healthcare.

N. Baum, M. J. Kahn, *Business Basics for your Healthcare Practice*,
https://doi.org/10.1007/978-3-032-25241-8_1

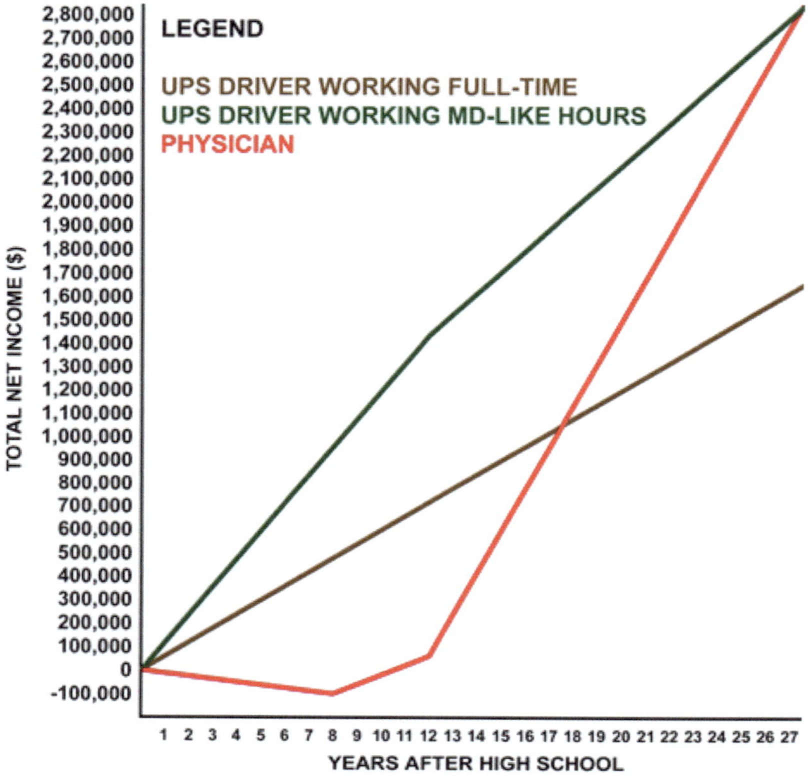

Fig. 1.1 Salary of UPS truck driver (brown line and green line) versus physician salary (red line)

The UPS driver is lifting heavy boxes all day and is at risk of early-onset back injury due to the daily heavy lifting they must do. Back pain is usually not considered an occupational hazard for physicians. (Exceptions are back and neck pain in interventional radiologists and cardiovascular surgeons.)

Take it from the scenario of the doctor versus the UPS truck driver, who can readily see that young men and women do not decide to become doctors for financial reasons. If we wanted to become wealthy quickly, we might consider becoming UPS truck drivers!

Nearly every physician who decides to become a doctor understands that they will have almost $250,000 of debt that will have to be repaid with interest [1]; and that they will have to get up in the middle of the night to go to work to care for sick patients; that they risk litigation and lawsuits during their career, and that will defer gratification and accumulation of wealth for many years.

Yet, thousands of bright, talented young men and women will enter the healthcare profession, and applications to medical schools are at an all-time high. We become doctors because we truly have a calling. We want to help people not only get well, but also stay well and avoid becoming sick, thereby reducing the need for doctor visits. We become physicians because we enjoy the gratification from patients who thank us every day for all that we do to make them better or keep them well. We don't believe there is another profession that offers such daily feedback from its customers or clients.

For the most part, physicians love what they do, and money is not the primary driver for joining the exclusive club of healthcare providers. However, this choice of profession does not negate the fact that we are small business owners and must be concerned with the business aspects of our practices, as well as be good clinical doctors.

Today, there are MBA/MD programs that provide business skills; however, most young physicians seldom enter medicine with the intention of becoming a businessman or woman. But nearly all doctors say they need practical, real-world guidance to run the business component of their practice. This book is for medical students, residents, fellows, and newly minted doctors (5–10 years in practice) to fill the void in most medical training programs. That void consists of providing the business skills necessary to become complete doctors.

Why Do We Become Physicians?

Doctors are in a field with a growing demand, as nearly 11,000 Americans turn 65 every day, and these Baby Boomers will need healthcare [2]. Along with the formidable barriers to entry, there are large numbers of physicians retiring, thus creating a decrease in the supply of physicians [3]. Every other industry or profession would envy this supply–demand advantage. If you believe healthcare is difficult, imagine working in an industry such as digital cameras or print newspapers. Can you imagine working in a profession for which demand is declining, where there is an oversupply of competitors, or if almost anyone can gain access to the field with minimal or no barriers to entry? The economic dynamics in our profession assure us that there will always be work and future employment.

Doctors have instant status as soon as the initials "M.D." or "D.O." appear after their name. With these two initials following your name, you immediately gain credibility with your patients. Doctors should never take this instant status for granted. For example, if a patient sees a doctor for the first time, they will divulge the deepest secrets of their medical history, including urinary symptoms, bowel habits, and even their sexual history. No other profession guarantees its young members such instant credibility. Doctors must uphold a high standard of confidentiality and ethical behavior and should never take their lofty status with patients for granted.

Medical doctors are in the top 5% of wage earners in the United States. If we compare the average physician's salary with those of other jobs, our incomes are at the top of the income chart. Additionally, most of the other salaries in the rare top 5% do not have the same upside potential as physicians [4].

Some successful physicians earn two to three times the average physician's salary [5].

Physicians are fortunate not to be compelled to retire at a certain age. Because the practice of medicine is not physically demanding, many physicians can continue working into their 80 s if they so desire, as most hospitals and groups do not have mandatory retirement policies. Only recently have older doctors, especially aging surgeons, been asked to submit a voluntary evaluation and consider accepting an assistant for specific surgical procedures [6].

Doctors, compared with many other professionals, have a wonderful lifestyle. The practice of medicine allows most men and women to spend time with their families, taking 2–4 weeks of vacation each year and having the option of working 8- to 10-h days. This book will provide numerous examples of becoming more efficient and productive, allowing doctors to be home for dinner with their families. Except for the hours when physicians are on call, they have a reasonable lifestyle. Younger physicians today are opting to work fewer hours per week, even if it means a lower income. Doctors can also select a geographic location and the type of practice they wish to have, a choice that is not as readily available to other professionals. Many career choices have geographic limitations regarding where employees can live or are at risk of suddenly being transferred anywhere at the whim of a superior. Still, physicians can work almost anywhere they choose. They can determine where they would like to live before starting their careers.

There are more opportunities for physicians than in other professions, especially for those entering practice within 7 years of graduation from training programs. Doctors can choose to work independently, join an extensive group practice, or be employed by a hospital or academic healthcare center. Although employed physicians must answer to a superior, starting salaries for employed physicians have increased, and they function relatively independently compared to other types of professionals employed by a large group, company, or organization.

This book reveals how young doctors can sculpt the kind of practice they wish to have. Doctors can tailor their practice to the exact type that makes them most comfortable. If a doctor is interested in seeing only patients with specific diagnoses or providing only a limited number of treatment options, they can easily do so. If the doctor wishes to see patients who speak a language other than English, this can be easily achieved. Suppose you only want patients who pay cash or are interested in establishing a concierge practice, where a limited number of patients pay an annual fee for 24/7 access to your practice. In that case, this is also a possibility.

There isn't a day that goes by that most physicians don't receive a compliment or accolade about the care they provide. Most physicians hear almost daily how terrific they are, unlike the UPS driver. If ego satisfaction and gratification are your primary motivators, you have chosen the right profession.

The practice of medicine offers job security and a promising future with guaranteed employment opportunities. Everyone who graduates from medical school and a training program can find a job. It may not be a perfect job, but it is a profession in demand and will undoubtedly provide a future of job security. It is a sad commentary that so many graduating lawyers cannot find a job practicing law and have thousands of dollars of debt [7].

Even though we face the challenge of declining reimbursements and higher overhead costs, a different career track wouldn't have eliminated these detractors. These same challenges exist in every industry and every profession. These challenges in other industries have resulted in extinction because competition has created ways to use robots and artificial intelligence to do the same things, either better or more cost-effectively. Companies, organizations, and medical practices have done so because they have found ways to be more efficient and productive.

Ultimately, they have done things better and more efficiently. Healthcare is one of the industries that focuses on creating greater efficiencies and lowering operating costs, thereby becoming more efficient and productive, while preserving patient satisfaction and improving clinical outcomes. This presents an opportunity to improve quality, maintain patient satisfaction, and, yes, enhance the bottom line (i.e., increase productivity).

Despite all the obstacles and detractors associated with modern healthcare, doctors have much to be thankful for. Those working in other industries have their lists of complaints, but they are often powerless to make changes because they are neither owners nor partners in the business. If physicians are members of a large organization, then numerous layers of bureaucracy must be navigated to implement changes. Doctors enjoy the opportunity to have significant control and the tools to implement change and refine our practices to improve the services we provide to our patients. If we put our problems and complaints with modern medicine on a scale and weigh those issues and concerns against the benefits of being a doctor, in that case, we will find that the scale weighs heavily in favor of the pluses, and we should be thankful to be a member of this wonderful profession.

The Three Stages of Medical Career

Every physician experiences three distinct career stages, each associated with its own set of challenges and adventures. Unfortunately, there are no courses in medical school and postgraduate training on navigating the three stages of a physician's career. Although most readers of this book will be in the first stage, it is essential to understand all three stages to carefully manage each one and achieve enjoyment and success at each stage.

Stage 1: Age 20–39—Time and Energy, but No Money

Despite the cost of an education—the average medical student graduate has more than $250 K in student debt—interest in medicine has not declined, with over 50,000 applicants for half as many seats [8]. Managing the first stage of a physician's career requires financial discipline, and unfortunately, not every medical student, resident, or fellow has had a proper education in personal finance.

We strongly recommend that physicians establish relationships with financial planners early in their careers. Such a relationship leads to years of prosperity and a comfortable retirement (Stage 3). Even without formal business training, a few fundamental principles are critical [9].

Markets ebb and flow over time. A diversified portfolio enables investors to mitigate financial risk. For example, an airline stock will fall in value as fuel prices increase. Conversely, the stock of oil and gas companies will rise in value as fuel prices increase. Investing in these stocks mitigates the risk of the other.

Investments with a higher rate of return also carry a higher risk. That means that over time, they are more volatile and can just as easily decrease as increase. A fundamental principle of investing is that the average investor earns an average rate of return over time.

For early-career physicians, the best advice is to hire a professional financial advisor to manage finances, invest early into a diversified portfolio, and minimize long-term investment risks.

Stage 2: Age 40–59—Money and Energy, but No Time

This second stage requires physicians to contend with the ever-present issue of burnout. Physicians can enhance their efficiency to have more time and a better work–life balance. We use the word "equilibrium" rather than "balance" because physicians work hard, and there is seldom a balance between work and life outside of our medical practices; rather, it is an equilibrium that tips toward work in the early years, excluding lives outside of medicine.

Burnout has many negative consequences for physicians. Burnout can lead to depression, anxiety, chronic stress, irritability, decreased self-esteem, and even an increased risk of suicide. It is noteworthy that the suicide rate among physicians is more significant than in other professions, and higher rates of suicide than in the general population [10]. It is also of interest that there are higher rates of alcohol and substance use among physicians experiencing burnout [11].

Burnout can lead to decreased job performance, increased absenteeism, and reduced enjoyment of our practices. It can also lead to increased medical errors and an increased risk of a malpractice suit. Burnout will ultimately affect patient satisfaction and can damage our online reputation. This decrease in enjoyment also motivates physicians to leave the practice of medicine at an earlier age.

Finally, burnout can have a profoundly negative impact on our health and well-being. Burned-out physicians are at an increased risk for cardiovascular disease and other health consequences, including hypercholesterolemia, type 2 diabetes, coronary heart disease, hospitalization because of cardiovascular disorders, musculoskeletal pain, fatigue, headaches, gastrointestinal disorders, and respiratory problems [12].

The concept of burnout is discussed in greater detail in Chap. 20.

Stage 3: Age 60 and Beyond—Money and Time, but No Energy

This third stage is when physicians start considering their exit from their practices.7 Often, this is a difficult time for physicians who have spent 40+ years working 50–60 h a week and suddenly have nothing to do. This situation leads to boredom, lack of exercise, poor diet, and mental health issues.

There are two certainties in life: death and taxes. To that we add another: retirement. Unless you fall dead at work, you *will* retire. With careful planning, the process can be easy and enjoyable. Retirement timing is usually a personal choice, usually without outside pressures. Regardless of their employment status, it's up to the physician to decide when and how to retire.

Being a physician is often at the core of who we are, and we worry about how we will feel without the work and the status that accompany our work. Most physicians want to retire while still healthy and enjoy physical activities such as travel. There is no magic date or time for physician retirement. Doctors spend their careers learning to diagnose and treat medical conditions, but they often lack clear guidelines on when and how to retire.

When the decision to retire is made freely, as in most cases, the first issue for most physicians is, "Will I have enough money to retire?" This question is best answered by your financial adviser, whom we hope you obtained in Stage 1 of your career. If that metric is not met, then retirement must wait.

The transition to retirement can be daunting and frightening, but it requires planning. When physicians leave the security of a medical practice and give up a regular job, money, and prestige, it is common for them to go through a grieving process. However, physicians who have a retirement plan in place and have begun the retirement process in the early stages of their careers often find that retirement is delightful and rewarding. The take-home message is that understanding the basic principles of savings, investments, and risk minimization early in your medical career will make the third stage just as enjoyable as the first stage of your career.

Why Doctors Need to Understand the Basic Principles of Business?

Most physicians will earn between $10 million and $12 million over the course of their practice lifetime. However, physicians will control that amount multiple times by directing healthcare for their patients. With the mere signature of a physician, they control almost 100% of all healthcare expenditures, yet physicians receive only 18% of the total $5+ trillion in healthcare expenses [13]. Using basic business skills and outstanding clinical management, individual physicians or groups must understand that to be successful, they must deliver a better product at a lower cost than their competitors. This focus on adding value and reducing healthcare costs is the direction of the future of American healthcare. That may be why 40% of the enrollment in US business schools is physicians [14]. The authors don't believe that an MBA will be necessary for new physicians to survive in the future. However, a minimum knowledge of the business is required, and we think that is the purpose of this book: to help young doctors cross the bridge between practicing medicine and running a business. How doctors understand the business of medicine will determine their future success.

Few physicians have any training in the business of healthcare. Our training teaches us how to diagnose and treat medical conditions. We must understand and accept that healthcare is a business. It is no different than Coca-Cola, Microsoft, or Apple, but on a much smaller scale. Those companies must be concerned about profit and loss, as well as expenses, including overhead, just as a medical practice must do regularly. One difference is that healthcare is a very regulated industry. We have laws established by the federal and state governments that we must adhere to closely or face fines and penalties.

The nature of medical practice has placed a price tag on nearly everything a doctor does or orders. The patient in this millennium often has high deductible insurance, expensive premiums, and often co-pays, making the patient have skin in the game. The days of transparency have arrived, and when a patient asks how much a CT scan costs or what the price of a BRCA gene test is, the doctor needs to know the answer or be able to provide it quickly for the patient.

Bottom Line

The importance of business in healthcare appears in the title "A Doctor by Choice, a Businessman by Necessity," which appeared in *The New York Times* by Dr. Sandeep Jauhar [15]. It will be necessary for all physicians to have a basic understanding of business fundamentals to achieve a successful practice. This book provides the basic business principles and metrics that will put you on the road to a practice that you will enjoy, ensure your productivity, and ultimately lead to your happiness.

Back to the Case

Sally was despondent about her experience after her rotation with the internist in private practice. She discussed her experience with the medical school dean, and she recommended that other students not be assigned to a physician harboring such negative attitudes about the medical profession. The dean placed Sally in touch with a more encouraging and constructive physician to shadow. Sally also decided to try to understand the role of business in medicine. Out of her negative experience, she understood that becoming a complete physician means being a good clinician and becoming knowledgeable and competent in the economics of the practice of medicine.

Key Takeaways

- The practice of medicine is a business, and as such, it requires doctors to understand the basic principles of business.
- It takes a doctor nearly 24 years to earn an income equal to that of a UPS truck driver.
- There are three stages of a physician's career: Stage 1, ages 20–39, Stage 2, ages 40–59, and Stage 3, age 60 and above. It is necessary to understand each stage to have an enjoyable and successful career.
- There are great joys and benefits of becoming a physician. There's magic in the initials M.D./D.O.

References

1. Rajapuram N, Langness S, Marshall MR, Sammann A. Medical students in distress: the impact of gender, race, debt, and disability. PLoS One. 2020;15(12):e0243250.
2. Kennedy HL. Aging and health for the US elderly: a health primer for ages 60 to 90 years. University of Missouri Press; 2021.
3. More students are entering medical school. AAMC. 2020. https://www.aamc.org/news/more-students-are-entering-medical-school
4. Duff-Brown B, Just how much do physicians earn-and why. Stanford Institute for Economic Policy Research, July 2023. https://siepr.stanford.edu/news/just-how-much-do-physicians-earn-and-why
5. Conover C. Are U.S. doctors paid too much. Forbes. 2013. https://www.forbes.com/sites/theapothecary/2013/05/28/are-u-s-doctors-paid-too-much/.
6. Span P. When is the surgeon too old to operate? The New York Times. 2019. https://www.nytimes.com/2019/02/01/health/surgeons-retirement-competence.html
7. Choyke B. ABA legal education section releases employment data for graduating law class of 2016. Chicago: American Bar Association; 2017. https://www.americanbar.org/content/dam/aba/administrative/legal_education_and_admissions_to_the_bar/statistics/2017_employment_data_2016_graduates_news_release.authcheckdam.pdf
8. The Hospital + Healthsystem Association of Pennsylvania. A New Record for Medical School Enrollments. HAP News, January 13, 2025. https://www.haponline.org/News/HAP-News-Articles/Latest-News/a-new-record-for-medical-school-enrollments
9. Baum N, Kahn M, editors. The business basics of building and managing a healthcare practice. Springer; 2020. https://doi.org/10.1007/978-3-030-27776-5.
10. Haque OS, Stein MA, Marvit A. Physician, heal thy double stigma – doctors with mental illness and structural barriers to disclosure. N Engl J Med. 2021;384(10):888–91. https://doi.org/10.1056/NEJMp2031013.
11. Haas K. Mental health challenges among physicians in the United States. Ballard Brief. 2023;3:3.
12. National Academies of Sciences, Engineering, and Medicine; National Academy of Medicine; Committee on Systems Approaches to Improve Patient Care by Supporting Clinician Well-Being. Taking Action Against Clinician Burnout: A Systems Approach to Professional Well- Being. Washington: National Academies Press; 2019.
13. CMS.gov. National Health Expenditure Fact Sheet. https://www.cms.gov/data-research/statistics-trends-and-reports/national-health-expenditure-data/nhe-fact-sheet
14. Viswanathan V. The rise of the MD\MBA degree. The Atlantic. 2014. https://www.theatlantic.com/education/archive/2014/09/the-rise-of-the-mdmba-degree/380683/
15. Jauhar S. A doctor by choice, a businessman by necessity. The New York Times. 2009. https://www.nytimes.com/2009/07/07/health/07essa.html

2 Time Value of Money

Case Study: Martika
Martika graduated from college 5 years ago and took a job with Bond Enterprises, a holding company, as her first job. As an economics major, Martika always envisioned a career in business. After her mother'sdeath from breast cancer 2 years ago, Martika began to have doubts about her career choice and volunteered at the hospice that cared for her mother prior to her mother's death. After speaking with friends and doing some research, she began to explore medicine as a potential career. She took premedical science classes at a local college, did well, studied for the MCAT, applied, and got accepted to her state medical school.

Because of her business background, Martika wondered if medical school would be a good move financially. Her current job at Bond paid well. Going to medical school would involve borrowing money for tuition and living expenses and she would not be able to work while a student. Although she would be paid for residency, her salary would be significantly less than that of a practicing physician. Over her lifetime, would her eventual salary as a physician compensate for her medical school debt and lost income? Would she be able to practice the specialty of her choice or would she be limited to higher paying specialties? Is medical school worth it?

One of the most basic principles of finance is the time value of money. Conceptually and simply, money is worth more now than at some time in the future. Stated another way, given the choice, you want your money sooner rather than later. This is because invested money earns interest and because you can use the money you have now for things that may not be available later. As an example, the time value of money dictates that if you are lucky enough to win the million-dollar lottery, you want the million dollars now, not 250 thousand dollars a year for the next 4 years. Why is this so?

Money has an opportunity cost. For example, suppose you want to buy an antique clock. If you have the money now, you can successfully negotiate the price and buy the clock. But, if you don't

N. Baum, M. J. Kahn, *Business Basics for your Healthcare Practice*,
https://doi.org/10.1007/978-3-032-25241-8_2

have the money now, you would have to wait until later to purchase the clock and the clock may have already been sold to someone else and no longer be available. Similarly, if presented with an investment opportunity, having money on hand allows you to make an investment that may disappear at a future date. Obviously, having money on hand provides a financial advantage for the holder to use the money for purchases, to lend, or to invest.

In addition to opportunity costs, money has more value in the present because most of us do not hold our money in a basket under our beds. Rather, we either put the money in the bank for safekeeping or invest the money. Either way, our money can earn interest. Interest is the money paid for the use of your cash. When you borrow money from a bank, or through your credit card, the bank charges interest, a fee for the use of their money. Similarly, if you put money in a bank, or lend money by purchasing bonds, you are compensated with interest payments for the use of your money.

Interest can be simple or compounded. As an example of simple interest, if you invest \$100 at 6% annual interest, at the end of the year, you will have \$106. Compounded interest allows for you to effectively earn "interest on your interest." When Benjamin Franklin died, he left approximately \$5000 to each of the two cities, Philadelphia and Boston. He required that the money be invested and that there would be two withdraws, a partial withdraw at 100 years and a final withdraw at 200 years. Because of compounded interest, at 100 years each city received a payment of \$500,000 and at 200 years, each city received approximately \$20 million. Franklin described compounded interest as, "Money makes money. And the money that makes money makes money" [1].

Going back to the example of a \$100 investment at 6% interest, if the interest was compounded monthly, at the end of the year, you would not have \$106 but \$106.17. If interest was compounded daily, at the end of the year, you would have \$106.18. The extra 17 or 18 cents arises from earning interest on interest. Although a mere 17 cents may seem trivial, suppose your initial investment were \$100 million. Now your compounded interest would be over \$6,170,000—a substantial sum indeed!

Compounding can also be illustrated by the following fable:

A peasant shepherd comes upon a young girl who has become ensnared in a bear trap. He hears her cry out and frees her. The young girl is so thankful that she promises the peasant a large reward as her father is King of the empire. Upon meeting the King, the peasant is offered 100 lbs. of wheat. Noticing that the King has a chessboard displayed on a table, the peasant offers an alternative reward. The peasant suggests that the king put one grain of wheat on the top left square of the chessboard and then doubles the number of grains successively throughout the 64 squares of the chessboard. The King quickly agrees to this alternative assuming that the uneducated peasant has made a silly concession. Understanding compounding, the wise peasant has actually struck a great deal. If the number of grains of wheat doubles on each successive square, then the sum of grains is $1 + 2 + 4 + 8 + 16 + \ldots, + 2^{64}$ for a total of over 18×10^{18} grains of wheat that would weigh more than 1645 times the global production of wheat in modern times! The amount of wheat placed on an individual square is "compounded" by the amount on the previous square. Certainly, compounding is important if you are borrowing or lending money. For the borrower, compounding costs money and for the lender, compounding allows money to grow.

In addition to the interest rate, the number of times compounding occurs in a given period can also affect the total interest. The more compounding periods there are, the greater the total interest. For example, \$1000 borrowed at 6% annual interest would cost \$60 of interest if the interest were simple or not compounded. If the interest were compounded monthly, the total interest payment would be \$61.68, daily compounding yields a total payment of \$61.83, and we can even calculate continuous compounding, meaning that the compounding is continuous and ongoing, which would yield a total annual payment of \$61.84.

Many commercial loans including credit cards display interest as APR (annual percentage rate). For example, if you were considering taking out a business loan of $300,000 with an interest of 6%, your annual interest payment would be $18,000 or $1500 per month. However, the actual payments on such a commercial loan are typically higher as they include not only the cost of interest but also the additional fees attached to the loan. The APR includes these extra costs. In the above example, if the loan also includes closing costs, insurance, and origination fees totaling an additional $5000, then your original loan amount would be $305,000. At 6% interest, the new annual payment would be $18,300 for an APR of 6.1%. The APR gives a better estimate of the actual cost you pay to borrow money because the APR includes the cost of interest plus the cost of additional fees. When shopping for loans, the APR gives a good sense of the monthly costs of borrowing money and can be used to compare loans. However, borrowers need to be cautioned that it is not only the APR that is important in choosing a loan, but also the duration of the loan. A 10-year loan spreads out the additional fees associated with the loan over a much longer time period than a 24-month loan, lowering the APR substantially. However, a borrower would pay more total interest on a longer loan. Therefore, when borrowing money, it is important to consider not only the APR but also the total number of payments to determine the better loan for a given situation.

In addition to interest (also called the cost of capital or discount rate), understanding a business opportunity requires an understanding of the present and future value of money that is intertwined with the time value of money. As is now obvious, the future value of money is greater than the present value because of opportunity costs and the cost of capital. Put mathematically, Future Value (FV) = Present Value (PV) × $(1 + r)^t$, where r is the interest rate or cost of capital and t is the number of pay periods between the present and the future.

Net present value is a business tool used to determine the financial benefit or detriment of business opportunities, and it relies heavily on the concept of the time value of money. Essentially, if costs or payments occur in the same time period, they can be simply added to or subtracted from each other. However, because of the time value of money payments or costs accrued at different time periods cannot be simply added or subtracted because their true value depends on when these transactions occur. To calculate net present value, all costs or payments are brought to the present value, using the present value equation, and can then be summed. In general, from a business perspective, any opportunity presenting positive net present value is beneficial, whereas any opportunity with negative net present value is not advisable.

Back to the Case

Going back to our introductory case with Martika, the financial value of an MD degree can be summarized as.

Value of MD = total change in salary with an MD less the cost of medical school attendance less the wages lost during training. These costs and payments must all be corrected for the cost of capital and calculated at the present value.

Using several assumptions in our model including an annual interest rate of 3%, a cost of medical school attendance of $70,000, a salary increase of $130,000 after residency with 3% growth per year, and a 4-year residency duration, the net present value of Martika's MD is over $1.7 million [2]. Certainly, this is a hugely positive net present value, making the decision to go to medical school financially advantageous and something that Martika should do from a financial perspective. Obviously, the above analysis does not begin to take into account career satisfaction, self-actualization, social status, and other nonfinancial gains that Martika might derive from a long career as a physician. In fact, there is probably no more valuable degree in the world than a US MD degree.

Key Takeaways

- You want your money sooner, rather than later.
- Early investing can compound earnings, leading to a greater net value.
- Getting an MD is a terrific financial investment.

References

1. Malkiel BJ, Ellis CD. The elements of investing: easy lessons for every investor. Hoboken: Wiley; 2013.
2. Kahn MJ, Nelling EF. Estimating the value of medical education: a net present value approach. Teach Learn Med. 2010;22(3):205–8.

3 Basic Accounting and Interpretation of Financial Statements

Case Study: Bryce

Bryce is in his second year of faculty at an academic medical center. He was asked to serve on the Board of Directors of his school's faculty practice plan, a role he desired because of his interest in practice management and because of his desire to become involved in academic leadership. When it came time to present the financial statements, Bryce felt at a loss. What is EBITDA? What is AR? Why are there multiple statements distributed to the group, rather than a simple table? Why does it appear as if there are different ways to account for the same transaction? Bryce wonders if anyone, other than the business folks in the room, really understands what these statements mean. Bryce wishes he had taken an accounting class in college or at least paid more attention to his roommates, who were business majors.

Basic Accounting

Basic accounting is predicated on the simple equation that *Assets = Liabilities + Equity.* In simple terms, looking at personal wealth, this means that your total wealth, your equity, is equivalent to what you own less what you owe (rearranging the equation: Assets—Liabilities = Equity). When balancing our own bank account, we typically perform this arithmetic automatically. Each month we have an account balance (Equity) to which we add our monthly paycheck (Asset) and subtract our payments (liabilities) such as mortgage payments or car expenses. Such a system of bookkeeping may be fine for an individual with a few transactions per month, but makes error detection difficult. Suppose you entered the wrong payment or the wrong salary amount? Would your account be overdrawn?

Double-entry accounting, which dates back to the eleventh century, is a system of bookkeeping where every entry into one account requires an opposite, yet equal, entry into another account. These two entries, termed debits and credits, allow for error detection as the sum of all debits must equal the sum of all credits for all accounts. The terms "debit" and "credit" are not foreign as we are used to having debit and credit cards in our wallets. A *credit* card allows us to make purchases that are later paid for, whereas a *debit* card represents a bank account from which funds are drawn. For the bank issuing the card, the credit card payments are recorded as credits as they increase the fund balance of the bank once paid, and the debit card payments are recorded as debits, as they create a negative fund balance in the bank when paid out. The system of double-entry accounting gives the two cards their respective names.

N. Baum, M. J. Kahn, *Business Basics for your Healthcare Practice*,
https://doi.org/10.1007/978-3-032-25241-8_3

As a simple example of double-entry accounting, say an opthalmologist's office sells a pair of glasses for $250. This could be recorded both as a debit of $250 to an account named "assets" and a credit of $250 to an account named "revenue." This is because the glasses represent an asset to the opthalmology office that is lost during the sale, whereas the payment for the glasses represents a gain in revenue for the office. Generally, from a bookkeeping perspective, there are five types of accounts: assets, liabilities, income (revenue), expenses, and capital accounts. Each of these has subaccounts that are recorded as a series of debits and credits.

Bookkeeping using the principles of double-entry accounting results in financial statements that are used daily in all businesses. The three basic financial statements used by businesses are (1) the income statement, also called the profit and loss statement or P&L, which demonstrates the "bottom line" of net gains or losses; (2) the balance sheet, which uses the basic accounting equation and lists assets, liabilities, and retained earnings (equity); and (3) the cash flow statement, which shows the outflow and inflow of cash related to operations, investments, and financing. Sometimes a fourth statement is produced, called the equity statement, which represents changes in the retained earnings (savings) of the company. We will not be discussing the equity statement further. Analysis of financial statements can provide an estimate of the financial health of an organization and can be used in planning future business strategies.

The main financial statement of interest to most physicians, and the one distributed on a monthly basis, is the income statement that typically covers a range of time such as the previous month, the fiscal year to date, the previous quarter, or all three time periods. The "bottom line" of an income statement is the net profit or loss for the given time period. Typically, income statements include information for the preceding period and the previous year for comparison. Income statements usually include entries for both budgeted and actual revenues and expenses. Figure 3.1 shows the income statement for Bryce's academic group practice.

From the income statement, looking directly at the bottom line, we can see that for August 2019, the group practice is "in the black" by $14,706, meaning they have income that exceeds expenses by that amount. Looking further at the income statement, in spite of a small positive bottom line, the practice is behind budget by $184,850. This may be of concern if such a trend continues. Looking at both expenses and revenue, the income statement tells us that the practice is behind budget due to both low revenue and increased expenses. Certainly, were this to continue, this would be a problem as the practice may not be able to pay its bills. From a historic

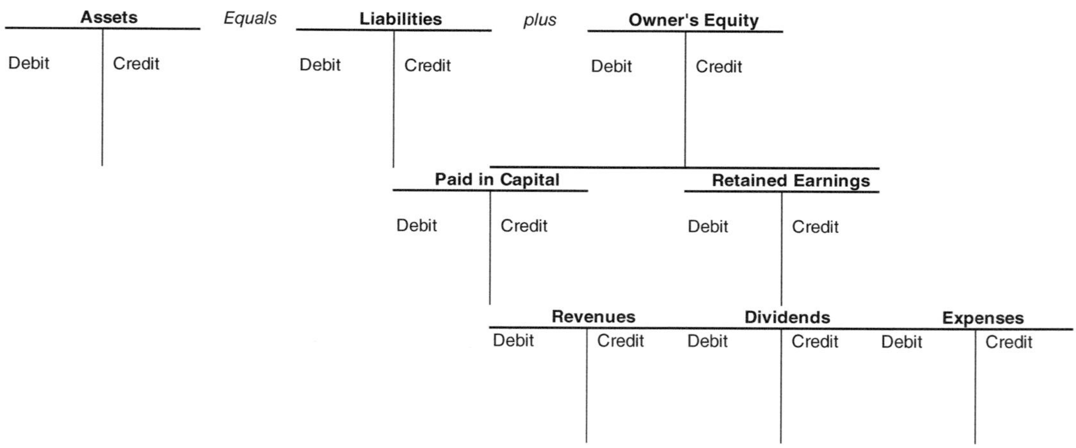

Fig. 3.1 Basic T-accounting 2022

perspective, the practice is doing better financially than the previous month where the net earnings were only \$379, but the practice is not doing as well as the previous year where net earnings were \$114,706. From a year to date perspective, the practice is \$129,412 in the black, but is still below budget, but much better than this point last year, where the practice was "in the red" for \$212,478. Bryce practices at Site E. Looking at the top of the income statement, Bryce can see that his site is doing the best of all of the sites financially and is above budget. This may mean a bonus for Bryce in the future! Certainly, looking at just a few areas of the income statement, we can learn a lot about Bryce's practice.

The balance sheet (Fig. 3.3), unlike the income statement, represents a snapshot in time. The balance sheet provides information on how assets are funded: through debt, equity, or other capital. Assets are generally listed in order of how easily they can be converted to cash, also known as liquidity. Liabilities are listed in the order that they need to be paid from first to last. Accounts receivable refers to money owed the practice by patients and insurers that has yet to be paid. It is an asset as it provides positive value to the practice. Accounts payable represents money that the practice has to pay out. This may be due to patients who were overcharged or for patients who were charged for a service that was later paid by an insurance company. Accounts payable is a liability because it is money that needs to be paid out. Again, for the balance sheet, from the basic accounting equation, *assets* = *liabilities* + *equity*. Equity is that money left over that adds value to a company. Let's look at the balance sheet for Bryce's practice in Fig. 3.2. First, the balance sheet must obey the accounting equation, or Assets must equal Liabilities plus Equity. For Bryce's practice, this is the case. He has both assets and debt plus equity of \$770,000. Sometimes, the financial health of an organiza-

BRYCE'S MEDICAL GROUP
STATEMENT OF ACTIVITY
Aug-19

1-MONTH (MTD)						2-MONTHS (YTD)			
BUDGET	ACTUAL	FAV (UNFAV)	Jul-18	Aug-18	DESCRIPTION	BUDGET	ACTUAL	FAV (UNFAV)	Aug-18
46,47,325	39,66,168	-6,81,157	41,09,613	38,98,084	SITE A INCOME	88,90,534	78,64,252	-10,26,283	77,36,099
2,58,703	1,52,674	-1,06,029	1,18,978	1,15,425	SITE B INCOME	5,17,405	2,68,099	-2,49,307	2,09,341
30,09,639	19,05,153	-11,04,486	19,24,358	31,01,420	SITE C INCOME	60,19,278	50,06,572	-10,12,705	44,44,469
8,08,428	6,20,808	-1,87,620	1,00,230	95,308	SITE D INCOME	16,16,857	7,16,116	-9,00,741	2,81,561
4,45,608	6,57,427	2,11,819	5,46,321	6,32,577	SITE E INCOME	8,91,217	12,90,004	3,98,788	10,33,651
29,917	32,108	2,191	1,036	21,875	OTHER INCOME	59,833	53,983	-5,850	3,650
91,99,620	**73,34,338**	**-18,65,282**	**68,00,537**	**78,64,688**	TOTAL INCOME	**1,79,95,124**	**1,51,99,026**	**-27,96,098**	**1,37,08,770**
-78,34,158	-60,58,899	17,75,259	-55,20,796	-66,79,667	LESS: Practice -REALTED COSTS	-1,55,25,502	-1,27,38,566	27,86,936	-1,16,74,289
13,65,461	**12,75,439**	**-90,022**	**12,79,740**	**11,85,022**	NET COST OF PRACTICE ASSESSMENTS	**24,69,622**	**24,60,460**	**-9,162**	**20,34,481**
					COST OF PRACTICE:				
5,38,291	6,01,893	-63,602	5,39,745	5,15,602	NET SALARIES & WAGES	10,76,582	11,17,494	-40,913	9,54,284
1,43,535	1,62,839	-19,304	1,66,758	1,33,518	FRINGE BENEFITS	2,87,070	2,96,357	-9,287	2,95,592
7,519	7,515	4	6,544	4,455	OPERATING SUPPLIES	15,038	11,970	3,068	9,041
2,46,905	2,44,385	2,521	2,81,058	2,20,831	PURCHASED SERVICES	4,93,811	4,65,215	28,595	5,00,977
12,873	15,223	-2,350	72,045	13,704	UTILITIES & POSTAGE	25,747	28,927	-3,180	74,257
44,652	33,740	10,912	31,368	39,009	OTHER EXPENSE	89,304	72,749	16,555	55,607
85,417	74,070	11,347	85,400	82,470	FACILITY FEES	1,70,833	1,56,540	14,293	1,64,730
10,79,192	11,39,665	-60,473	11,82,918	10,09,588	TOTAL OPERATING EXPENSES	21,58,384	21,49,253	9,132	20,54,489
					NON-OPERATING EXPENSES				
1,25,858	1,33,316	-7,458	1,24,691	1,28,771	MALPRACTICE EXPENSE	2,51,717	2,62,087	-10,370	2,49,317
-39,145	-12,248	-26,897	-28,248	-68,042	LESS: RECOVERIES	-78,290	-80,291	2,001	-56,848
86,713	1,21,068	-34,354	96,443	60,728	NET MALPRACTICE EXPENSE	1,73,427	1,81,796	-8,369	1,92,470
11,65,905	**12,60,733**	**-94,827**	**12,79,361**	**10,70,316**	TOTAL COST OF PRACTICE EXPENSES	**23,31,811**	**23,31,049**	**762**	**22,46,958**
1,99,556	**14,706**	**-1,84,850**	**379**	**1,14,706**	NET EARNINGS	**1,37,811**	**1,29,412**	**-8,400**	**-2,12,478**

Fig. 3.2 Income statement 2022

tion can be determined by the Debt-to-Equity Ratio. This gives us a measurement of risk as it can tell us how well debt is managed. Lower numbers are better. For Bryce's practice, this ratio is calculated as total liabilities divided by Equity, which gives a ratio of 1.66. This is not very high, suggesting that the practice is prudent in its borrowing practices. Another thing to look at is how the equity has changed over time. Looking at balance sheets for the past several years can show if the business is growing or contracting. Finally, return on equity (ROE), defined as net income divided by equity, can give a sense of how well the equity is being used to produce income. For example, if the practice purchased colonoscopes with their equity, the ROE could be an indicator of the success of that strategy.

The cash flow statement shows where cash comes in and goes out of a business in three areas: operations, investments, and financing. As an interesting example, let's look at Ford Motors. We may logically assume that Ford Motors is in the business of making cars. However, looking at the cash flow statement for Ford Motors on Yahoo Finance for 12/31/21 [1], we see that the total cash flow for Ford from operations was $15.8 billion, the total cash flow from investments was a $2.7 billion, and the total cash flow from financing was $23.5 billion lent out. Based on an analysis of cash flows, Ford Motors is as much a lending company as they are a car manufacturing company!

In addition to the basics of the three financial statements that we have discussed, there are other terms and additional information that can be derived through analysis of financial statements. One commonly used line item in an income statement is EBITDA. EBITDA stands for "earnings before interest, taxes, depreciation, and amortization." EBITDA is sometimes used as an alternative to net income. EBITDA is used in income statements as it eliminates the effects of financing (interest) and capitalization (depreciation and amortization). Do not let this term confuse you. EBITDA and net income are very closely related.

Additionally, analysis of financial statements can help us know how well the practice is doing at collecting owed money. This refers to "days in AR." Although not specifically spelled out in financial statements, this can be calculated if you know the charges for the past year and divide that number by the days in a year. Because most health expenses are discounted by insurance companies and other third-party payors, charges are very different from revenue in healthcare, so, in addition to the income statement, you would need to know total charges to make this calculation. Additionally, many third-party payors will not pay bills that are older than 180 days. Days in AR is an important number to know!

Finally, the health of a practice can be assumed by the *liquidity* of the practice, which gives an impression of the amount of money the practice has on hand in case of emergency. This can be presented as "working capital," which is the difference between current assets and current liabilities. For Bryce's practice, his working capital, from the balance sheet, is $89,000 minus $61,000 or $27,000. A company with negative working capital could not pay off short-term debts if required to do so and would be considered "illiquid." Another commonly used indicator of liquidity, or ability to pay debt, is the *current ratio*, the ratio of current assets to current liabilities.

Although there are many other calculations based on financial statements used by businesses, these are the major ones used and understanding these will go a long way toward being able to analyze financial statements.

Back to the Case

Bryce went to the business manager of his practice to learn more about the data presented. His manager was quick to point out that she worked for Bryce, and not the other way around. She explained the accounting used in his practice and gave him a much better understanding of the financial wellbeing of his practice. Bryce was satisfied that he was working in the right place and also felt more confident the next month when the group's financial statements were presented. He even knew enough to ask about days in AR and was pleased that it was only 28 days and improved from last year. Bryce wondered if getting an MBA would be valuable in the future (Fig. 3.3).

BALANCE SHEET
31-Dec-19

ASSETS	
Current Assets	
Cash	$ 2,100.00
Petty Cash	$ 100.00
Temporary investments	$ 10,000.00
Accounts receivable	$ 40,500.00
Supplies	$ 34,800.00
Prepaid insurance	$ 1,500.00
Total Current assets	$ 89,000.00
Investments	$ 36,000.00
Property, Plant & Equiptment	
Land	$ 12,000.00
Buildings	$1,80,000.00
Equiptment	$2,01,000.00
Less: depreciation	$ (56,000.00)
P,P,E net	$3,37,000.00
Other Assets	$3,08,000.00
Total Assets	$7,70,000.00

LIABILITIES	
Current Liabilities	
Notes payable	$ 5,000.00
Accounts payable	$ 35,900.00
Wages payable	$ 8,500.00
interest payable	$ 2,900.00
taxes payable	$ 6,100.00
unearned revenues	$ 2,600.00
total current liabilites	$ 61,000.00
Long-term liabilites	
notes payable	$ 20,000.00
bonds payable	$4,00,000.00
Total long-term liabilites	$4,20,000.00
Total Liabilities	$4,81,000.00
OWNER'S EQUITY	
Retained earnings	$2,80,000.00
accumulated other income	$ 9,000.00
total equity	$2,89,000.00
Total liabilites & Equity	$7,70,000.00

Fig. 3.3 Balance sheet 2022

Key Takeaways

- Assets = Liabilities + Equity.
- There are three basic financial statements: the income statement, balance sheet, and cash flow statement.
- Understanding basic principles of accounting allows physicians to understand the financial health of their practice and allows for strategic planning.

Reference

1. https://finance.yahoo.com/quote/F/cash-flow?p=F

4 Contracts and Negotiation

> **Case Study: Sherri**
> Sherri is in her final year of her Maternal Fetal Medicine Fellowship and has received her first job offer in a large inner-city Obstetrics and Gynecology Practice. Sherri first learned of this position through a recruiting firm that sent her an email 3 months ago. Sherri spoke on the phone with the recruiter who connected her with the Medical Director of the Practice. Following her interview, Sherri felt that this practice was a good fit for her; it was large enough that call would not be onerous, the patient population included medically underserved patients who she like to care for, she liked the other physicians and office staff and had a good vibe about the work environment, and the practice was in a city where she had friends and family. In reviewing her job offer, she was a bit overwhelmed. Although the salary was more money than she thought she would ever earn, was it fair? Sherri had over $300,000 in educational debt and there was no provision to help her pay for some of her loans, a benefit that she knew others in her fellowship program had been offered with other practices. There was no provision for CME and license expenses. Sherri wondered what was negotiable? She was not real comfortable asking for more money. Should she hire an employment lawyer? Sherri wished she were in the NFL, where at least she would have an agent to help her negotiate.

Contracts

A contract is a legal agreement, typically between two parties. Although contracts can be verbal, they are almost always written such that all parties in the contract are protected legally and so that there are no misunderstandings between the parties of the contract. The parties of the contract are the entities involved in the agreement. The Terms and Conditions of the contract spell out the rights and responsibilities of each party in the contract. Terms and Conditions often include legal remedies that parties can use if there is a suspected breach in the contract.

Basically, a contract has three parts: offer, acceptance, and consideration. An offer is a promise to provide something to a promisor, acceptance is an agreement by the promisee to abide by the contract, and consideration is a legal

N. Baum, M. J. Kahn, *Business Basics for your Healthcare Practice*,
https://doi.org/10.1007/978-3-032-25241-8_4

concept that involves the bargaining for a quid pro quo that provides a benefit to the promisee and a detriment to the promisor. For example, if I tell you that I am going to give you $100 and then renege, this is not a contract as there is no consideration. There is no exchange of promise. On the other hand, if I tell you that I will give you $100 for cleaning my gutters and you accept my offer, then this is a contract. If you do not provide the services agreed upon, then I have legal recourse. In this example, there is the offer to clean gutters; acceptance of my proposed fee; and consideration, the exchange of fee for services.

Very few physicians enter solo practice nowadays. Because most physicians are employed by a group, hospital, or educational institution, most physicians receive and negotiate an employment contract. Physician employment contracts are both similar and different from other employment contracts. Because most physicians have limited experience with contract law, it is always prudent to have employment contracts reviewed by a legal expert who is representing your best interests. This is firm advice, and hiring an attorney is money well spent. In many academic practices, an "offer letter" is substituted for a formal contract. From a legal perspective, assuming verbiage in the offer letter spells out that the letter is binding, offer letters are really a type of contract. Academic practices sometimes use offer letters because of the assumption that they are less formal and less subject to close legal scrutiny. Be careful, however, with offer letters and make sure that, as with an employment contract, you do not agree to something that you will later regret. Alternatively, some offer letters may not be binding and are sometimes more like "letters of intent" that merely propose initial terms for the eventual formal contract. In this case, physicians should use caution in accepting the offer prior to seeing the formal contract.

Employment contracts should stipulate a start and end date and should specify the renewal process. The process for terminating the contract should be clearly articulated. Provisions for malpractice insurance after the physician has left the practice should be clearly articulated. This is called *gap* or *tail insurance*. Sometimes this type of insurance is provided by the employer, sometimes it requires the physician to pay out-of-pocket for such coverage. In any rate, it is important for physicians to understand how they are covered for possible malpractice cases arising after the employment term has ended.

The major focus of a physician employment contract is the stipulated compensation. Compensation takes the form of salary, benefits, and incentive pay. Physician salaries depend on specialty, location, experience, demand, and a host of other factors. This makes comparison between offers difficult and may limit the ability to negotiate a salary. Typically, after the first year of employment, physician salaries include some portion that is "at risk" in the sense that it is related to productivity. This at-risk portion is typically dependent on work relative value units (RVUs), charges, and/or collections. Because collections depend on a number of variables, including payor mix, ability of the practice to bill and collect for services, and contracts signed with third-party payors, incentive pay based solely on collections may not accurately reward hard work. As such, inventive pay that also includes work generated (RVUs) is preferable. Benefits typically include health insurance, vision and dental insurance, malpractice insurance, money for CME and licenses, vacation, sick leave, and disability insurance. Additionally, maternity and paternity leave may be offered as a benefit. More recently, because of the student debt that young physicians have acquired, loan repayment can be benefit. Many practices also offer a signing bonus and money for relocation. Because this money may be considered salary, there may be tax implications that should be understood prior to signing the contract.

One peculiarity of physician employment contracts is the issue of *restrictive covenants*. These are also called non-compete clauses and are used to prohibit a physician from practicing in a certain geographical area for a set period of time in the case of termination or separation. Restrictive covenants are important to a group practice because they prevent a former employee to leave and take patients away from the practice to then compete with the original group.

Restrictive covenants can be difficult to enforce in some jurisdictions as they represent restriction of trade. The laws surrounding restrictive covenants continue to change and evolve. Therefore, it is important to have restrictive covenants closely reviewed by an employment lawyer and, if part of the final contract, the geographical limitation should be limited in radius and the time restriction should be as short as possible.

The five aspects of restrictive covenants that must be reviewed and discussed before signing a contract are geographical limitation and duration of the restriction, termination agreements, ownership of files, and final negotiations.

Duration and Geographical Scope

Restrictive covenants specify the length of time the restriction is in place and geographical area where a physician is restricted from practicing after their employment ends. The duration and geographical scope of these covenants must be reasonable and not impose an undue burden on the physician, allowing them to earn a living.

Many states have enacted legislation to limit the duration of restrictive covenants. You can access each state's status on restrictive covenants at https://www.acc.org/-/media/Non-Clinical/Files-PDFs-Excel-MS-Word-etc/2022/07/Appendix-1%2D%2DRC-status-by-state-71822%2D%2Dfinal.

Termination and Enforcement

Restrictive covenants become enforceable if the physician voluntarily terminates their employment or is terminated for cause, such as breaches of the employment contract, practice policy violations (e.g., HIPAA violations), or conduct that causes significant harm to patients or the employer. Other causes for termination include when the physician loses their license or hospital privileges, and the employer is unable to obtain malpractice insurance for the physician.

Some states prohibit employers from enforcing non-compete agreements if the employer terminates the physician without cause or if the departing physician terminates employment for cause. For example, if a layoff or practice merger occurs and the physician has done nothing wrong, there should be no penalty applied to the departing physician. Additionally, the restrictive covenant should not apply if the employer fails to pay the physician in a timely manner, as stated in the contract.

Ownership of Patient Files

This is a contentious issue for physicians, regardless of where they work, whether it's in a hospital or a private practice. When a physician leaves a medical practice, the issue of ownership of patient files is a concern for both the departing physician and the practice where the departing physician was previously employed and provided care for the patients. The departing physician would like to notify their patients that they are leaving and inform them of the new location and telephone number.

If this issue is not addressed in the employment contract, conflict is likely to occur. There should be an understanding of who will provide notice to patients. The contract should stipulate who will write the letter and precisely what the letter will say. Finally, the agreement should specify that the former employer will notify patients when they call the practice of the new arrangements and provide the departing physician's contact information. The employment contract should stipulate that the departing doctor will retain access to patient lists and records.

Ownership and Business Transactions

Physicians with an ownership interest in the practice may be subject to enforceable restrictive covenants under certain circumstances, such as.

Sale of the physician's ownership interest or of the practice's assets.

Transfer of control of the business entity through merger or consolidation.

The contract must clearly define the terms and conditions of the restrictive covenant and ensure compliance with state laws.

Negotiation and Review

Before signing any contract, every employee physician should consult with legal counsel to understand the implications of the agreement. Our medical training does not provide education or advice on restrictive covenants. Since physicians are usually not familiar with the legal nuances of restrictive covenants, seeking legal advice from a knowledgeable counselor who specializes in this area is worthwhile, especially when considering the cost of employing a legal professional. By understanding the legal framework surrounding these agreements, physicians can make informed decisions before signing an employment contract and navigate the complexities of restrictive covenants.

Another issue specific to a physician employment contract is the issue of partnership. Partnership is a commitment to partial ownership of the practice. Unlike having equity in a commercially traded company, partnership is illiquid in that it is difficult to value, nearly impossible to sell, and may carry the obligation on the part of the physician partner to cover any shortfalls in practice income with personal income. Typically, partnership is a benefit offered after several years of employment and typically becoming a partner involves a series of payments or salary offsets over several additional years until partnership is achieved. Another complication of partnership is the distribution of ownership. Is it equal across the group, or is the majority of the ownership held by those who entered the partnership first, the senior partners? The compensation differences and distribution of equity in the partnership between junior and senior partners should be clearly articulated prior to signing a contract.

Finally, the employment contract should specify what happens if the group is acquired by another party or in the event of a merger or consolidation. This type of clause is called "assignability." If the employment contract remains in place after merger or acquisition, then it is assignable. If the contract is null and void in case of such an event, then it is non-assignable. The contract should offer a remedy to the physician in the case of non-assignability. This could include release from the non-compete clause or a financial payout to the physician whose contract was voided by a change in ownership.

Negotiation

Most physicians have had little training in the art of negotiation. Some physicians assume that nothing is negotiable and accept an initial contract as is, whereas some feel that everything is negotiable. Basic negotiation skills are obviously important, especially when negotiating your starting salary as this is the amount that all future increases will be based upon. A 3% increase on $300,000 is more money than a 3% increase on $200,000.

More than anything else, a successful negotiation depends on having *information*. If you know what others are getting paid for the same job, you know your negotiation point. Luckily, especially in academic medicine, salary information is available. The Association of American Medical Colleges (AAMC) publishes annually salary information divided by specialty, geographical region of the country, public/private medical school, and faculty rank. This data is not self-reported but is gathered from business offices of medical school ensuring its accuracy. Additionally, many states such as Nevada have sunshine laws making all salaries of public employees available to the public. As such, the salary of any faculty member at a state school may be available online. For non-academic jobs, Medscape publishes salary information that is gathered from survey responses. Other survey-derived data comes from the American Medical Group Association (AMGA), the Medical Group Management Association (MGMA), Merritt Hawkins, and the US Bureau of Labor and Statistics Occupational Employment Statistics. Care should be used when interpreting self-reported data as physicians who report salaries are more likely to be those on the higher end of the spectrum. Obviously, this type of salary information is absolutely critical at the beginning of any salary negotiation. It is also important to gather other information about the practice prior to negotiation, including the degree of competition for patients from other groups, the patient payor mix, and expected work schedules including call.

A successful negotiation involves give and take on both sides and results in an outcome that is usually not perfect for either side, but is mutually beneficial to all parties. As such, be prepared to make concessions, and when asking the other side to do so, treat people with respect, be patient, and have logical reasons for your requests. Again, use the information you have gathered before the negotiation to make your points. When you are negotiating, set priorities. Identify your limits and identify those things that you could concede if necessary. Develop a strategy. What could you give up and in exchange for what else? Start off with an easy issue, like office space. Then build up to harder negotiating points such as salary or partnership. Finally, return to issues that are likely not to be contentious like vacation time so that both you and your employer can feel good about the negotiation. After most of the bargaining is done, return to those last unresolved issues like restrictive covenants. These trickier issues will be easier to negotiate once both sides have a feeling for each other and both sides have a vested interest in a successful resolution.

Lastly, in the interest of all parties, get your final negotiated contract in writing, including all concessions on both sides. Although both sides may negotiate in good faith, anything not written is difficult to prove, especially if there is a change in personnel in the group.

Back to the Case

Sherri gathered information, including the salaries offered by other practices to the three other fellows completing her program. She was able to find cost of living conversions for different cities in the United States and was able to derive a fair range of salary for a starting Maternal Fetal Medicine specialist in her new city. She also was able to get information from her specialty society about benefit packages offered to new graduates. Sherri was not able to negotiate her starting salary, but was able to negotiate a signing bonus. The practice had never offered a loan repayment program and was uncomfortable about the tax ramifications of such a benefit. Sherri conceded this issue but was able to negotiate a more generous family leave arrangement, important to her as she thought about starting a family. When Sherri reviewed the contract, she realized that little things like money for CME and licenses were included. She got her contract in writing and hired an attorney friend to review it. Sherri really wanted the job offered as it met so many of her personal and professional needs, so she was less in charge of the negotiation, but at the end she felt satisfied and comfortable that her first job would be a good fit.

Key Takeaways

- A contract is a legal document. Get everything in writing and have a legal professional review prior to signing.
- Do not be afraid to negotiate. Gather information, stay calm, and have a rationale for your asks.
- Negotiations involve compromise. Identify your limits from the onset. Use your ability to compromise to get the things you really need.

5 Basic Personal Finance and Investing

Case Study: Jamal

Jamal is 40 years old and about to complete his neurosurgery residency. Jamal was a nontraditional medical student, starting medical school after working for a start-up in the biotech industry for nearly a decade. During medical school, his wife worked as a labor and delivery nurse. He and his wife had a baby daughter when medical school started. Although Jamal has a medical school debt of nearly $300,000, he does have $40,000 saved in a 401 K from his previous employer. He already signed a contract for a job with a large multispecialty group practice. His contract includes a signing bonus of $50,000 along with $10,000 to be used toward moving and other related expenses. His initial salary is guaranteed for 1 year at $550,000. After 1 year, and for the next 3 years, his salary includes a $400,000 guarantee and bonus to be paid based on his clinical productivity. Although his employer will not be contributing toward his retirement for the first 2 years, after 2 years, his employer will match his contributions up to 10% of his take-home pay to a retirement plan. The benefit package provided by his employer includes life and disability insurance, health insurance for him and the ability to purchase health insurance for his family at a reasonable cost, and an allowance for CME. Jamal is happy to be finally finishing residency and earning real money. He is concerned that he has not really paid attention to things like life insurance and how to put money away for retirement and wants to make sure that he can retire by age 65. He is anxious and in need of advice.

Physicians are typically in the top 5% of wage earners in the United States, and physicians in specialties, like neurosurgery, can easily be in the top 1% of wage earners. Despite this fact, many physicians find themselves ill-equipped to manage their money due to the lack of expertise and training. It is very prudent, if not essential, for physicians to solicit the help of a financial planner. The earlier a physician establishes a relationship with a financial planner, the better because of compounded interest that was discussed in Chap. 2. In addition to a financial planner, it is also important for a physician to have an accountant. Even though doctors can do their own taxes, the time spent doing this is probably worth more than an accountant will cost. Additionally, an accountant signature on a tax return is reassuring. Even with a financial planner, understanding some basic investment strategies will allow for a more fruitful relationship with a financial planner.

N. Baum, M. J. Kahn, *Business Basics for your Healthcare Practice*,
https://doi.org/10.1007/978-3-032-25241-8_5

One of the fundamental tenets of investment is the relationship between risk and reward. This means that the *greater risk an investor is willing to take, the higher the potential reward, and the higher the potential loss*. An example of the relationship between risk and reward is the story of the Beardstown Ladies who were featured in both the lay press and television [1]. This group, composed of older women in Illinois, formed an investment club known formally as the Beardstown Business and Professional Women's Investment Club in 1983. This group achieved notoriety for its returns on investment of over 23% per year for their first 10 years of activity, greatly exceeding average market returns. These women even wrote a book titled *Beardstown Ladies' Common-Sense Investment Guide*. Based on the concept of risk and reward, returns this high would suggest that this investment group assumed a high level of risk, or that they were extremely lucky. However, neither explanation appeared to be the case in a review of their portfolio. Rather, when audited, it appeared that the group did not properly account for returns, as they included new contributions to the fund by members in the group in their calculation of total return on investment. When properly audited and accounted for, the group was found to have a rate of return of only 9%, which is nearly 5% less than the return on the S&P for that same time period. This finding is consistent with another investment concept, which asserts that the average investor will earn an average rate of return. This means that the only way to consistently beat the market average in an investment portfolio would be to either have unusual luck, to have improperly accounted for earnings, as in the case of the Beardstown Ladies, or to have insider information that will land you in jail. In fact, in a perfect market, factors affecting stock prices are already figured into its cost. When Amazon first started operations, the financial benefit to FedEx who shipped their products was theoretically already accounted for in the FedEx stock price. For those who have trouble believing that over time, they cannot beat the market average, because they have a "better broker" or because they are a "better investor," Consider 100 people standing in a room each holding a penny. They flip their coins in unison and sit down when the flip landed on tails. At some point, someone is left standing. Are they a "better" coin flipper than all of the others? Certainly not!

Another important tenet of investing is the concept of diversification that can help to mitigate risk. For example, consider an investor who owns stock in an airline company. This investor is at risk if oil prices rise, because then his stock will lose value since the major expense of an airline is its fuel costs. To diversify, this investor may want to also purchase stock in an oil company. This will provide a hedge against rising oil prices, thus decreasing the value of his airline company stock. If he invests in oil companies, he will be financially protected due to the increased value of his oil company stock. Similarly, if oil prices fall, the value of his oil company stock will decrease, but his airline stock will provide a financial hedge against such a rise in oil prices. Diversification can be accomplished by owning stocks in multiple economic sectors or by owning stocks in different areas of the world.

We have spent time using stocks as examples, but what exactly is stock? Simply stated, stock represents ownership or equity in a company. Suppose your family owns a company that makes chocolates. The shareholders in this family business are you and your relatives. Suppose further that the chocolate business is becoming increasingly successful such that the company wishes to expand to a national market. This is going to require a significant amount of cash for additional equipment, supplies, employees, and marketing. Where can you obtain the additional funds? You could ask the shareholders to contribute personal money toward the expansion. Alternatively, you could sell part ownership in the company to investors. This part ownership is stock, and when companies do this on a large scale, it is known as going public. Shareholders are able to vote on company policies as they are part owners.

Stock price is dependent on many variables, but because stocks are traded publicly, there is a market that determines the stock price. The return on investment for a stock purchase is related to the riskiness of the stock itself, with the rate of return being the same for all stocks of equal risk. Owning stock carries financial risk because if a company goes bankrupt, the stock may be worth nothing. Some stocks pay dividends that are periodic cash payments to shareholders. Some stocks never pay dividends. As with all stock prices, the value of a stock that pays dividends is incorporated into the stock price. This particular type of stock is known as common stock. There is another type of stock called preferred stock, which obtains its name because in case of bankruptcy, preferred stockholders are paid before common stockholders. However, unlike common stock, preferred stockholders do not really have equity (ownership) of the company and do not have voting rights. As such, preferred stock can be thought of as a type of debt. Because preferred stock is less risky, its rate of return is generally less than common stock.

Generally, if a stock is undervalued, you should buy it. On the other hand, if a stock is overvalued, you should sell it. But suppose we believe the stock is overvalued and we do not own it? A short sale refers to selling overvalued stock that you do not have at a later date. This type of investment is legal but risky because if you are wrong, and the stock price increases, you have to provide the stock at the higher price even though it was priced lower at the time of the transaction. The finance pages often include stories about people who made money in the stock market in the face of a steep decline. Typically, these people are said to have shorted the market. What they did was to sell stock that they did not own at an inflated price only to later purchase the stock at a discounted price, then sell the stock to the buyer at the higher price, and pocket the difference as a profit. As an example, in 1992, George Soros was said to have made $1 billion in 1 month by shorting the British pound or betting that it would decrease in value [2].

Most investors diversify their stock portfolio through the purchase of mutual funds or exchange traded funds (ETFs). Mutual funds are companies that pool money from many investors and purchase many stocks to make up the fund. This allows the investor to have a diversified portfolio without having to personally purchase many individual stocks. There are several indicators (indexes) of the strength of the US economy based on stock prices. The Dow Jones Industrial Average (DJIA) is calculated as the sum of 30 representative stocks divided by a number called the Dow Divisor. The Dow Divisor is formulated such that stock splits or other structural changes do not alter the DJIA. The divisor also corrects for inflation. Another commonly used index is the Standard and Poor 500 (S&P 500). The S&P 500 is a weighted sum of the prices of 500 large common stocks actively traded in the United States. Index funds are mutual funds that follow a given index. These are also called ETFs. An ETF is like a mutual fund but typically includes all of the stocks contained in an index. Owning ETFs is like owning a piece of the Dow or a piece of the S&P. ETFs are diversified due to the varied industries and economic sectors represented in the index.

Another way that your family chocolate company could raise capital to expand would be to borrow money from the public. This type of business debt is called a *bond*. Bonds are less risky for investors than stocks because in the case of bankruptcy, debt holders are paid first. Based on what you have learned, it should not come as a surprise that bonds generally have a lower rate of return than stocks as they are less risky. Bonds typically pay interest on the borrowed money several times a year. These payments are called coupons. Bonds are also sometimes called fixed income investments because their value is predetermined at the point of sale. Bonds have a maturity date that designates the date when the bond principle is to be paid. Bonds also have a face value dictating the payment due at maturity, and bonds have a coupon rate. As an example, a 10-year $10,000 US Treasury Note with a 6% coupon rate. We know that this bond will mature at 10 years at which point the holder is entitled to full payment of $10,000. The bond holder is also entitled to two $300 coupon payments per year for the life of the bond. Many of us have received US savings bonds as gifts from an aunt or uncle. These are called zero coupon bonds as they do not have biannual interest payments. Rather, they are discounted at the point of sale. For example, currently you can buy (online) a $100 US savings bond for $50. The bond reaches face value at 20 years and will continue to earn interest for up to 30 years. Aunt Sally purchased that bond for you for your first birthday because it only cost her half the face value and she wanted to provide money for you when you reached 21 years of age. Your aunt also felt good about contributing to the US economy, and she knew that savings bonds carry no risk as they are backed by the US government.

Another major type of financial instruments includes derivatives or options. Derivatives are investments whose value depends on the value of an underlying asset. Fire insurance is an example of a derivative. If you purchase fire insurance for the total value of a $400,000 home, the insurance policy is worth nothing unless your house burns to the ground at which point it is worth $400,000. Fire insurance can therefore be considered a derivative investment on your house.

Generally, there are two types of options called "puts" and "calls." A put is the right to sell, and a call is the right to buy. Physicians are familiar with options without realizing it. Take a salary structure that includes a salary guarantee and a salary cap. The salary guarantee is an option provided to you that is a derivative of your salary. A salary cap is a benefit to your employer and is also an option. In the above example, the salary guarantee is a put because it protects against low earnings, whereas the salary cap is a call as it sets an upward limit. The value of options can be calculated where the value of the put is set to be equivalent to the value of the call. In options lingo, this is called a zero premium collar and such a strategy may be better at setting physician salary caps and guarantees than trial and error [3].

Options are traded on the Chicago Board Options Exchange. For example, on December 14, 2018, an investor could purchase a call option on Apple stock for $5.25 for a strike price of $165 with an expiration date of December 28. At that time, Apple stock was trading at $167. This means that any time prior to December 28, the holder of the call option could purchase a share of Apple stock for $165. Obviously, this option is worthless at the point of purchase because the option costs over $5 so the holder would have to spend $170 for something worth $167. Suppose the price of Apple stock rose to $175 prior to December 28th? Then the option would be profitable as the holder could purchase for $170 something worth $175. Puts work the same way but are a right to sell so are profitable when a stock price falls below a certain value.

Why are options important? Obviously, they are speculative investments as they require some prediction of the future and they are zero sum as for every seller, their needs to be a buyer so someone always wins and someone always loses in an options transaction. Stock purchase, in contrast, can provide a net gain for both seller and buyer if the stock price goes up after purchase.

Like fire insurance, options can be used as insurance for stock purchases. Say you purchased 100 shares of Apple stock at $165. You would be out of pocket $16,500. If you wanted to reduce your out-of-pocket expenses, and have an immediate return on investment, you could sell call options on your stock. Let's say you sold 100 calls for $5 each with a strike price of $170 and an expiration date in 6 months. You would immediately receive $500 for the options sale. Assuming the stock price prior to expiration was $175, you would be forced to sell your shares at the strike price of $170, and would receive $170 × 100 = $17,000. Your net profit on the transaction would be $1000, $500 from the option sale, and $500 from the $5 increase in price per share. On the other hand, if the stock price never went above $160, the options you sold would be worthless, but you would still have the $500 from the sale and would effectively recoup the money lost on the stock price drop. This investment strategy is called selling covered calls. The calls are covered, because you own the underlying stock. There is nothing illegal about selling calls on stock you do not own (uncovered calls), but this is extremely risky because there is theoretically no upward limit to the stock price, and if the stock price increases, you would have to provide the stock at the strike price regardless of the cost. For example, if something remarkable happened to Apple and the stock price went to $1165, and you owned no shares, you would have to provide 100 shares for this price, even though at the time of the option purchase, shares were trading for $165. You would have to pay $116,500 for stock that was only worth $16,500 at the time of the option sale for a net loss of $116,000!

Another way to use options as an insurance policy on a stock is the concept of a protective put. In this instance, you buy a put to protect you against an unexpected drop in stock price. Using the above example, suppose you bought 100 puts on your Apple stock that you bought for $165 a share. Suppose the puts cost $5 and suppose the expiration date is in 6 months and that the strike price is $160. This strategy would mitigate any drop in stock price that is more than $5 because if the price drops to, say, $150, you still have a right to sell it at $160.

These examples show how options can be used to protect stock investments, but also show how selling uncovered calls can be quite risky indeed.

What gives US currency value? Many physicians are shocked to learn that US currency is not backed by gold or silver since 1933. Currency backed by gold or silver is called commodity currency. A great example of the definition of money and the concept of commodity currency occurred on the tiny island of Yap in the South Pacific (Yap is also known for being the highest per capita consumers of Budweiser beer!). On Yap, instead of gold or silver, several hundred years ago, money came in the form of large limestone discs, often weighing several tons, which were traded in exchange for goods and often transported on small bamboo canoes. Because of the sheer girth of these stones, the concept of money on Yap became abstract and the coins or large stone discs could often not be moved at all. Interestingly, there is a story about one large stone that ended up on the bottom of the sea due to a huge storm that capsized a canoe. Even though the stone was under hundreds of feet of water, the stone was still considered currency and was traded as any other stone. This abstract notion of money should not be unfamiliar as we never see our money in a bank, but believe that it is there based on pixels that produce account information on our computer monitors. This is another definition of faith.

What gives the US dollar value? The US dollar is fiat currency, meaning its value is backed by the US government. One US dollar is valued at the amount of US goods and services that can be purchased for that dollar. A dollar bill in your wallet has the seal of the U.S. Federal Reserve System. The Federal Reserve System is a bank for banks. The Federal Reserve does not print money; that is the job of the Bureau of Engraving and Printing. Rather, the Federal Reserve can loan money to banks. Why would banks need to borrow money? When you deposit $100 into a bank, they do not store the $100 in a vault. Rather, the bank lends the money to others and collects interest on the debt. This greatly increases the total supply of money in the United States. In fact, for large banks, only 10% of deposits must be held in reserve. When banks fall below this level, they have to borrow money from the Federal Reserve. As such, the Federal Reserve controls the economy. Although it does not print money, it sets interest rates for short-term loans to other banks, which in turn affects interest rates on car loans, mortgages, and other bank loans. The Federal Reserve can also buy and sell US government bonds. If the Federal Reserve wants to slow the economy, the Federal Reserve will increase interest rates and will sell bonds to reduce the amount of money available for spending. If the Federal Reserve wants to stimulate the economy, it can decrease interest rates to encourage spending and the Federal Reserve can buy bonds to put more money into the economy.

Back to the Case

Jamal took the advice of others and found a financial planner who was highly recommended by his brother-in-law. Jamal and his financial planner discussed his short- and long-term financial goals, including providing for his family, providing for his daughter's education, and his desire to retire at 65. Jamal bought additional life insurance and invested in mutual funds and worked out a monthly purchase to dollar average.

With dollar averaging, if the market dropped, Jamal's mutual funds were cheaper that month, and if the market rose, his current funds were more valuable but the funds he bought were more expensive. Jamal comfortably invested the most he could each month based on his budget. Jamal also hired an accountant.

Key Takeaways

- Get a financial planner and an accountant.
- Reward is related to risk. There is no free lunch!
- The average investor earns an average rate of return.

References

1. Gongloff M. Where are they Now: The Beardstown Ladies; 2006. https://www.wsj.com/articles/SB114596682916135186. Accessed 31 Jan 2019
2. Topstep Trader. How George Soros made $1 billion shorting the British pound; 2017. https://blog.topsteptrader.com/story-of-george-soros-breaking-the-bank-of-england. Accessed 31 Jan 2019
3. Kahn MJ, Long HW. A real options approach to clinical faculty salary structure. J Health Care Finance. 2012;39:87–96.

6 Organized Medicine

> **Case Study: Amber**
> Amber is in her second year of residency training in physical medicine and rehabilitation at a major academic medical center. Amber became interested in how to better make changes for populations of patients from a policy perspective. Amber has received emails from the AMA, inviting her to attend an AMA sponsored meeting in Chicago. Amber has never considered herself much of a joiner. What should she do?

The power and voice of a group are stronger and louder than those of individuals. As healthcare is a major part of the US economy, physicians often join groups or associations to advocate for their patients and for the profession.

History of Organized Medicine in the United States

Prior to the establishment of the American Medical Association in 1845, *anyone* could publicly place a sign stating they were a doctor as there was no national standard for physician training. In 1845, Dr. Nathan S. Davis called for the first national medical convention, which led to the establishment of the American Medical Association (AMA) in 1847. Their first charter was focused on scientific advancement, setting standards for medical education, launching a program of medical ethics, and improving public health. These were the initial goals of the AMA more than 150 years ago, and they are still the aspirations of the organization today. The AMA is the first organization of its kind in the world to establish uniform standards for medical education, training, and practice, as well as the first to develop a national code for ethical medical practice. Ever since its inception, the AMA Code of Ethics dictates professional conduct for all practicing physicians. The AMA, with the Association of American Medical Colleges, sets the standards for medical education today through the Liaison Committee on Medical Education, the accreditation body for allopathic medical schools in the United States.

The AMA provides health and scientific information to its members and to the public and carries out a broad range of health education programs via mass media and lectures. It keeps its members informed of significant medical and health legislation, and it represents its profession before Congress and other governmental bodies. The AMA sets standards for medical schools and internship programs, and it alerts the public to quack medical remedies, snake oil salesmen, and other medical charlatans.

Publications of the AMA include the highly rated *Journal of the American Medical Association (JAMA)* and 11 other journals

N. Baum, M. J. Kahn, *Business Basics for your Healthcare Practice*,
https://doi.org/10.1007/978-3-032-25241-8_6

devoted to such medical specialties as internal medicine, psychiatry, and pediatrics. In addition, the AMA publishes the online journal *JAMA Network Open*, which focuses on original medical research in an open-source format.

Just a few decades ago, it was not unusual for physicians to be members of their county medical society, specialty society, state medical association, national specialty society, and the AMA, but physician participation is steadily decreasing. While the practice of medicine seems to be changing almost daily, support for organized medicine as a whole seems to be decreasing during a time at which patients and their physicians need help more than ever. Let us not forget that there is strength in numbers. It would be very difficult for one doctor to create changes in healthcare policy alone. Whereas if doctors join together in support or protest of legislation, it becomes a much more powerful display of force and much more can be accomplished.

Historically, just as the economy expands and grows during war, physician membership in organized medicine usually increases during difficult times—times in which medicine is facing more intrusion by government regulation and restriction on how physicians can and do practice medicine, often without consideration for the protection of patients' rights. In the 1950s, about 75% of all practicing physicians in the United States were members of the AMA. According to recent statistics in 2025, membership in the AMA is only about 15% of the nation's physicians.

So, where are all the physicians going? Today, there appears to be apathy for participation in organized medicine. Certainly, membership costs are one constraint, especially if a physician joins local, state, national organizations plus one or more of the specialty societies. Many practices and hospitals that employ physicians will cover the costs of these annual dues to these organizations. However, this provision must be in the physician's contract. (See Chap. 5) In addition to cost concerns, doctors today have time constraints that might preclude going to additional meetings and time away from their families. Finally, there are concerns as to the actual value of membership.

It has not been easy for organized medicine. Some of the consequences may be worth noting. Physicians are no longer the powerful force in society they once were. Their opinions and recommendations no longer go almost unchallenged. Although the AMA's use of political action committee (PAC) dollars can be used to assure that legislators at least listen to physicians' views, the effectiveness of such a strategy is mitigated by underfunding.

There was a time, more than half a century ago, when organized medicine played a key role in physicians' lives and held enormous sway over US healthcare policymaking. During that time, three-quarters of physicians were simultaneously members of their county and state medical societies and the American Medical Association (AMA). Physicians spent many hours of their free time in these three groups, dealing with clinical learning, running for elected offices, holding forums, and hammering out positions on all kinds of issues. For most older physicians, that era is long gone.

In contrast to the AMA, specialty societies enjoy very high membership rates and do not seem to have a problem staying relevant to doctors. However, each specialty society has developed its own particular position on healthcare issues, replacing the once-unified voice of the House of Medicine with a chorus of sometimes conflicting views.

Meanwhile, doctors seem to be following the growing trend among all Americans of moving away from groups. The 2000 book *Bowling Alone*, by Robert D. Putnam, demonstrated this trend by showing that even as the number of bowlers continued to rise, the number of people in bowling leagues had markedly fallen.

What Are the Reasons to Consider Joining Organized Medicine?

Organized medicine consists of groups of physicians categorized into three groups: (1) practicing physicians, (2) young physicians, and (3) resident and medical student sections. Each group or section works together to advocate collectively on behalf of the physician–patient relationship, patients' rights, and medicine as a whole. Each individual group also works together to advocate for their section's interests. Giving physicians and medical students a voice in the business of medicine allows physicians to advocate for the best quality of care for their patients and ensures physicians are also treated fairly on the state and national levels.

Organized medicine has been front and center in confronting the problem of physician burnout, which is impacting nearly 50% of all healthcare providers (See Chap. 22) Burnout is a complicated issue complicated by physician feeling of irrelevance in a complex healthcare market. Organized medicine has recognized that medicine is a business and doctors are in dire need of guidelines on suggestions for running an efficient, productive, and, yes, profitable practice that is relevant to the care of patients. These organizations are providing young doctors with the necessary tools and resources to run a cost-effective medical practice and to hopefully feel less burned out.

Compliance with national imperatives is a major problem that impacts nearly every practice. There are compliance regulations that are onerous, time consuming, and difficult to interpret. Recent reports looking at HIPAA and Meaningful Use audit findings have shown that most organizations do not retain the necessary supporting documentation of completion of core set objectives and measures. This puts the practice at increased risk of decreased reimbursement, costly fines, and prohibition of certain patient populations, such as those covered by Medicare and Medicaid, from using the practice. Many organizations offer audit solutions that help practices verify and validate that privacy and security programs meet compliance and business objectives. Billing and coding have become increasingly more complex. Organized medicine can help physicians understand these complexities and be properly reimbursed for their work.

Organized medicine has played, and will continue to play, a major role in the education and training of young physicians. You can plan on accessing the latest in technology and education through your national, state, local, and specialty organizations.

Our national medical societies and organizations have taken a leadership role in confronting and managing the American opioid crisis. This has been a crisis that the medical community is culpable, and we have taken responsibility for solving this crisis and reducing the use of opioids and providing services for those who are addicted to these drugs. Organized medicine, as a national voice, had the clout to affect change through education and through their ability to direct local and national resources toward solving this crisis.

One of the best examples of the effectiveness of organized medicine was a report in the *New England Journal of Medicine* in 1991 authored by Lucien Leape, who reviewed 30,000 randomly selected patients' hospital records. The study shocked the medical profession. This report demonstrated that nearly 4% of patients admitted to a hospital suffered an injury that prolonged their hospital stay or resulted in measurable disability and that nearly 14% of those injuries were fatal. Further, the study found that 70% of those injuries were clearly preventable. The study extrapolated that data of 30,000 patient records to the entire nation and estimated that 120,000 people were dying from preventable medical errors. The study showed medication errors accounted for the largest group of preventable medical errors. Leake estimated that there were 1 million preventable medical errors in the United States each year, and the cost of these errors added to the already bloated healthcare budget by $33 million every year. This report in the *NEJM* generated front-page coverage in nearly every major American newspaper. This was an unacceptable blemish on American healthcare that galvanized organized medicine (AMA) as this was such a large problem that one person or group could not possibly solve. The AMA demonstrated that error prevention systems were in place in other industries such as the airline industry. The AMA recommended that the healthcare profession adapt the same systems that were accomplished in other industries and that errors could be reduced and the quality of medicine improved.

Shortly after the publication of the Leake report, the AMA, Joint Commission on the Accreditation of Healthcare Organizations, and the American Association for the Advancement of Science hosted a conference on errors in medicine where a prevention, education, and research agenda was established. It was through this pioneering work on part of a group of organized physicians that patient safety was recognized as the sine qua non of quality. Thanks to these doctors and organized medicine, there were, for the first time, sophisticated and efficient methods of measuring quality that could compare institutions and doctors through the quality lens. The take-home message is that change can occur in medicine, albeit slowly, but when we put the patient first and recognize that we are fallible but that we can correct our errors, we are, indeed, making progress.

Medical associations provide unparalleled networking opportunities, allowing young doctors to connect with their peers, mentors, and other industry leaders. As a member, you are in the unique position to attend conventions, seminars, and other related events with like-minded professionals in the field. Medical associations will provide you with not only clinical collaboration but also socialization with like-minded colleagues.

A medical association's annual meeting represents an incredible opportunity for you to meet and network with the largest gathering of your peers every year. Networking with professionals outside your place of employment can give you a broader perspective on the market and healthcare in general. Listening to the experiences of others may even leave you feeling energized and refreshed with the feeling you are not alone in the fight to change the course of American medicine.

The field of medicine is always in a state of change. Healthcare professionals can keep up with the newest developments and scientific breakthroughs through their associations' seminars, journals, CME courses, and other educational opportunities. Additionally, many associations, especially the specialty societies, offer all of the certification courses you will need throughout your entire career. Your professional organization also provides access to mentors, giving you an opportunity to participate in mentoring others as well. Having a mentor in any field will help your career grow and thrive. As an association member, you are in the unique position to gain a competitive edge by utilizing of all of the educational resources and marketing materials available to you.

Associations are always looking for young doctors to help organize their annual meetings, workshops, CME courses, and legislative committees. Helping your organization work to improve your profession as well as to help improve the overall state of healthcare can be a very rewarding opportunity. Working on these projects will also be a great introduction to organized medicine and will often serve as a springboard to reach higher levels in the organization.

To fully receive the benefits of membership, you need to be engaged with the association. With any membership you get what you put into it. Get involved early in your career and as often as possible and you will reap the benefits offered to you as a member.

Healthcare associations are great places to find the latest jobs in your field! Looking for a new position during your training? Most organizations collect positions available throughout the nation, and you can submit areas where you would like to work and find available jobs in your specialty and location where you would like to work. An excellent resource is www.healthecareers.com. This site allows you to submit your name and email, and you can be notified electronically as new jobs become available.

There are several special examples of organized medicine besides the AMA, state organizations, and specialty societies that you may consider joining. These include the American Medical Women's Association (https://nmanet.org/), which is an organization that functions at the local and national levels to advance women in medicine and improve women's health.

The National Medical Association (NMA) (https://nmanet.org/) is the voice of African American physicians and the leading voice for parity and justice in medicine and the elimination of disparities in healthcare for all Americans regardless of ethnicity. The NMA represents the interests of more than 50,000 African American physicians and the patients they serve. The NMA is committed to improving the quality of health among all minorities and disadvantaged people through its membership, professional development, community health education, advocacy, research, and partnerships with federal and private agencies.

The American Medical Student Association (AMSA) is the oldest and largest independent association of physicians-in-training in the United States. AMSA members are medical students, premedical students, interns, residents, and practicing physicians. AMSA is focused on future physicians who believe that patients and health professionals are partners in the management of healthcare and that access to high-quality healthcare is a right and not a privilege. The AMSA annual convention is the largest gathering of medical students and regularly draws an attendance of more than 1500 physicians-in-training, medical educators and health policy innovators. AMSA continues to search for new and innovative ways to improve healthcare, healthcare delivery, and medical education.

AMSA remains a leader in the campaign for resident work hour reform—authoring the Patient and Physician Safety and Protection Act of 2003. The passage of this act by Congress limited the work week of residents and fellows to 80 hours per week.

AMSA publishes an excellent magazine, *The New Physician*, available to all students and new physicians, which will provide the information you need to enrich your medical training and launch your career as a physician.

AMSA local chapters continue to reach out to serve the health needs of their communities. Annually, local chapters contribute over 1 million hours of community service.

Back to the Case

Amber's trip to Chicago was "mind-blowing," allowing her to serve as an alternate delegate for the first time. Because the AMA trip to Chicago was her first introduction to organized medicine on a national stage, she did not know what to expect, which made for an even better experience.

She experienced collegiality of residents from all different walks of life and all different types of programs, from multiple geographic areas all coming together for one specific cause. She decided to become involved in organized medicine because she knew that there were strengths in numbers and that a group of doctors could advocate better for patients than one doctor alone could possibly accomplish.

Key Takeaways

Organized medicine has the objective of promoting the science and art of medicine and also to enhance public health. Let us not forget that there's strength in numbers. It is highly unlikely that one person can produce significant changes in healthcare policy. However, when we work together through the auspices of organized medicine, we can improve American healthcare. By standing together, united in vision and commitment, we physicians can shape the healthcare system this country needs.

7 Transitioning from Training to Private Practice

Case Study: Phil the Neurosurgeon

Phil is a fellowship-trained neurosurgeon. He had 13 years of training and is about to complete 5 years of military service, including several tours in Afghanistan and Iraq, to repay his education. Fortunately, Phil did not have any appreciable debt upon entering private practice. Phil has expertise in midbrain surgery, utilizing stereotaxic localization for brain tumor treatment. He is a highly skilled surgeon, but due to his extensive training and the lack of mentors during his military experience, he is uncertain about how to transition into private practice.

Medical doctors spend the first third of their lives in preparation for their medical career. They undergo intensive schooling, face stressful examinations, and often incur hundreds of thousands of dollars in debt. The day you enter practice is the day you leave the womb of the training program and the day you become a real doctor who is held responsible for the decisions you make. The newly minted doctor can no longer hide behind teachers, professors, and mentors.

Unfortunately, most medical training focuses on the diagnosis and treatment of diseases and medical conditions. Few training programs offer any guidelines on starting or managing a medical practice. Starting a medical practice is also viewed as one of the most rewarding accomplishments for a physician. Having your own practice or joining a small group practice offers young physicians the opportunity to make decisions and provide treatment that directly impacts the quality and standards of care delivered to patients. That's the good news. However, private practice comes with a multitude of obstacles to overcome, including hardships, start-up costs, and common mistakes to avoid.

There's no denying that starting your own practice, even if you are an employed physician or going into small group practice, can be overwhelming. However, there is nothing as exciting as finally entering this exclusive Club Medicine and being able to treat patients and enjoy the fruits of the long labor required to become a doctor. Nearly every doctor will tell you that it's worth the long, arduous journey.

Ideally, you would like to have everything in order and ready to start caring for patients on your first day of practice. The first recommendation is to start early, typically 6–9 months before the end of your training. Starting early will require a significant time commitment.

Everything takes time to prepare for practice, and that is often more time than you anticipate. Obtaining a license in another state can take months of correspondence, copying transcripts from undergraduate and medical

N. Baum, M. J. Kahn, *Business Basics for your Healthcare Practice*,
https://doi.org/10.1007/978-3-032-25241-8_7

school, proof of citizenship, and a copy of your medical degree issued by a medical school approved by the state board. This vetting process by state boards of medical examiners can be very frustrating. In training, you are accustomed to having patient care-related documents and forms readily available at the click of a mouse. However, working with other people, such as bureaucrats in state medical societies, insurance companies, lenders, real estate agents, lawyers, contractors, third-party payers, and technology firms, can be a source of anxiety and frustration. Remember, no one is as eager to start a practice as you are.

Even when everyone is on board, much of the preparation for practice takes time, and there is not much you can do to speed up those processes. For example, the credentialing process for most hospitals requires at least 6 months.

Most successful physicians who make transitions use a checklist. Figure 7.1 is an excellent checklist provided by Physician Practice Specialists (https://physicianpracticespecialists.com/practice-start-up/step-by-step-practice-start-up-guide-checklist/).

Once you have finished your training program, signed your contract or lease, had business cards and stationery printed, and your name is on the door, what do you do next?

Healthcare Start-Up Issues

The following is an abbreviated list of items* to consider when contemplating the opening of a new practice. This list is not comprehensive and should be viewed only as a general guide. Actual needs will be dictated by specific markets, programming, and strategic goals of the principal(s) involved.

Strategic Planning

1. Select a Qualified Consultant to Develop:
    1. Business Description and Goals
    2. Market Assessment
    3. Financial Feasibility Study: Assumptions, Proforma Financial Statements, and Capital Requirements
    4. Operational and Marketing Strategies

Facilities

1. Select Office Site/Negotiate Lease
2. Design Office Layout/Tenant Improvement, Needed vs Desired
3. Design Office Signs (Interior/Exterior)
4. Design Employee Workstations
5. Investigate Structural Alterations/Regulatory Issues/Infection Control Issues
6. Address HIPAA (Privacy Regulation) Facility Design Issues
7. Design Patient Flow (Incl. Privacy) Issues
8. Lay Out Exam Rooms/Procedure Room/ Patient Areas/Staff Areas
9. Select Phone Systems: Design and Layout
10. Plan EHR & EMR system I Billing, Accounts Receivable & Practice Management Information Systems
11. Select Information System Hardware and telecommunications equipment
12. Procure Office and Clinical Equipment
13. Select Supply Vendor and Order Initial Inventory
    a. Medications
    b. Supplies-gloves, bandages, centrifuge, microscope
    c. Exam tables

Practice Management

1. Select Legal Counsel and CPA
2. Develop Legal Structure
3. Create Corporate Documents
4. File a Business Name
5. Establish a Tax ID Number
6. Obtain a Business License
7. Obtain Business Liability, Malpractice, And Workers' Compensation Insurance
8. EHR: Selection and Implementation of an Electronic Health Records System (practice management and electronic medical record)
9. Prepare for Health Plan(s) Participation
Including Medicare/Medicaid to meet All Relevant Requirements Established in Federal/State Guidelines and Demonstrate Compliance *(Physical Plant, Equipment, Supplies, Written Clinical and Administrative Policies/Procedures, Forms, Staff Qualifications, Traceable Systems, Chart Note Review, OSHA,* Etc.*)*
10. Negotiate Payor Contracts

Fig. 7.1 Healthcare start-up issues

11. Identify Clinical Services/Develop Special Program/Services
12. Write Clinical and Operations Policies, Procedures, and Protocols
(a) Office Systems and Information Flows
(b) Appointment Scheduling
(c) Patient Registration
(d) Check-In/Reception
(e) Medical Records
(f) Nursing/Back Office
(g) Check-out Reception
(h) Referrals/Follow-Up Care
(i) Pharmacy
(j) Supplies (Clinical/Non-Clinical)
(k). Conduct a HIPAA Risk Assessment for Privacy, Security, and Breach Notification Rules
(l). Establish Practice Management Benchmarks and Indicators to Judge Success
(m). Develop a Medicare Fraud and Abuse Compliance Program and Evidence of Implementation
(n). Conduct Ongoing Operational Reviews and Strategic Planning

Financial Planning

1. Establish and Implement and Operating Budget
2. Set Up Billing and Collection Protocols/Policies
3. Open Bank Accounts
4. Establish Working Capital Line of Credit
5. Establish Credit Card Processing Capability
6. Determine Outsourcing Needs/Establish Contracts (e.g., Billing, Payroll)
7. Establish and Implement Proper Purchasing Policies and Procedures
8. Establish Accounting and Reporting Systems for Effective Cash Management
9. Develop Financial Management Policies and Procedures
10. Establish Proper Internal Control Measures

Human Resources

1. Develop Personnel Policies and Initial Staffing Plan
2. Establish Proper Orientation and Training Programs
3. Establish an Internal Safety Program
4. Set up Payroll and Quarterly Tax Reporting Systems
5. Post Federal/State Mandated Employee Postings
6. Develop Position Descriptions
7. Develop A Compensation and Benefits Plan
8. Recruit Employees

Marketing and Generating Referrals

1. Develop Collateral Material, (i.e., Practice Brochure)
2. Establish and Implement a Marketing/Referral Development Plan
3. Develop a Public Relations Program
4. Plan and develop an Online Presence Program (i.e., website)
5. Obtain Stationery and Business Cards

*Checklist for Transition from Training to Practice (Used with permission from Provider Services Nationwide (https://www.physicianpracticestartup.com).

Fig. 7.1 (continued)

Credentialing with Insurance Companies

Begin the credentialing process early, as it may take 4–6 months to obtain permission to see their patients covered by their insurance. We have seen doctors start practicing with a state license, but they are not included in insurance plans. They, therefore, cannot be reimbursed for their services. Being excluded from insurance plans can be frustrating for a young doctor starting their practice.

Credentialing is a process used to evaluate physicians' qualifications and practice history. This process includes reviewing a doctor's completed education, training, residency, and licenses. This also includes a review of any certifications issued by a board in the doctor's specialty.

You do not have to be board-certified, but if you are going to practice a specialty, you must demonstrate that you are at least board-eligible.

Credentialing with insurance companies, otherwise known as provider enrollment or achieving in-network status, can be challenging, especially if this is your first foray into that process. Even with experience and every tool at your disposal, credentialing can be a daunting task. Here is a brief overview of how to complete the provider enrollment or insurance credentialing process to become an in-network provider. Keep in mind that each payer may be slightly different [1]. Start by obtaining your CAQH ID. The Universal Credentialing Data Source is designed to simplify the credentialing process for providers by consolidating data in a single repository. This data may be accessed by participating health plans and other healthcare organizations. The CAQH ID enables providers to update their information. Commercial payers will require this information for your application. Ensure CAQH has a valid W-9 and malpractice certificate uploaded. You can easily register for your CAQH ID online at https://proview.caqh.org/PR/Registration.

Next, request to join the network on the insurance company's website. Sometimes it is not easy to find a network site, so always contact the payer to follow up with your request, or call them if you cannot find the join network request. Many insurance companies have credentialing hotlines set up; hence, check out their website for this number.

If the panel is open or the insurance company needs doctors in your specialty, or if they need additional primary care doctors, the credentialing process can begin. The panel will request specific information, such as the CAQH ID, NPI, and practice EIN. The practice EIN is an Employer Identification Number (EIN), a nine-digit number assigned by the IRS. The EIN identifies the tax accounts of employers and others, even if there are no additional employees. The IRS uses the number to identify taxpayers who are required to file various business tax returns each year. You need to verify that the practice EIN you provide matches the one listed on the W-9 that should already be in the CAQH system.

You must follow up on the material you submitted. Your request may fall through the cracks at the payer level. Information and documents may be lost or misplaced, and you will receive a notice that the file is incomplete. Therefore, we suggest that you contact the payer frequently to ensure everything is proceeding correctly. If a document or form is missing, you can promptly submit or resubmit any required or missing information.

Contracting with Insurance Companies

Once credentialing or primary source verification is complete, you will move to contracting. The contracting phase is the all-important part of determining how much you will get paid for your services to the payers' members. A contracting representative will be assigned to you, and that representative will draft your agreement. Your agreement will be drafted by the payer, typically 3 months after you initiate the credentialing process. The contracting department will then review it. At this time, your fee schedule is created. You should follow up every week or two to check the status with the payer regarding your fee schedule. You must review the fee schedule before signing, as they may submit a lousy initial agreement. The fee schedule is not always included, so you may need to request a fee schedule and provide the payer with your top 20 codes or the procedures you perform or plan to perform most often.

After signing the contract, plan on an additional 30 days for them to load your name, contact information, and the fee schedule into their system. You will be issued a provider identification number (PIN) and a letter of participation that indicates your effective date of having permission to see their patients.

You are still not done! You must verify payer participation and save the email or letter received from the payer confirming participation. Finally, ensure your billing system is updated with payer information (EDI enrollment), and only then can you start submitting claims.

It is now evident why this process takes so long. Obtaining credentials and contracting takes time, and you cannot receive compensation unless you have a self-pay practice where credentialing is not required.

Use of Technology

If you are an employed physician or decide to open your own practice, you will depend on technology to support your practice. Effective use of modern technology will enhance the care of your patients. Pay attention to selecting, installing, training, and supporting the technology used in your practice.

Currently, technology is relatively inexpensive compared to the cost of employee salaries, which range from 18% to 25% of gross income. You need to get comfortable with that technology that is constantly changing. The technology that you purchase will soon become obsolete. Therefore, your technology selection should include the necessity to upgrade, expand, and replace your existing technology. If you are starting your practice, consider the intended purpose of the technology. Consider the needs and requirements before contacting a vendor. List your technology requirements and present them to a vendor, asking how their product supports the essential needs of your practice.

Look at the reliability of the product you are considering. Nothing can bring your practice to a screeching halt like a power outage, and all the technology is out of commission. With that in mind, check the performance record of the technology. We also recommend purchasing devices that preserve your data in the event of a power outage. This includes a surge protector and battery backup that powers down to protect hardware, software, and sensitive data.

In recent years, cloud storage has become an increasingly popular solution for medical practices to store sensitive data, offering numerous benefits, including enhanced accessibility, improved data security, and cost efficiency. However, it is crucial for healthcare providers to carefully evaluate and manage cloud storage solutions to ensure the protection of sensitive patient information.

When considering cloud storage, medical practices must ensure that the cloud service provider complies with the Health Insurance Portability and Accountability Act (HIPAA) regulations and other applicable data privacy laws. Selecting a vendor that provides encryption, secure data transmission, and multifactor authentication can help protect sensitive information. Additionally, medical practices should implement internal policies to regulate access to cloud-stored data and monitor usage to prevent unauthorized access or data breaches.

Furthermore, it is essential to maintain a contingency plan for data recovery in the event of unexpected incidents, such as power outages or security breaches by hackers attempting to access your sensitive data. Regularly backing up data and developing a disaster recovery strategy can help ensure business continuity and minimize disruptions to patient care. By taking these measures, medical practices can confidently leverage the advantages of cloud storage while maintaining the privacy and security of sensitive patient data. (See Chap. 19 on Crisis Management for more information regarding practice disruptions.)

One size does not fit all. Consequently, be certain that your technology acquisition can be easily integrated into your workflow and meets

HIPAA regulatory requirements. Choose a flexible program that can be tailored to meet your specific practice needs. The best example is your electronic medical record program and practice management system.

An essential requirement for any technology purchase is the service reputation of the equipment. It is necessary to be aware of the technical support for the program. You will want to know if help is available early in the day, on weekends, and after your practice closes. Additionally, you want to know how quickly the vendor's support team responds to problems you encounter with their product. It is reasonable to expect a response from your practice within 1–2 h when you need assistance.

You will need to decide whether to use your insurance billing software program or outsource the billing to a service that will handle it on behalf of your practice. There are caveats for using a billing service. The billing service is unfamiliar with the patients and may be rude and insensitive when requesting payment for services. Additionally, many of these services lack coding experts and may inflate their collection statistics by down-coding your services. A billing service means one less employee, but you may be leaving significant amounts of money on the table.

The age of telemedicine has arrived, a positive side effect of the 2020 pandemic. Now, many patients, especially Millennials, are expecting to have virtual visits with their physicians. For telehealth sessions, you will need to select a HIPAA-compliant platform. (For more information on telemedicine, see Chap. 22)

Finally, we suggest that you investigate the security of any technology system you decide to use. Sensitive information must be encrypted. A recent concern is the ability of hackers to obtain access to your data and then hold it hostage, demanding payment for its return.

Our best advice is to obtain references from users of the technology. We suggest that you visit practices that have already implemented the technology and "kick the tires" of the technology, which means watching the program in use in a similar practice. Most physicians and office managers will provide you with their opinions on the program and discuss its benefits and drawbacks.

Suggestions for Getting Started

We provide 10 suggestions to facilitate the transition process. Although not all of these suggestions may apply to you and your practice, we assure you that most of them will be helpful.

Find a Mentor

Your senior partner may not be able to help you—chances are, they entered private practice more than 10 years ago. Although the senior partners may be excellent clinicians, we can assure you that their clinical skills will probably not help you in your transition from training to practice. Finding a career mentor is a vital step after finishing your residency. A senior physician who knows the ropes or the politics of the medical community in which you plan to practice can be an invaluable resource. A senior physician will likely be flattered that you have asked them for guidance and counsel. Pick their brains about practice and the realities of the real world of medicine.

For a career mentor, we recommend selecting a senior, well-established physician with a high level of visibility within your medical community. Examples might include an executive in your local medical society, the previous chief of staff at your hospital, or even a family friend in the medical profession. It is not necessary to select a mentor in your specialty. If you are a surgeon, consider an internist or a medical specialist. If you are in sports medicine, consider selecting a cardiologist or rheumatologist. Your primary purpose in choosing a mentor is not to develop a referral source, but to learn the unique aspects of your medical community. The mentor should introduce you to physicians with whom you share common interests and who could become your future professional allies. Your mentor may also invite you to social functions at the hospital that you might not have otherwise been included in. Ask to join the mentor at the first few hospital staff meetings, requesting that they introduce you to their colleagues and contemporaries. You will find that the advice from a mentor is priceless. The mentor will be instrumental in helping you achieve a rapid career advancement.

Learn How to Write or Create an Effective Referral Letter

Most residency programs focus on the diagnosis and treatment of disease. They provide little training on the techniques of communicating with other physicians. Therefore, most new physicians unknowingly give the referring doctor too much information. Like you, today's doctors are too busy to read two- to three-page letters. They will be unimpressed by a lengthy letter, and chances are, they will not even read it. Referring doctors appreciate short letters, those that are to the point, and those that are timely. What information are primary care doctors looking for in a letter from a referring doctor? The working diagnosis, the medications you recommend prescribing for the patient, and the treatment plan you wish to initiate are most often cited as the key elements. (For more information on communicating with referring physicians, see Chap. 10.)

Meet the VIPs

As soon as you begin your practice, you should introduce yourself to several key individuals within your hospital. They are

- The medical director.
- The hospital administrator.
- The chief of staff.
- The chief of your department.
- The emergency room physicians and staff.
- The business/admitting office staff.
- The physician services representative.
- The marketing/PR staff.
- The director of MCE.
- The head of physician referral services.

Meet Other Physicians

You need a core group of physicians to refer patients to you. Probably 10–15 physicians who will refer to you regularly is all that is required initially. Block out time each week for calling upon doctors you think could send you referrals. Initially, you will find that doctors in practice for less than 5 years and older physicians near retirement are the best contacts to make. Look beyond your specialty when courting referring physicians.

Do not neglect your specialty, as you may find colleagues in your specialty who do not perform the procedures that you do as a result of your recent training. Consider sending a brief letter to the doctor you plan to meet a few days before the scheduled appointment. The letter could mention your training, areas of interest, and expertise, as well as why you moved to the community, and any personal information that may be of interest to the doctor you are approaching. Sending a brief thank-you letter after the meeting is also a nice gesture. Invite this colleague to assist you. For example, suppose you are a recently trained plastic surgeon, and an older plastic surgeon is not trained in breast reconstruction. In this case, the older doctor may be happy to send you their patients. This way, the more senior physician remains involved in the patient's care and is assured of getting their patient back.

Remember, you do not always need to meet a potential referral source in the doctor's office. Visit the physicians' lounges and dining rooms, and attend social events organized by the hospital, such as sporting events and health fairs. Today, it is possible to introduce yourself virtually; however, an in-person meeting remains the best way to establish a professional relationship.

The Buddy System

Most medical staff offices have programs to orient new physicians to the hospital. Be sure to find out if the hospital has a "buddy system," in which an assigned physician will serve as your guide and show you around the hospital and the medical community. Request a copy of the medical directory and the names of other new physicians on the staff. Learn about the schedule of staff meetings and the committees you may be eligible to join. Be sure to contact the chairpersons of committees that interest you or provide opportunities to meet new physicians.

Contact Nonphysicians

Please introduce yourself to the nurses in your hospital to discuss your area of expertise and share your interests with them. Meeting the community's pharmacists is also a good idea; patients often ask them to recommend a physician. Other worthwhile contacts include podiatrists, chiropractors, lawyers, social workers, beauticians, barbers, and manicurists.

Especially for Surgeons

To have your first cases go smoothly, consider the following:

1. Introduce yourself to the operating room supervisor and staff.
2. If you are performing procedures new to the OR staff, consider offering an in-service program to the operating room nurses.
3. Before leaving your residency, obtain copies of your instrument cards to present to the operating room staff to have the appropriate instruments on hand for your first cases. This measure will ensure that all the necessary instruments, sutures, intraoperative medications, and any additional equipment required for your surgical procedures are available for the early cases you schedule in the hospital.
4. Before starting your first few cases, meet with the scrub nurse and the circulating nurse to discuss your plans, preferences, and needs, including your glove size. Educating the operating room personnel before surgery begins is the best way to succeed for your first few cases. Your first few cases must be seamless. There will be people evaluating your behavior, skills, and outcomes, so ensure that the early cases accurately represent your personality and talents.

Keep in Touch

Rolodex cards may be a thing of the past. Yet, many offices still collect cards of colleagues, pharma, device companies, and other essential contacts, using a Rolodex file. Address/file cards are an effective way to keep your name in front of the physician and the staff. Your card will contain not only your name, address, and phone number but also an email address, a direct line to your cell phone, and even your home number. Additionally, you can include your office hours, an answering service, a professional information number (PIN), partners, and the names of your office manager, secretary, and nurse. Also, include any other information you think might be helpful, such as the insurance plans you are currently on. For those who are more technologically savvy, consider using one of the electronic file card apps. CamCard (https://www.camcard.com) is a business card reader that utilizes a smartphone's camera to capture, store, and edit business cards using optical character recognition (OCR).

Pharmaceutical Contacts

Physician services departments will have the names and telephone numbers of the contacts who can help you. Knowing pharmaceutical representatives and medical manufacturing companies can also be helpful. Pharmaceutical representatives have the necessary materials and resources to help new physicians establish their practices. Some pharmaceutical companies even have divisions dedicated to assisting new physicians to start their careers.

Setting Fees

Lastly, you will want to consider how much to charge for your services. Few areas will impact your practice more than the fees you charge for your services. Most studies indicate that few patients choose doctors based solely on fees. If you join a group or have partners, this task will be easy, as their fees are your fees. Occasionally, a colleague will share this information with you. Another technique is to use the relative value unit. These values are in "Relative Values for Physicians" [2].

Take a Vacation

And our final piece of advice—do not go to work the day after you complete your training on July 1! Why? There will never be a time when you can have a long vacation with very little responsibility. We understand that you may have significant debt and are eager to reduce your financial obligations (see Chap. 9 on debt reduction). We recommend a 4- to 6-week hiatus between the completion of your training and the commencement of your practice. The practice or hospital you are joining managed without you for months or years. In that case, a few additional weeks will not make a significant difference. Yes, you may be eager to begin, but you should take advantage of this gap and take an extended vacation with your significant other and family. We can assure you that you will not have 6 weeks off from your practice until 35–40 years later, when you retire. We have never encountered a doctor who has regretted this decision (see Appendix).

Back to Neurosurgeon Phil

Phil went online and obtained a checklist for the licensing and credentialing process. He spent nearly 6 months preparing for the transition to private practice. He joined a single-specialty neurosurgery practice and had partners help with the hospital credentialing process. Phil admits that there was nothing easy about the move from training to practice, but starting early was his best advice. He also took a much-needed vacation after being discharged from the service and was delighted that he did.

Bottom Line

Medicine has indeed undergone significant changes since the first day you started medical school or even began your residency. Many young physicians are discouraged about the prospects in healthcare, or find starting a practice daunting, and opt for becoming an employed physician instead. However, there are still excellent opportunities available to every physician, regardless of their practice experience. The transition from residency to private practice can be less daunting when you know and implement the proper steps for success. Our final advice: Start early, 6–9 months before you complete your training, as the credentialing process takes longer than expected.

Key Takeaways

- Transitioning from training to practice can be a source of anxiety and tension.
- This pressure can be alleviated by using a checklist.
- The more lead time you have, the faster you can become credentialed and start billing for your services.
- Find a mentor, an established physician who will help you in the transition process.

Appendix: Practice Transition List

Task	Task complete	Contact person	Remarks
Finance & General Ledger			
Identify staffing requirements			
Develop job descriptions			
Hire Staff			
Identify Hardware Needs			
Purchase and Install Hardware/Software			
Determine how lock-box accounts will be transferred to the practice			
Create Financial system format in system			
Input opening balance sheet			
Determine how financial statements will be completed/outsourced to CPA?			
If internal—Develop policies and procedures			
Download chart of accounts from PeopleSoft (if desired)			
Create chart of accounts in new system			
Determine fixed asset accounting requirements			
Plan to transfer any depreciation associated with capital items			
Accounts Payable			
Develop policies and procedures			
Determine A/P process (approval levels, etc.)			
Set—up vendor master tables			
Set—up A/P disbursement bank account			
Update credit applications with vendors			
Notify Vendors of change of mailing address			
Practice to obtain new general accounting application			
Determine cut off date and plan for any open (unpaid) invoices			
Update AP system to address any recurring payments (rent, utilities, etc) for specific business units			
Review to verify nothing set up for pre-pay			
Payroll			
Develops Policies and Procedures			
Determine payroll process (who will approve pay rates)			
Determine benefit structure (from HR section)			
Obtain W-4's for all employees			
Set—up employee tables			
Build deduction tables			
Set—up P/R disbursement bank account			
Human Resources			
Group Benefits: Practice selects broker			
Group Benefits: Designs welfare benefits (insurance, cafeteria, and reimbursement account plans)			
Group Benefits: Practice selects insurance company and plans			
Group Benefits: Practice selects providers to administer COBRA and reimbursement accounts			
Practice conducts welfare benefits enrollment for active employees and physicians and for current COBRA participants			
Practice selects provider for 401(k) Plan			
Practice conducts 401(k) enrollment for participants who are eligible, but not enrolled			

(continued)

Task	Task complete	Contact person	Remarks
Reimbursement			
PRACTICE MANAGEMENT SYSTEMS			
+Medic (NC, Jacksonville, VA, OH)			
Determine plan to find vendor (Perot) to host +Medic application or have practice assume responsibilities			
Legal review of contract to transfer resp. to practices			
Order and implement circuits for new environment			
Determine if any issues associated with multiple databases on same hardware for practices			
Adjust monthly billing to transfer to each practice			
Terminate phone lines for EDI and Support			
PRACTICE OPERATIONS			
Develop and Implement Reimbursement Operations Policies and Procedures			
CODING AND BILLING UPDATES			
Subscribe to periodicals such as: Part B News Letter, Part B Answer Book, etc.			
Determine individual responsbile for monthly review of carrier's newsletters and web sites			
Determine individual responsible for interpreting and disseminating information to sites			
Develop process for training of both clinical and administrative staff—as needed			
Develop/implement process for monitoring utilization of new codes			
Determine individuals responsible for updating practice management system—as needed			
Determine individual responsible for review of annual ICD9 updates and changes			
DOCUMENTATION AND CODING COMPLIANCE			
Develop/implement internal chart audit program			
Develop/implement process for random review of charge tickets and charge entry process			
REVENUE CYCLE MONITORING			
Develop process and individual responsible for quarterly review by site of all functions			
Develop training materials and implement on going training program			
IT			
Preliminary Tasks			
Confirm local site project team members			
Identify corporate project team members including legal, operations, and IT			
Practice Web Sites			
Practice contract with 3rd party hosting service			
Practice contract with 3rd parties for content and vicinity mapping			
Migrate contracts for domain name registration			
Orchard Lab Systems (AR, IA, MN, OK, IN, NY, OH, NC, SC, VA, TX, CO, OR)			
Verify all contracts in local practice name			
Transition support directly to site/vendor			
Impac Radiation Systems (Austin, Baylor, Ft. Worth, IN, SC, AZ, CO, NV)			
Determine infrastructure requirements			
Implement infrastructure requirements per vendor including redundancy			

(continued)

Task	Task complete	Contact person	Remarks
Transition support to agreed upon plan			
Varis Radiation Systems (IA, El Paso, OR)			
Determine infrastructure requirements			
Implement infrastructure requirements per vendor including redundancy			
Transition support to agreed upon plan			
Research (eRT and CTMS)			
Verify site will have internet connectivity			
Create user accounts with USON to limit access to CTMS server			
Work with USInternetworking to change IP addresses of sites connecting to eRT			
Network Tasks			
Analyze network maps to determine scope and impact. Include the number of sites affected.			
Confirm date to transition network connections and equipment from the US Oncology network			
Identify who will have ownership of networking equipment after the transition			
Inventory data circuits including contract terms			
Inventory networking equipment including maintenance terms			
Verify/Change billing information for data circuits at the local practice			
Change passwords on networking equipment			
Transfer ownership and support to practice			
Telecommunication Tasks			
Inventory voice circuits including contract terms			
Inventory telecommunication equipment including maintenance terms			
Verify/Change billing information for voice circuits at the local practice			
Identify who will have ownership of any telecommunication equipment after the transition			
Transfer ownership and support to practice			
Security Tasks			
Identify all practice employees			
Confirm data to remove application access from the US Oncology network			
Remove access to all applications for employees transitioning including Domain access, remote access, PeopleSoft, clinical applications, practice management applications, email, internet access, etc.			
Engineering Tasks			
Inventory computer equipment including desktops, laptops, printers, software, and servers through site survey			
Determine which equipment will transition to the practice. Included in this will be cost for any equipment transitioning from the USON network			
Remove US Oncology configuration and passwords			
Transfer ownership and support to practice			
IT Contract Tasks			
Identify all contracts affected by the departing practice (Microsoft, SBC, Perot Systems, etc.)			
Determine if contracts can be transferred to the practice			
Transfer ownership and support to practice			
Risk Management			
Affilation Transition			
All open compliance issues have an agreed upon resolution			
All open Hotline calls have an agreed upon resolution			
All open Internal Audits have an agreed upon resolution			
Transfer responsibility of the Self-Assessment Action Plans			

(continued)

Task	Task complete	Contact person	Remarks
Compliance Program Requirements			
Designation of Compliance/Privacy/Security Officer			
Designation of a Compliance Committee			
Development of a Sanction Screening Program			
Code of Conduct Development/Implementation			
Annual compliance training program development/implementation			
Implementation of a Hotline Process			
Development of a Compliance Issue Tracking System			
Development of a Compliance Inquiry Tracking System			
Policies and Procedures development and implementation			
Design of a Self Audit Program			
Method of disseminating Compliance Communication Updates			
Risk Management			
GENERAL			
1. Identify personnel responsible for coordination of risk management		Executive director	
2. Determine which of the following insurance programs will require policy changes:		Executive director	
Workers' Compensation Insurance			
Property Insurance			
Primary General Liability Insurance			
Excess General Liability Insurance			
Professional Liability (Malpractice) Insurance			
Owned and Non-owned Auto Insurance			
Crime (Employee Dishonesty) Insurance			
Employment Practices Liability Insurance			
ERISA Bond for 401(k) Plans			
3. Identify insurance broker for each of the above programs		Executive director	
WORKERS' COMPENSATION INSURANCE			
(Currently all admin employees are covered by a master policy with Virginia Surety; certain practices are covered by individual policies with Virginia Surety)			
4. Determine the employer for each employee in post-transition period		Insurance contact	
5. Identify current worker's compensation carrier		Insurance contact	
6. Identify changes needed to current policies in post-transition period		Insurance contact	
7. Obtain premium quotations for any new coverage		Insurance contact	
8. Bind insurance changes effective on the transition date		Insurance contact	
PROPERTY INSURANCE			
(Currently all locations are covered by a master policy with Industrial Risk Insurers)			
9. Obtain list of current insured locations		Insurance contact	
10. Identify ownership of locations to be insured in the post-transition period (corporate vs practice)		Insurance contact	
11. Determined insured value of each site of service (corporate vs practice)		Insurance contact	

(continued)

Task	Task complete	Contact person	Remarks
12. Obtain premium quotations for new coverage		Insurance contact	
13. Bind insurance coverage effective on the transition date		Insurance contact	
GENERAL & EXCESS LIABILITY INSURANCE			
(Currently all locations are covered by a master policy with PHICO Insurance Company)			
14. Obtain list of current insured locations		Insurance contact	
15. Identify ownership of locations to be insured in the post-transition period (corporate vs practice)		Insurance contact	
16. Determine square footage of areas of ownership and shared responsibility by location (corporate vs practice)		Insurance contact	
17. Obtain premium quotations for new coverage		Insurance contact	
18. Bind insurance coverage effective on the transition date		Insurance contact	
PROFESSIONAL LIABILITY (MALPRACTICE) INSURANCE			
(Current coverage provided by a number of carriers)			
19. Identify current insurance carrier		Insurance contact	
20. Identify what changes, if any, are necessary		Insurance contact	
21. Obtain premium quotations, if needed		Insurance contact	
22. Bind insurance coverage, if needed		Insurance contact	
OWNED & NON-OWNED AUTO INSURANCE			
(Current coverage provided by a master policy with the Hartford)			
23. Identify existence and ownership of owned autos		Insurance contact	
24. Obtain premium quotations for new auto liability coverage and owned autos, if any		Insurance contact	
25. Bind insurance coverage effective on the transition date		Insurance contact	
CRIME (EMPLOYEE DISHONESTY) INSURANCE			
(Current coverage provided for the network by a master policy with Zurich)			
26. Identify the nature and extent of cash disbursement, cash receipts, etc. in the post-transition period		Insurance contact	
27. Obtain premium quotations for new coverage		Insurance contact	
28. Bind insurance coverage effective on the transition date		Insurance contact	
EMPLOYMENT PRACTICES LIABILITY INSURANCE			
(Current coverage provided for all network employees by master policy with National Union)			
29. Determine if this coverage will be continued in the post-transition period		Insurance contact	
30. Obtain premium quotations for new coverage, if any		Insurance contact	
31. Bind insurance coverage effective on the transition date		Insurance contact	

(continued)

Task	Task complete	Contact person	Remarks
ERISA BONDS FOR 401(K) PLANS			
(Current 401(k) plans are covered by individual ERISA Bonds provided by the Hartford)			
32. If employees are shifted from one employer to another and their 401(k) funds are moved from one plan to another, the amount of the bond may need to be changed		Insurance contact	
Banking Checklist			
1. Determine and/or setup bank account to be used for A/P disbursements		Controller	
2. Determine and/or setup bank account to be used for payroll disbursement		Controller	
3. Initiate changes through APD to redirect corresponding payroll charges		Controller	
4. Deliver all remaining check stock to US Oncology for accounts that will no longer be used		Controller	
5. Return all remaining check stock previously issued for Emergency A/P disbursements		Controller	
6. Determine lockbox arrangements that will be used going forward		Controller	
7. Notify all payers of any applicable changes to remittance address or banking instructions for electronic payers		Controller	
8. Update authorized signers on local deposit accounts		Controller	
9. Determine where merchant payments (credit card transactions) are to be deposited and initiate any required changes		Controller	
10. Review petty cash funding procedures to ensure appropriate separation		Controller	

References

1. For practice start-up and credentialing. https://www.physicianpracticestartup.com/
2. Physician fee schedules. https://www.cms.gov/cms-guide-medical-technology-companies-and-other-interested-parties/payment/physician-fee-schedule

8 Managing Student Debt

Case Study: Dimitri

Dimitri is a fourth-year medical student who is about to graduate from a private medical school in the northeast. Dimitri has borrowed money to cover his medical school expenses and has additional loan debt from college. His total educational debt is over $300,000. Dimitri is fortunate to have matched into his first-choice spot for his Family Practice residency. He is going to a small town in the southeastern United States. He has just met with his financial aid counselor to do his exit interview to review his total debt, and is astonished by the amount of money he will be expected to repay. What are his repayment options?

In 2024, the mean indebtedness of all medical school graduates was $203,606, with debt being higher for graduates of private medical schools when compared with public medical schools [1]. Twenty-three percent of medical school graduates reported debt of over $300,000, and 67% of graduates reported some medical education debt. Certainly, Dimitri is not alone. The cost of attendance at US medical schools has increased at a pace surpassing that of inflation, with a median 4-year cost of attendance for private schools for the Class of 2021 at $390,848 [1].

Despite the high cost of attendance, going to medical school is financially advantageous with a net present value of over $1.6 million [2]. This means that someone would have to give you $1.6 million prior to starting medical school for you to be in the same financial position at retirement as if you went to medical school! A medical education is an investment with an excellent return. Even for students planning careers in lower paying primary care specialties do well financially as physicians. A study investigated whether or not students could afford a career in primary care using financial planning software [3]. The authors concluded that a primary care field remains financially viable for medical school graduates with median levels of debt. The study further concluded that graduates with high levels of debt needed to consider extended payment plans, loan forgiveness programs, or living in a lower cost area of the country in order to cover their educational debt.

In spite of the fact that going to medical school is a good financial move, the amount of debt accrued by graduates can be onerous, and because physicians have a high earning potential they have little choice but to pay back their loans. They cannot default. Generally, monthly loan repayments include both a portion of the amount borrowed (principal) and a portion of the interest accrued over the life of the loan. Remember, you have to pay for someone to lend you money. For new graduates, or in the case of financial hard-

N. Baum, M. J. Kahn, *Business Basics for your Healthcare Practice*,
https://doi.org/10.1007/978-3-032-25241-8_8

ship, most loans allow for a period of forbearance where payments can be suspended or delayed with the accrual of additional interest. However, if a physician delays paying their loans, they will be penalized with additional interest payments. As such, it is generally not advisable to delay the start of educational loan repayment.

Basically, there are three types of traditional loan repayment models for physicians: (1) standard repayment; (2) extended repayment, and (3) graduated repayment. Standard repayment requires the borrower to make fixed monthly payments that include both principal and interest. Typically, the borrower is required to pay off the principal and interest in 10 years, with interest payments being the majority of the payment during the first few years. If a borrower has multiple sources of loans (federal government and private loans), all of the loans can be consolidated through a third party who basically "buy" the individual loans and package them as one larger loan. Typically, consolidated loans are paid off over a longer period of time (20 or 30 years). Generally, this reduces the monthly payment, but increases the total amount of interest paid over the life of the loan, raising the overall total amount paid back by the borrower. Standard repayment is the "default" if no other type of repayment plan is chosen.

Extended repayment, like consolidation, allows the borrower to spread out the payments over a longer period of time (20 or 30 years), with an increase in the total interest accrued. As such, the monthly payments are lower, but the total amount of money repaid is increased due to interest charged on the loan during the extended repayment period.

Graduated repayment allows the borrower to make smaller payments initially, with increases in payments after several years. As with extended payment, the borrower pays for this benefit with higher interest payments.

In addition to the three typical repayment models, borrowers can enter income-driven repayment plans. In these types of repayment models, the amount paid per month in repayment is closely tied to income earned. These loans are generally divided into those that are income contingent and those that are income based. Income contingent plan payments are based on the lesser of either 20% monthly discretionary income or a calculated amount based on a 12-year repayment plan and a multiplier based on income. Income-based plans allow borrowers to make monthly payments based on family size and adjusted gross income. Typically, payments are capped at 10% of discretionary income. For a typical resident earning $60,000 per year, the income-based repayment would be between $370 and $440 per month. In addition to income contingent and income-based repayment plans, borrowers can enter pay as you earn (PAYE) or revised pay as you earn (REPAYE) plans, both of which require payments that are calculated as a percentage of discretionary income with some consideration for family size. REPAYE plans differ from PAYE plans in limiting interest payments to 50% if the monthly payment does not cover the entire interest payment. As with all financial decisions, it is best to discuss loan repayment strategies with a financial advisor before making any final decisions. Each repayment plan has its own tax implications, including whether or not the payments of principal and/or interest are tax deductible. Additionally, some repayment plans may allow for loan forgiveness after a certain number of payments.

Are there ways to have someone else pay off your educational debt?

In 2007, the College Cost Reduction and Access Act was created to provide indebted college, graduate, or professional school graduates a way to reduce their federal student debt burden by working in public service. Loans considered eligible for public service loan forgiveness (PSLF) included any loan issued under the federal Direct Loan Program, including subsidized and unsubsidized Stafford Loans, PLUS loans, and Federal Direct Consolidation Loans. Unfortunately, private loans were not deemed eligible for forgiveness.

To qualify for PSLF, the borrower has to make 120 monthly on-time payments in a qualifying plan and has to work full time for 10 years in a government or not-for-profit (501c) organization. Qualifying repayment plans for PSLF include any one of the previously described income-driven repayment plans (income contingent repayment, income-based repayment, PAYE, or REPAYE). The huge benefit of PSLF is that after making 120 payments, the remainder of the loan balance is forgiven. When originally established, there was no cap or maximum amount of loan debt that could be forgiven. As such, under PSLF, it really does not matter how much you owe. Your payment is only dependent on your income. Those with higher debt have a larger amount of debt forgiven at the end of the loan period. Over the past few years, attempts have been made to cap the amount of PSLF at $57,000. More recent proposals include eliminating PSLF entirely. The future of PSLF remains uncertain, but as of the time of this writing, PSLF remains intact under law.

In addition to PSLF, there are several other federally based loan forgiveness programs. All three branches of the military (Army, Navy, Air Force) offer medical school scholarships through the Health Professions Scholarship Program (HPSP) that cover medical school tuition, fees, and provide a stipend for living expenses for medical students in exchange for military service. What is often not recognized is that the military also offers loan repayment opportunities after graduation from medical school. Loan repayment does require active military duty and/or reserve status in a branch of the US military. The amount of repayment can be substantial (up to $275,000) and may also include sign-on bonuses for practicing physicians that range between $220,000 and $400,000 depending on specialty.

Like the military, the Indian Health Service offers loan repayment, paying up to $40,000 per year for service in Indian Health Service facilities providing care of American Indians or Alaska Natives.

For physicians involved in research careers, the National Institutes of Health (NIH) offers a competitive loan repayment program where successful applicants who agree to a 2-year minimum contract to engage in research funded by a nonprofit organization are provided $35,000 per year to repay undergraduate, medical school, or graduate school debt. The NIH also offers loan repayment programs for clinicians from disadvantaged backgrounds or for physicians engaged in health disparity research.

The National Health Service Corps (NHSC) offers loan repayment for those physicians who commit to working at least 2 years at an NHSC-approved site. These are typically in rural communities or in the inner city. Physicians who practice primary care or mental health are eligible for up to $50,000 that is tax free and extendable for an additional 2 years.

In addition to the above federal programs, many states have programs that repay medical school loans for physicians who agree to practice in medically underserved regions or federally designated health professional shortage areas.

Finally, many practices and hospitals offer a sign-on bonus for new hires, if not a direct stipend for loan repayment. For a $25,000 bonus, assuming a 25% tax rate, the signing bonus would net $18,750. That sum could be used to make an extra bonus payment on student loans, saving thousands of dollars in interest over the life of the loan.

In addition to loan repayment, it may also be advisable to refinance debt at a lower interest rate. Depending on the interest rates on loans and interest rates offered by consolidation companies, this may be an attractive way to decrease the total money paid on a loan. As with other decisions, careful consultation with a financial advisor is important before making any decision regarding loan repayment.

Back to Case

Dimitri met with a financial advisor and decided to enter an income-dependent repayment plan during residency. He hoped to be able to use loan repayment during his time spent in residency, in a small not-for-profit hospital, toward qualification for the PSLF program. He planned to remain in the small community and to work for a federally qualified health center. After 10 years, he hoped that the PSLF program would still be in place when he would become eligible for loan forgiveness. Dimitri felt comfortable with the $370 per month repayment schedule. He remained optimistic that as a physician, even one engaged in primary care, he would enjoy his lifestyle and career and that financially he would be secure.

Key Takeaways

- Most medical students in the United States graduate with educational debt.
- Physicians will be able to pay back their debt.
- There are many opportunities for loan forgiveness, including federal and state programs.

References

1. Medical Student Education: Debt, costs, and loan repayment fact card for the Class of 2024. Association of American Medical Colleges, October 2024
2. Kahn MJ, Nelling EF. Estimating the value of medical education: a net present value approach. Teaching Learn Med Int J. 2010;22:205–8.
3. Youngclaus JA, Koehler PA, Kotlikoff LJ, Wiecha JM. Can medical students afford to choose primary care? An economic analysis of physician debt repayment. Acad Med. 2013;88(1):16–25.

9 Obtaining and Maintaining Referrals from Physicians and Other Sources

Wishing to be friends is quick work, but friendship is a slow ripening fruit. –Aristotle

> **Case Study: Omar**
> *Omar is a fellowship-trained urologist who joined an academic practice. His practice consisted of hundreds of patients from the previous urologist. However, he complained of having few physicians in the area refer patients to his practice. What should he do?*

The mainstay of any successful practice is the patients you already have and the ability to attract new patients, which includes referrals from other physicians. Maintaining positive relationships with both patients and colleagues is key to a successful healthcare practice. Specifically, establishing and preserving connections with physicians is essential to creating a strong referral network and a steady patient inflow. This chapter will the discuss methods and techniques to enhance referrals from your colleagues.

Talks on medical marketing often begin with the three As of marketing: availability, affability, and affordability. Since all physicians probably think of themselves as available, as likable, and as offering appropriately priced services, how do you differentiate yourself from the competition?

One of the biggest misconceptions about marketing is that to do it well you must spend lots of money on peripherals. There are many other steps that are far more effective and essential to marketing than logos and gifts you send out at Christmas. The most essential element of your marketing plan is to make your practice user-friendly. Nowhere is this more important than in working with your referring physicians.

The traditional methods of obtaining physician referrals usually involved trial and error. They were seldom discussed, and some were almost intangible. Perhaps you went to school with another physician in the area and later he or she referred patients to you. Perhaps you joined a group practice and got the overflow patients. Maybe you went to emergency rooms and made yourself available to treat patients who did not have their own physicians.

One of the cardinal rules, especially for new physicians, was to always be available. If a new physician did an excellent job with every new patient who was referred to him/her, gradually the word-of-mouth method would start working and new patients would be forthcoming. The word would get back to the referring physician that the new physician was truly competent. The new physician could slowly build a good reputation in this way.

N. Baum, M. J. Kahn, *Business Basics for your Healthcare Practice*,
https://doi.org/10.1007/978-3-032-25241-8_9

By relying on word of mouth and outstanding service, it could take from 2 to 3 years to get a practice up and running. These methods worked in the past because there were enough primary care doctors, enough patients, and enough referrals to go around. Today we are seeing fewer physicians start out by themselves in private practice. Many physicians are opting to join large group practices or are employed by hospitals or are joining with mega groups consisting of large numbers of physicians all in the same specialty and may have physicians who are fellowship trained and are sub-specialists with unique, specified areas of medical interest. That means you must be a lot more organized about getting those physician referrals.

This chapter will take the concept of physician referrals out of the realm of hit or miss—you will not have to use the shotgun or scattershot approach but can focus your efforts like a laser to obtain physician referrals. If you follow the steps outlined in this chapter, you will have a guaranteed plan for making your name visible and your reputation known within the medical community in a shorter period than it takes for word of mouth to spread your name and reputation within the physician community. By targeting your efforts, your practice, in essence, will become user-friendly—your colleagues will want to refer patients to you and will enjoy doing so. And, as the quote from Aristotle makes clear, this is a deliberate process that also requires patience and persistence.

The main strategy for getting physician referrals is to have your name cross the minds and desks of referring physicians and their staff members frequently and in a positive fashion. If you can do that, physician referrals will come your way. This strategy derives from the tactics of William Wrigley, the chewing gum magnate, who, at the turn of the century, set down this dictum: "Tell 'em quick, and tell 'em often."

All 26 techniques outlined in this chapter, from prompt reporting to gift-giving, are designed with this strategy in mind. There should be good chemistry between you and your referring physicians. If they have good feelings about you, they will want to refer patients to you. You can make yourself more attractive to referring physicians by making it easy to do business with you and your staff.

Almost all the techniques require minimal amounts of time and energy and negligible expense, yet their effectiveness in generating physician referrals is quite significant. Remember, you must have a staff capable of handling patients, and you must ensure follow-up and develop excellent communication with referring physicians.

1. Report to referring physicians promptly. The adage for selling real estate is location, location, location. When it comes to increasing your attractiveness to referring physicians, the mantra is communicate, communicate, and communicate. If you are looking for the best way to make yourself accessible to your referring physicians, consider prompt reporting. When primary care physicians were surveyed about why they make referrals, prompt reporting was at the top of the list. You must always keep your referring physicians informed about their patients' progress. You need to make them feel that they are the captain of the patient's healthcare ship.

When you see a patient by referral, follow this cardinal rule: Never allow the patient to return to the referring physician's office *before* your report does. Nothing is more embarrassing to the primary care doctor than to be in the dark about what is going on with the patient. If the patient or the patient's family calls the referring physician before he or she has had a full report from you, it makes you both look bad.

The following story is a prime example of what must never happen. A primary care physician called his patient's relatives at home to tell the family that the grandfather, in the intensive care unit, was not doing too well. The family said, "Yes, we know, he died last night!" This was a gross lapse in communication that resulted in embarrassment for a primary care physician. You must avoid communication failures with your referring doctors as well.

When a physician sees a patient referred by a primary care physician, it is often 7–10 days before the primary care physician receives the referral letter. Even with electronic medical records, primary care physicians will not receive follow-up communication for several days that increases the possibility that the patient will contact the primary care doctor before the referral letter arrives. The older method consisted of report being dictated, transcribed, and mailed. Frequently the patient will beat the referring letter back to the primary care physician.

How user-friendly are you when a patient returns to his or her primary care physician and the referral letter has not arrived? The physician asks the patient what the specialist said or did. The patient responds, “I don’t know, but he gave me a large yellow pill and now I have a rash and am itching all over.” Now the primary care physician must ask his nurse to tell the receptionist to call your office, have your receptionist or nurse locate the chart, and then track you down if you are not in the office to discuss your management of the patient. That scenario does not endear you to the referring primary care physician.

A solution for avoiding this scenario is to use the lazy person’s referral letter. This is a referral letter that requires absolutely no dictating. Here’s how it works: as soon as you have seen the patient, write down, at the end of your office notes, your impressions, the medications you prescribed, and the plan of treatment. For instance, if I see Mrs. Smith for cystitis, recommend that she take a course of sulfa, and suggest that I see her again in 2 weeks, I circle these buzz words in the notes.

When my nurse goes through the electronic medical record after Mrs. Smith’s visit, she sees that I have circled these words. She calls up a boilerplate referral letter on the computer screen, which has blanks to fill in (see Exhibit 12–1). The nurse types in the appropriate physician’s name, the diagnosis, the medications, and treatment plan. The letter closes with the statement, “I will keep in touch with you regarding her urologic progress.” We then print out the letter and fax it directly to the physician’s office.

This letter delivers the essentials to the referring physician. What are primary care physicians looking for? Most will tell you that there are three ingredients of an effective referral letter: the working diagnosis, the medications you have prescribed, and the treatment plan. You can bank money on this one—they are not interested in the depth and detail of your history or the fine nuances you detected on the physical examination. For the most part, they are as busy as you are and do not have the time to read a lengthy two- to three-page report that you dictated and conduct a treasure hunt to find the diagnosis, prescribed medication, and treatment plan. You can create a user-friendly referral letter that meets the three necessary criteria and that lands on the primary care physician’s desk before the patient returns for an office visit. If your practice is using an electronic medical record, sending a copy of the EMR notes that can often be coded to an E & M of Level 4 or 5 does not constitute an effective letter. The typical length of these notes—three to four pages—is too long. Often, the vital information, that is, diagnosis, medication, and treatment plan, is hidden in the notes and not easy for a busy primary care doctor to locate. Today, most EMRs allow you to create a template where there are fields that include diagnosis, medication, and treatment plan. Then, with a few mouse clicks or taps on a touchscreen computer, you can generate a very effective referral letter that can be faxed immediately to a referring physician while the patient is still in the exam room. Now it is virtually impossible for the patient to be seen by the primary care physician before the referral letter has arrived. This level of communication with the referring doctors is so effective that if a patient is seen by the specialist and then goes directly from the office of the specialist to the referring physician, the letter is in his/her office before the patient arrives. You and your practice become very user-friendly by telling the patient that a letter has been sent to the referring physician and that he/she should mention this to the receptionist when he/she checks in with the referring doctor (Fig. 9.1 is an example of a referral letter created on EMR.)

January 22, 2017

Dr. Alfred Colfry
4224 Houma Blvd
Metairie, LA 70006

RE: XXXX

DOB: XXXX

Date of Visit: XXXX

Dear Al,

XXXX was seen for a problem of: XXXX

Chief Complaint: Urinary retention after hernia surgery. The catheter was removed and he was able to void with a weak urinary stream.

Current Impression:

Retention of urine unspecified (788.20; New Without Added Workup)

BPH with obstruction or lower UT symptoms (600.01)

XXXX request transfer of his urologic care to this office because he is elderly, and it is difficult for him to travel to your Metairie office. I told him you have an office on Napoleon Avenue, and he was going to speak with you about those days you are in that office. I also told him that he had to speak with you before he could make an appointment with me, and he told me he would give you a call.

Sincerely,

Neil Baum, M.D.

Fig. 9.1 Physician referral letter from the electronic medical record

Because the letter is sent out immediately, if the patient calls with any questions, the referring doctor can answer any questions without having to contact the specialist. Furthermore, the letter can usually be generated without any dictating. For those who must dictate the two- or three-page traditional referral letter, consider underlining or boldfacing the essential information, including your impressions, the medications, and your recommendations. Nearly all referring physicians indicate that they prefer a timely computerized referral letter over a delayed three-pager. Doctors may be concerned if referring physicians are upset when they receive a computerized, impersonal form letter. Surveys indicate that referring physicians prefer timely information as opposed to a delayed personal letter.

Although most visits can be handled in this manner, some of your examinations will uncover a problem that is complicated or has ominous implications. If your examination turns up a significant finding or you need to decide regarding the patient's treatment plan, you should contact the referring physician by phone and notify them of your findings. Failure to do so can potentially result in embarrassment for both you and the referring physician. If the patient calls the referring physician to discuss your suggestions, and you have not yet informed the physician about your treatment plan, it makes him or her appear uninformed or even uncaring. The referring physician will likely think of you as unprofessional and will probably stop referring patients to you.

Neil Baum, M.D.3525 Prytania, #614New Orleans, LA, 70115 Phone: (504) 891-8454

Date: ________

Your patient __________ had the following procedure: ________________

The pertinent findings included: ______________________________

I recommended____

You will be receiving the dictated operative note. Please call me if you have any questions.

Dr. Neil Baum

Fig. 9.2 Sample of stat operative note

If you operate on a patient, call the referring physician's office immediately afterward. Notify the physician's nurse that the surgery went well, and everything was successful. A stat operative note that notifies the referring doctor of the outcomes of the patient's surgery, the pertinent findings, and what postoperative treatment will be instituted is very appreciated by the referring doctor. This stat operative note is faxed to the referring physician and arrives long before the dictated operative note from the hospital or ATC (Fig. 9.2 is a sample of the stat operative note.) Also, if you realize before or during the procedure that the surgery is going to be significantly delayed, notify the primary care physician's office. The doctor will then be up to date on the patient's progress in case he or she runs into the family on the way over to the hospital. However, if a complication develops during surgery or if the patient has changed rooms or has been sent to the intensive care unit, notify the referring physician via a phone call or text the doctor if that is a preferred form of communication. If there is a significant lab or pathology report, call the referring physician and let him or her know what has been found. In those situations, the patient or the patient's family may contact the physician immediately. If you have not apprised the physician of the situation first, then he or she will not be well informed.

There are other economic considerations involved in using the lazy person's referral letter. Do you know that the typical referral letter can cost you anywhere from $13.00 to $25.00 or more every time you pick up the tape recorder to dictate a referral note? How can this be, you ask. Let's do the math: Today most physician time is valued at $300–350 an hour. The typical referral letter requires 3–5 min of physician time. So, for your time alone the cost for each referral letter would range from $25 to $30. The charges of a transcriptionist who makes $25,000–35,000 a year plus benefits and charges you $2–3 a page must be added to the equation. Finally, there are costs for stationery and postage, adding $3 or more per letter. Using the lazy person's referral letter, you reduce your costs to under $1 per letter. Plus, it satisfies the needs and wants of your primary care physicians—the letter arrives before the patient returns.

You will find that most of your colleagues will be delighted with the letter and often say they "hoped that my colleagues would learn to use the same technique." However, if you find a referring doctor who does not wish to receive the lazy person's referral letter, then send the longer version referral letter to one of those doctors. Should you decide to send the longer referral letter, then underline the three necessary areas consisting of the diagnosis, medications, and treatment plan. Remember, one size *does not* fit all. The best way to identify what kind of a referral letter to use is to ask your referring physicians which kind of letter, the brief letter that lists diagnosis, medications prescribed, and treatment plan, or the longer, detailed letter.

2. Make your referring physicians look good. Your objective should be to keep the referring physician involved and functioning as the captain of the healthcare ship. I am reminded of the story of a patient who went to see an orthopedic surgeon. During the history and physical, the doctor asked the patient, "What have you done for your problem?" The patient said, "I've been to a chiropractor." The doctor asked, "What did that fool tell you?" The patient responded, "He sent me to you!"

Whenever possible, compliment the referring physician. Of course, you do not want to appear unnatural or superficial. When the referring physician's name comes up in conversation with the patient, you can make a comment such as, "He is such a fine doctor and is very knowledgeable about your medical problem," or "She is one of the best doctors in our community."

Sometimes I get complimentary notes from patients referred to me by other physicians. I photocopy each note and send it back to the referring physician with an accompanying note that reads, "Thought you might like to see that your patient had a positive experience at my office." After all, the kind of experience the patient had reflects on the referring physician.

If a patient tells me, "Boy, I sure am glad that Dr. Jones sent me to you," I have a response. "Do me a favor," I say. "The next time you see Dr. Jones, mention that you had a good experience at my office." The patient is more than happy to oblige, which increases the positive feedback received by the referring physician. Also, if the patient gives you a compliment, ask him/her if she would submit that compliment to the online reputation review sites such as Healthgrades.com, yelp.com, or RateMDs.com.

Also, remember that the patient's perception of you is partly determined by how the patient perceives the referring physician. If you make the referring physician look good, then you are really enhancing your image as well.

3. Vary your referral patterns. Today, the number of patients referred to specialists is decreasing. One of the reasons for this is that certain specialists (for instance, gynecologists and general surgeons) are doing more primary care and keeping the patients in their practices. When patients go to a multispecialty group practice or preferred provider organization (PPO), they are kept there and do not circulate in the community looking for other healthcare providers. Also, primary care physicians are treating more medical conditions that were once referred to specialists. Finally, there is an emphasis on cost-containment means that many primary care physicians now treat adult-onset diabetes, arthritis, benign enlargement of the prostate, urinary incontinence, and even common dermatological conditions.

Often referral patterns are cut in stone, and specialists refer to only one or a few groups of primary care doctors. One of the benefits of your marketing efforts will be that patients will come directly to you: You will become the primary care doctor and control the referrals. For example, if a patient comes to a urologist with urinary symptoms, and she needs to see a gynecologist or a cardiologist, the urologist becomes the referring physician and has the opportunity to direct the referrals.

It is important that specialists make every effort to send new patients to primary care doctors who have frequently referred patients to them. Now more than ever it is important to acknowledge referrals from primary care doctors and other specialists. The best way for you to do this is to take advantage of your marketing and send colleagues new patients. They will appreciate new patients more than a fruit basket at Christmas.

4. Provide courtesies to your referring physicians and do not inconvenience them. One of the best ways to prevent inconveniences for your referring physicians is to assist with the hospital paperwork for patients whom you share. For example, have your office notify the referring physician when you are admitting his or her patient. If you do this, the hos-

pital secretary will not be calling the referring physician late in the evening, which may require the physician to see the patient even later that evening or early in the morning. Likewise, contact the referring physician when you discharge his or her patient. By doing this, you ensure that the referring physician will not make a needless trip to the hospital to see a patient who has been sent home.

You can fill out the prescriptions that apply to your specialty and leave them in the patient's chart or with the patient so that the referring physician does not have to write all the prescriptions.

This also applies to hospitalists who are caring for referring doctors' patients in the hospital. Hospitalists are also marketing themselves to the PCPs and the specialists, and they want to be user friendly. Hospitalists also need to keep the avenues of communication open between the hospitalists and the referring doctors by being certain that what was done to their patient was sent to the referring doctor so that continuity of care will take place after the patient is discharged from the care of the hospitalists.

Remember, you want your referring physicians to feel that it is easy to work with you and that you will go the extra mile on their behalf.

5. Recognize your referring physicians' accomplishments and those of their children. There is no better way to enhance your relationship with your referring physicians than to acknowledge their accomplishments. It is a nice gesture to cut out articles from local newspapers that mention your referring physicians or their families. Whenever one of your referring physicians receives an appointment or promotion, acknowledge it with a written note.

A nonmedical story that emphasizes this concept. A doctor's son was 4 years old, and he rescued a bird from the backyard swimming pool. The family took the bird to the zoo, where it was saved. The family's rabbi, on hearing the story, sent the 4-year-old boy a letter:

> I just heard the story of your wonderful, good deed in saving the bird from drowning in the pool. You should be proud of yourself. I am proud of you for doing such a wonderful thing. Whenever you hear the birds chirping to themselves, you can be sure they're singing your praises.
> Well done, Craig.
> Rabbi Cohn

Can you imagine how much Rabbi Cohn's stock escalated when the 4-year-old boy received that letter? The parents could not wait to contribute to the synagogue's annual fundraising campaign!

Doctors like to hear positive comments about their children. Taking the time to find out about their children is a guaranteed way to let your referring physicians know that you are thinking of them. (This is also a nice gesture to do for your patients.) If a referring physician's child just received a scholarship or an athletic award, send a note. Your staff are usually familiar with the names of your referring physicians, and they can call them to your attention when reading the newspaper or finding evidence of accolades on the Internet. This is a simple little thing to do, but it is universally appreciated.

6. Send birthday cards. Sometimes it is difficult to find out your colleagues' birthdays. You can try calling their hospitals or the county medical society. Ask for the birthdays, not the birth years, and you should have no problem. You will not be given the years—that is confidential—but frequently you will find out the days. You might want to compile a list and ask for all the birthdays at the same time.
7. Don't intrude on your referring physicians' turf. Today, many physicians are trying to generate additional practice income by performing procedures or diagnostic tests in their offices. You need to be aware of who performs which tests. Avoid performing tests or procedures that your referring physicians are equipped to handle. For example, if you plan to admit the patient of a referring physician to the hospital, ask the patient to have the preadmission blood work, EKG, and chest X-ray done in the referring physician's office rather than at the hospital or a third-party lab.

If blood work is all you are requesting, have your office draw the blood, send it by courier to the referring physician's office, and ask for a copy of the results for your records. When you use the referring physician's facility or lab, you are being considerate and allowing the physician to maximize the use of his or her equipment and employees.

8. Show an interest in your referring physicians as people. Try to know about your referring physicians' nonmedical interests and hobbies. Whenever you see or read something that is of interest to one of your referring physicians, take the time to send it to them or call it to their attention. This is one way of saying that you are interested in your referring physicians even when you are not professionally relating to one another. For example, if one of your colleagues is a fly fisherman and you see a book on fly fishing offered in a catalogue or on Amazon.com, send him the book especially if you know he plans to leave for Alaska to go salmon fishing. This simple and inexpensive gesture will endear you to your referring physicians.
9. Invite your referring physicians to participate in support groups or seminars. This increases their exposure in the community and provides them with an opportunity to attract more patients.

If a referring gynecologic physician is an expert in hormonal issues in menopause, invite him/her to participate in one of your programs on women's health issues. This can be a plus for both of the doctors to increase their exposure in the community and will likely result in new patients for both doctors.

If you try to involve colleagues in your specialty, they will be less likely to criticize your marketing efforts. You will create allies, not adversaries, in the medical community.

10. Do not forget your referring physicians' staff. In addition to building a good relationship with your referring physicians, you must include their staff. Whenever you have contact with them, make it a point to be pleasant, cooperative, and interested in them as people. Learning their names will go a long way toward building a good working relationship. You will be surprised how many physician's staff have the ability and the permission to make referrals to other physicians.
11. Ensure that you are easy to contact. You can make it easier for your referring physicians and their staff to contact you and your office by supplying each office with a colored Rolodex card. The card can be made more visible by making it slightly higher than the standard Rolodex card. It should contain your telephone number; private line; office hours; answering service number; and the names of your office manager, secretary, nurse, and any other employees who may be requested by the referring physicians or their staff. Most practice management software programs contain physician directories where the contact information is located. You want to be certain that your information is correct in those directories. A nice gesture is to provide referring doctors with your cell phone number so they can easily reach. Remember, you don't want to make it difficult for a referring doctor to find you.
12. Start a journal club network. As every physician knows, it is no trivial pursuit to stay abreast of the medical literature. With the literature doubling or tripling every decade, it is nearly impossible for the busy practitioner to read all the journals in his or her areas of interest and expertise. There are over 5200 medical journals indexed on Medline, and the National Library of Medicine search service now has access to 10 million full-text articles.

By developing a journal club network with your fellow physicians, you maintain an awareness of the literature and help your colleagues at the same time. For example, there were reports in the medical literature on ophthalmic side effects of Viagra and other phosphodiesterase-5 inhibitors. If you come across these articles, send copies to your ophthalmologic colleagues and primary care physicians.

Here is how to start your network. Send a letter to about 10 of your colleagues. Explain what you are doing and what they can gain from participating. Exhibit 35–3 is an example of the letter that can be used to start a journal club.

The network is best kept informal—you do not want to add work to your colleagues' loads. The easiest way to accomplish this is to email the articles to your colleagues, and they can read these online or print a hard copy. Your staff can also be alerted to look for articles in newspapers and lay magazines that relate to your colleagues' specialties. This helps keep your colleagues informed on what their patients are reading.

13. Target your colleagues' reading. As with the journal club network, targeting their reading can facilitate your colleagues' continuing medical education and yours as well. If you send a referral letter that mentions a new diagnosis or treatment modality, attach an article that contains the new information. By doing this, you increase the likelihood that your colleague will read the article. Consider using a yellow highlighter pen and mark the one or two sentences most pertinent to the patient and the referral letter. For example, the use of thiazide diuretics is associated with the side effect of erectile dysfunction. The use of ACE inhibitors or calcium channel blockers is less likely to produce erectile dysfunction (ED). Before a patient starts on one of these antihypertensive drugs associated with ED or stops the thiazides because of the fear or presence of ED, try to educate your referring doctors by including a copy of the journal article with the referral letter. To ensure that referring doctor reads the article, underline the one or two sentences describing the efficacy of the medication you recommend.

To further direct a colleague's attention, you can apply a note to the front page of the article with a message (for example, "Please see page…"). Although this might seem like you are setting up a treasure hunt, you can be sure your colleague will appreciate being directed to the most important information. You have supplied new information and saved your colleague time,

14. Identify interests that you share with your referring physicians. Another way to let referring physicians know you care about them is to send them books, CDs, cartoons, and even nonmedical articles that may be of particular interest to them. For example, if one of your colleagues graduated from the University of Texas, you might send a link on YouTube (https://www.youtube.com/watch?v=pxBQLFLei70) to one of the greatest graduation speeches of all times by Admiral William McRaven, the Navy Seal who was the commander of Seal Team Six that took out Osama Bin Laden. The commencement speech has been viewed over 50 million times.

Suggested books you might send colleagues include Tim Russert's book, *Big Russ and Me*, Richard Carlson's *Don't Sweat the Small Stuff—and It's All Small Stuff*, and Rabbi Harold Kushner's *When Bad Things Happen to Good People.*

15. Hold on to old friends. When physicians retire, their former patients often continue to call them. They still have a lot of clout in the professional community. And, of course, their patients ask them for referrals to primary care physicians as well as to specialists. Acknowledge a colleague's retirement in some way by sending a note of appreciation or taking him or her to lunch. Then continue to remember your colleague on the same dates as before. This will help you maintain a referral source even after your colleague's shingle has been taken down.
16. Keep tabs on the movers. When a physician moves to another area of the country, it is important to maintain communication. If you send a "good luck" letter, cards at the holidays, and your blog/website information,

this will encourage the physician to send you patients when someone from the old community asks for a referral.

17. Develop intra-specialty referrals. You can do this by finding niches in the marketplace. Just because you are a specialist does not mean you cannot get referrals from other doctors in the same specialty. You may be doing procedures or diagnostic tests that they are not doing and that may be helpful to them. You may have equipment or training that they do not have, allowing you to develop referrals from colleagues in your specialty.

The key to these referrals is to make sure you send the patients back to your colleagues and that you do not operate on these patients for other problems that the original doctors can handle. Treat the patients only for the problems that the referring physicians requested.

Let your colleagues know that you are willing to see their patients and give their patients back. The easiest way to do this and make your colleagues feel secure is to offer to help at their institutions. In that way, the referring physician gets to see the procedure and has the security of knowing that you are not taking the patient away.

Another way to get referrals from specialists in your field is to refer patients who call when you are not available. Sometimes patients call out of the blue with a problem that cannot wait. Rather than have your staff say, "I'm sorry, the doctor is not available," and let that patient go back to the Internet to find a doctor, you can have them referred to one of your colleagues. For instance, if you are out of town, have your staff call the covering doctor's office to get an appointment for the patient. Your colleague appreciates getting a new patient and hopefully will return the favor.

18. Develop cooperative projects with referring physicians. For example, a urologist worked with a group of gynecologists who were interested in treating urinary incontinence. They did a project comparing the use biologic materials to synthetic materials for vaginal slings. It was a small project, but it created a nice opportunity to work together and learn what worked best for our patients with this condition. If you collect the data and write a paper, all the doctors receive recognition and publicity. This kind of collaboration also has the potential to bring all of the participants new patients.
19. Personally meet every physician who refers a patient to you. Many times, in the doctor's lounge, you may hear the following remark: "You know, I have a referring doctor down in St. Elsewhere. He's sent me two to three patients a month for the past five years, and I've never even met the guy!" If you do not go out of your way to meet that physician and invite him to your office, somebody else will, and that referral source will soon dry up.

If a physician refers two to three patients a month to you, you need to visit his or her office and meet him/her personally. Offer to give a talk at the physician's hospital. Try to make your paths cross. Otherwise, that golden goose (your referring physician) will cease laying the golden egg (referring patients to you).

20. Meet all new physicians in your area. Every July and August, when physicians announce they are starting their practices, you will receive announcement cards in the mail, or you will see these announcements in the paper. Most doctors throw those cards away. Some doctors write "congratulations" on the cards and send them back. It is best to take this gesture one step further.

Write a welcoming letter to each new physician. Offer to get together for breakfast or lunch. Then offer to share resources. If the new physician is in private practice, make a visit to the office with your office manager. Indicate that you would be more than happy to have your office manager assist the new physician's office manager.

Frequently, new physicians will have lots of questions even if they join a group or are employed by the hospital. You can offer to be of assistance, and this will be appreciated by your colleagues.

21. Refer patients to physicians new to the area, especially those just starting their practices. Send patients to new physicians as soon as possible. Everyone remembers who his or her first few patients were, and if you are the person who referred those patients, you will be forever appreciated by the primary care doctor. First patients make an indelible impression.
22. Offer marketing advice to new physicians. In addition to sending new patients to new physicians, you might consider referring them to one of the best books on ethical medical marketing, Marketing Your Clinical Practice—Ethically Effectively, and Economically (fourth edition, Jones and Bartlett, 2018). This book provides ideas for new physicians just starting their practices, and the marketing chapter discusses ethical but effective methods of practice promotion. An additional resource is Navigating the Transition from Residency to Physician Practice (https://resources.nejmcareercenter.org/article/navigating-the-transition-from-residency-to-physician-practice/).
23. Keep your referring physicians abreast of changes in your specialty or in your practice. If you attend a meeting or convention and there is new information that may be of interest to your colleagues, email a single-sheet informal newsletter about the latest developments in your practice and in your field. These short newsletters are often much appreciated by referring physicians. Samples of medical newsletters are available at https://wgcontent.com/blog/4-healthcare-newsletters-we-cant-get-enough-of.
24. Give your referring physicians useful and unique gifts. Giving gifts to your referring physicians is not the most effective method of generating referrals. However, there are techniques of giving certain types of gifts that will make you stand out from the others at holiday time. If you send wine or a fruit and cheese basket, it will most likely get lost among the dozens of similar gifts the physician receives.

For something a bit different, consider giving gifts that your colleagues will use or receive all year long. Membership with Harry and David's Fruit of the Month Club (harryanddavid.com) is a good choice since the physicians will receive a box of fresh fruit each month of the year.

If you know your colleagues' reading habits, you can consider giving them subscriptions to their favorite magazines such as Architectural Digest, Connoisseur, or National Geographic as gifts.

Another nice gift is a Lucite cube that could be used either as picture holders or as holders for motivational quotes by such people as Winston Churchill ("Never give in, Never give up, NEVER, NEVER, NEVER"), Vince Lombardi ("If you strive for perfection, you may not always reach it, but you will achieve excellence."), and Abraham Lincoln ("Success may come to those who wait, but they will receive only the things left by those who hustle."). Then each month send another motivational message to insert in the cube, as well as a story or comment about the author and how the quote applies to the contemporary practice of medicine. Experience has demonstrated that colleagues really seemed to appreciate this unique gift. You know that this is an appreciated gift when you visit the office of the referring physician that you spot those Lucite cubes with the motivational quotes on their desks.

One of the best gifts is laminated and personalized luggage tags. The tags are bright red with the colleague's last name in white type, and laminated, with gold-colored plastic cords to attach the tags to the luggage. The owner of the luggage with these tags will easily recognize their suitcase when it comes down the baggage chute at the airport.

By varying the time of year when you send your gifts, you can also make them stand out. For instance, consider sending your gifts and holiday wishes at Thanksgiving instead of during December. People are usually not as rushed at this time and chances are that they will remember your gifts.

One very generous and effective gift is to donate to a charity or civic organization in the name of one of your referring physicians. Of course, it really helps if you know your colleague well and choose a charity or foundation that they have worked for or supported.

We do not consider gift-giving essential to a successful marketing plan or effective physician referral program, but if you decide to give gifts, make them timely, unique, and one that will last the entire year.

25. Provide suggestions and indications to your primary care doctors for referral to your specialty. For example, not every UTI or enlarged prostate requires a consultation with a specialist. Provide the primary care doctor with a short monograph on suggestions for specialist referral. This monograph reviews the most common urologic conditions and gives evidence-based medical guidelines for management and referral.
26. Finally, go the extra mile for your referring physicians. Make it a pleasure for them to work with you. Find the little extras that make it a convenience instead of a chore. These little extras can make a big difference in your relationships with your referring physicians.

For example, a referring physician once asked about the office's unique uniforms. The office manager sent a copy of the catalog that was used to purchase the uniforms to the doctor and his office manager. Both were extremely appreciative of this gesture, and all it took was a little effort from us.

Facts of Life

All of us would like, whenever possible, to have a bilateral referral arrangement with our colleagues. Have you ever experienced a situation in which you are sending patients to another physician and getting no reverse referrals? Of course, you can change your referral source, hoping that the other physician will notice that there is a decrease in referrals and will call you to ask what happened, but do not hold your breath. Chances are the physician is busy enough and will not notice the decrease.

A better alternative is to discuss the facts of life with the physician. During your meeting, recall for the physician the number and names of patients you have sent him or her in the last 6–12 months. Ask whether the quality of patients was satisfactory and whether the physician would like to continue receiving your referrals.

If the physician answers yes to both questions, ask how he or she feels about your quality of medical care: "Do I enjoy a good reputation in our community? Have the patients I have sent you, as well as any others we may both be treating, been satisfied with my medical services?"

If the answers are again yes, then it is time to initiate the facts-of-life discussion. At this time, you should suggest that you would like to see some patients in return if you are to continue referring patients to that physician. If he or she does not agree, it is time to find another referral source.

A fact of life discussion story: An internist contacted a urologist when one of his patients from the intensive care unit was in urinary retention and need the insertion of urethral catheter. The urologist went to see these patients, often in the middle of the night, for several years, hoping to demonstrate that he was available to provide urologic care for all his patients. However, when this internist had patients with nonemergency urologic problems, the internist referred them to another urologist. After years of being inconvenienced in this way, the urologist requested a meeting with the internist. The urologist started the discussion by saying, "I am capable of seeing patients not only in the middle of the night but also between 8:00 AM and 5:00 PM as well!" The urologist did not request all his referrals, but he did ask for a few. If that was not acceptable, then he could get someone else to come in the evening hours to insert catheters. What was the worst that could happen? He would receive no referrals; however, he would have a good night's sleep!

As it happened, this discussion brought about a change in that physician's referral pattern and the urologist began receiving a few daytime referrals as well. This hard ball approach for everyone and in every circumstance, but whenever you feel exploited or that referrals are a one-way street, consider having a tactful discussion before abandoning the potential referral source. Remember not to go into such a discussion with a defensive attitude. It may be that there is a very simple reason for the physician's behavior, and that you simply were only seeing it from your point of view.

If you are worried that marketing is going to leave you all alone, perhaps even generating contempt from your colleagues, remember that effective marketing *includes* rather than excludes your colleagues.

Omar's Story and Physician Referrals

Omar recognized that staying in the office and not making an effort to meet the potential referring physicians in the area was the best place to start his marketing efforts to his colleagues. He visited all the physicians that were his age in the community and tried to know their staffs as well. He arranged to give several grand rounds of presentations on his areas of interest and expertise. Omar created an informal journal club with his fellow colleagues. He sent effective referral letters to the local doctors including articles he authored demonstrating his areas of expertise. He made every effort to be available when called for a consult or for a patient in the emergency room. Within a few months, he noted the fruits of his labor and started receiving referrals from the doctors in the area. In essence, he took the advice from Aristotle and recognized that obtaining physician referrals was metaphorically "a slow ripening fruit."

Key Takeaways

Marketing yourself to your colleagues does not mean that you are trying to take away "market share." When you open possibilities, you increase their business as well as yours. The way in which you do this does not take away, it just adds—to your stature in the professional community, to the respect you get from your peers, and to the bottom line.

- Building strong, professional relationships with other physicians is crucial for securing referrals. Networking, open communication, and mutual respect can foster these connections.
- Providing high-quality patient care is essential for earning trust and referrals from other healthcare professionals. Consistently delivering excellent outcomes and patient satisfaction boosts your reputation.
- Make your practice visible and easily accessible to referring physicians. This includes having a user-friendly referral process, clear communication channels, and a positive online presence.
- Keep the referring doctor "in the loop" and report back promptly to the referring physician.

Appendix

Exhibit 12–1 Boilerplate "Lazy Person's Referral Letter"

Date

Dear [Referring Physician],

[Patient] __________ was seen for a problem of [diagnosis], and he/she is being treated with [medication] __________ . I recommend that he/she have [treatment] __________.

I will see him/her again after he/she finishes the medication and will keep in touch with you regarding his/her urologic progress.

Sincerely,

Neil Baum, MD

Exhibit 12–2 Example of a Birthday Card Sent to Male Colleagues

Source: Designed by Barbara Dale. Reprinted by permission.

Fortunately, all subsequent birthdays
are celebrated with cake.

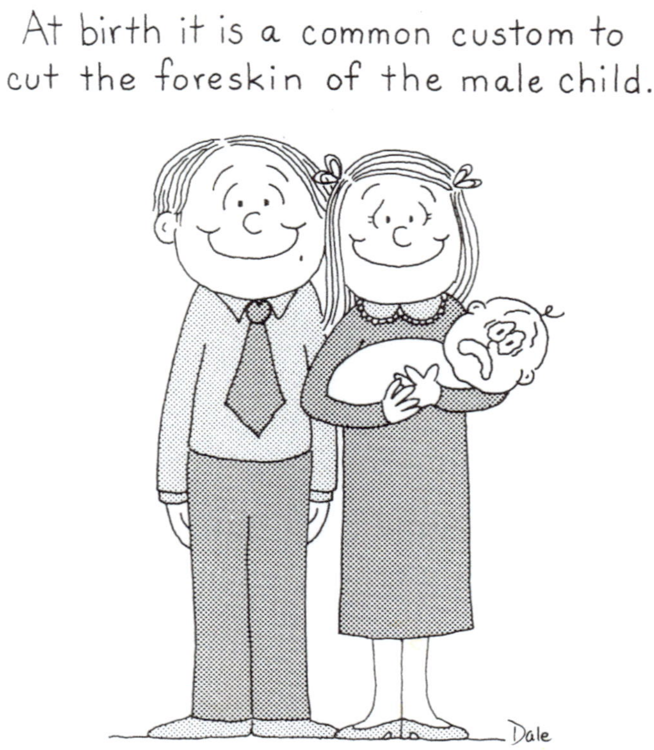
At birth it is a common custom to
cut the foreskin of the male child.
Dale

Exhibit 12–3 Sample Letter for Starting a Journal Club Network

[Date] __________

Dear [Physician] __________,

With the rapid pace of developments in medicine today, it is difficult for most physicians to keep up with the progress. To stay abreast of all the changes, I suggest that you and I establish an informal journal club.

I will be reviewing the urologic literature on a regular basis. If I see articles that are pertinent to [physician's specialty], I will make copies and forward them to you. I hope you will do the same for me.

Perhaps in this way we can extend and increase our coverage of the medical literature.

Sincerely,

Neil Baum, MD

1. National Library of Medicine. https://pmc.ncbi.nlm.nih.gov/about/intro/#:~:text=About%20the%20ContentAbout%20the%20Archive
2. Personalized luggage tags are available from Amazon. https://www.amazon.com/s?k=personalized+luggage+tags&hvadid=694616913764&hvdev=c&hvexpln=67&hvlocphy=9025150&hvnetw=g&hvocijid=8302849974175305573%2D%2D&hvqmt=b&hvrand=8302849974175305573&hvtargid=kwd-13853257&hydadcr=24629_13626730&mcid=ab92bc4a111e3867ae9b611b0a906cc0&tag=googhydr-20&ref=pd_sl_45l46fs7yf_b_p67

10 Branding Your Medical Practice: How to Make Your Practice Distinctive and Unique

> **Case Study: Kaila's Story**
> Kaila is a junior associate practicing primary care in a multispecialty practice located in a moderate-sized community. Kaila joined the multispecialty group practice immediately after completing her residency and receives most of her patients from specialists within her group. Kaila is interested in nutrition and weight loss, and she chose her residency because of its focus on wellness. Kaila would like to utilize those skills to expand her referral base. Kaila plans to attend some practice promotion and marketing seminars to learn how to brand her practice.

How does a passenger train differentiate itself from the behemoth airline industry and keep market share in the transportation market? One distinction is all it takes—Amtrak's singular competitive advantage against airlines: scenery. Flying to a distant destination certainly takes less time and may even cost less than taking a train. So why does passenger train travel still exist when an airplane ride takes less time and is cheaper?

As an example, the Northern Pacific rail line has a "Vista Dome" car, and passengers can marvel at a 360-degree view from inside the dome. Amtrak carefully schedules its rides to ensure passengers can enjoy the best vistas during daylight hours. Their subtle message is, "You can't see the same scenery from an airplane." This distinctive branding and their scenery message cannot be duplicated by multibillion-dollar airlines.

Another example everyone has experienced is the marketing and promotion of bottled water, such as Evian®, Fiji®, and Smart Water®, to name a few. In contrast to many areas of the world, in our country, most tap water is free and safe to drink. Yet, millions of Americans pay $1.69 or more for a liter of bottled water. The price of bottled water is 20% more than the same volume of Budweiser beer, 40% more than the same volume of milk, and three times the cost of gasoline! Now that's the power of branding: motivating people to pay more for water than what is available for free at the tap. Let us examine the examples of how physicians can make their practices the epitome of healthcare.

Most of our choices—from the coffee shop we frequent for our jolt of java to the company that supplies the medical office with its medical supplies—are based on a branding strategy. Doctors may not even be aware of it, because subliminal suggestions, social media, and word-of-mouth marketing can be as contagious as a multimillion-dollar advertising campaign.

N. Baum, M. J. Kahn, *Business Basics for your Healthcare Practice*,
https://doi.org/10.1007/978-3-032-25241-8_10

What Is Branding?

The American Marketing Association (the other "AMA") defines a brand as a "name, term, sign, symbol or design, or a combination of them intended to identify the goods and services of one seller or group of sellers and to differentiate them from those of other sellers." Branding is more than that. It is everything you do to attract and maintain quality patients. Branding allows a practice to attract the type of patient it wants. Such a "fit" creates patients who choose you over your competition.

Branding helps you differentiate your medical practice from others in the community. Branding considers the "look and feel" of your office, your staff, your educational materials, and every other detail that gives your patients clues as to who you are, what you value, and how they might be treated if they become a patient in the practice.

The business side of healthcare is undergoing rapid change. Both physicians and office managers are looking for new ways to connect with patients. In the not-too-distant past, a new physician would place an announcement in the paper and a listing in the Yellow Pages of the local phone book. Then they were ready to practice their craft. Physicians would promote themselves by meeting colleagues in the physician lounges, going to the emergency rooms, and waiting for patients to arrive. Today, with patients using the Internet and social media, it is much more challenging to build a practice using antiquated techniques that were effective just a few decades ago. It is now necessary to build a brand for your practice.

Questions you need to ask *and* answer include: what makes your medical practice unique and special? What is your sustainable competitive advantage? Everyone believes that they are members of a truly unique practice or organization, but how do we convey that to existing patients and potential new patients? Have you thought of yourself as the best in your field in your community? Or do you enjoy a reputation in your community of treating a specific disease or condition? Are you the best robotic surgeon in your area or region? Do your patients see you as a superstar, and, most importantly, do they know about your areas of interest or expertise? If not, you need to build a more cohesive brand image. Branding is the art of attracting your ideal patients using highly targeted messaging that captures their attention and motivates them to choose your practice for their medical care.

Branding is also an opportunity to create a name, term, symbol, or design that identifies and defines your practice, differentiating it from others. Branding is just as important as marketing or sales. Branding influences and changes the way people think. Branding appeals to desire and touches emotions. The goal of branding is to emotionally predispose potential patients to form a relationship with you, believing you are the best choice for them. With more medical information available to existing and potential patients at their fingertips, today's medical consumers are too sophisticated and skeptical to be sold. They want to arrive at their own decision on their own terms. Branding is helping them get there. Branding "pre-sells" your expertise, or your practice, before the patients even meet you or open the door of your office and enter the reception area. These potential patients call to make an appointment because of the reputation or impression you have created, indicating that you are indeed the best at what you do and the best fit for them. Your patients also believe they will receive outstanding care and attention from you and your staff. Branding offers you an opportunity to sculpt your practice exactly as you would like. Your brand can be created to attract patients who pay cash, those of a specific demographic, such as a particular age group or location, those with the disease or condition you wish to treat, and ultimately, patients who appreciate the value of your medical care and expertise.

Just as successful practices and businesses have a mission statement that serves as a roadmap or motivation for employees and a guarantee to customers or patients, a brand is your opportunity to declare your promise to your patients about the outstanding service that they will receive when they are part of your practice. Your brand can attract patients to the practice as long as you keep your promise and deliver on it. This ability to find a unique distinction applies not only to the healthcare profession but also to a medical practice, provided the practice can identify its unique distinction in its marketplace.

Benefits of Branding

Branding enables you to become your patients' first choice as their physician, even before they need one. Branding can attract and then maintain quality patients who have had a positive experience with you and your practice.

Attracting and retaining high-quality patients involves promising—and then delivering on that promise—to provide your patients with a stellar medical experience. Then, patients return to you again, and they brag about you and your practice to their friends, creating invaluable word-of-mouth buzz about you and your practice. If you are in a competitive environment, you need to attract patients by increasing your visibility and that of your practice. Frankly, your visibility attracts more prospective patients. Still, your ability to keep them depends on what you provide them with during their interactions with you and your staff. So, your name and face need to be circulating in the community in a tasteful, professional way that your preferred patient base will see.

Branding is all about perception and visibility, which builds credibility in the eyes of your prospective patients. If they see something in the media a few times, it sounds familiar to them, and they get the impression it must be good. When prospective patients recognize you and say to themselves, "he looks familiar," you are on your way to developing a brand. All things being equal, the more positive visibility you create, the more likely you will attract patients to your practice. Patients want to feel comfortable with their choices, and familiarity breeds that comfort.

Your patients' and prospective patients' perceptions are your reality, and they define their decision to see you versus the others due in large part to your branding. They have made this decision, not based on objective evidence, but on their perception that you are the best choice for them. They did not arrive at that choice using logic—they made the decision emotionally and then justified it with logic. Perhaps they saw you on the news, your photo in the social column at a fundraiser, or their friend passed along the informative newsletter you distributed to your patients. It can be the monthly column you wrote for a local magazine or publication, or your appearance on the local news where you are interviewed about a new procedure or treatment that you offer your patients. Branding also occurs when you sponsor a health-related event, such as a walk or run to raise awareness or funds for a specific type of cancer.

Another benefit of branding is when your website ranks at the top of search results on Google or Yahoo. Today's marketplace is too competitive and too crowded to rest on your laurels. Your name needs to stay in front of your preferred patient base, so they visit you when they have a medical need now or in the future. You cannot assume they will stay loyal to you if you do not maintain an active relationship with them. If you are not visible, you allow your competitors to redirect your patients to their practices. This situation must be avoided at all costs.

Getting Started to Brand Your Practice

Begin by letting your patients know what sets you apart, such as your specific fellowship training or your advanced medical skills. Inform your patients what you offer that differentiates your practice from your competitors—such as evening and Saturday morning appointments or a technology or treatment that others don't provide. Let your brand stand out—offer transportation for your patients to and from your office or the hospital (if permitted in your area).

- Show your personality in your marketing tools—You can portray yourself as the "Top Doc to the Stars," the physician to the high school, college, or professional team in your community, or "The Local Neighborhood Doctor."

- Specialize and be selective. It is not possible to be everything to everyone. Instead, select an area of interest or expertise that is unique and special, and that makes you and your practice special.
- Be where your prospective patients are—Have offices in various parts of the community or region where your preferred patients live. This means making it convenient for your patients to become part of your practice without having to travel far to receive their medical care.
- Build rapport and trust with every patient—Use the patient's name when speaking to them in person or over the telephone. Make the patient feel special, not just a diagnosis or medical condition. When a patient calls for an appointment, your receptionist should conclude the phone call by stating the patient's name before terminating the call: "Mrs. Smith, it is nice to speak with you. Dr. Strangelove looks forward to meeting you next week at 2:00 PM. Do you have any questions before that appointment?"
- Stay in contact with your patients throughout the year—Send them a practice newsletter, birthday cards, and thank-you notes when they refer a patient to you.
- Refine your patient relations processes—Have your staff introduce themselves using their name to new patients and then walk all new patients from the reception area to the exam rooms. Of course, make sure you see them on time!
- Stay consistent with your message. Don't try to be all things to everyone. Select an area or areas you deem worthy of your brand, and ensure you relate that message to both existing and potential patients.

For those physicians who take branding seriously, the payoff can be huge. The difference between good practice and great practice lies in the details. Please pay attention to every aspect of yourself, your staff, and your practice to ensure they align with your personality and the image you are trying to portray. Don't think of branding as taking patients from your colleagues or your competitors. Think of branding as the opportunity to have your existing patients and potential new patients have your name and the name of your practice come to mind whenever a medical problem that you treat, or you have as an area of expertise, comes up in any conversation.

To start the branding process, could you gather your staff and conduct a brainstorming session? You begin by writing down what you want to achieve and identifying your target market. For example, if you are an orthopedist and wish to specialize in sports medicine, then write down the ages of patients you want to treat, the injuries that you want to treat, and the ability of this patient population to pay for your services.

Be as specific as possible to define not only the medical condition(s) but also the patients' demographics, payer mix, and what you can reasonably deliver consistently. It is this consistency that is vital to the success of your branding process.

Your branding must remain in sync with your skills, staff, facility, operating systems, and principles. Set aside at least an hour for a branding brainstorming session with your team. Ask your staff to write down as many concise core messages they can think of that pertain to your practice in each of these categories:

- Courtesy (how you will treat patients, their families, and your fellow providers).
- Punctuality or your commitment to being on time. Being on time is a fundamental element of branding, which involves providing patients with access to the practice and ensuring they are seen on time. You can be the most outstanding expert in the field, but if patients wait 4–6 weeks to get an appointment and then wait 60 min to see the doctor, all your branding efforts will be wasted.
- Expertise or what you specialize in. Your expertise is what differentiates you from others in the community.
- Referrals or how you will accept or forward communications and recommendations for care or services. For the most part, this means sending a referral letter within 24 h of seeing a patient referred by a colleague. (See Chap. 9 on writing an effective referral letter.)

Next, consider what your target market needs. If you are an obstetrician specializing in infertility, you need to establish a reproductive laboratory. In that case, you need to think about the technicians and other specialists who you will need to have in place to achieve these goals so that patients can conduct all of their infertility care at one facility and not have to go to the reproductive endocrinologist in one building, a lab in another location, and then undergo the IVF in still another office.

You'll need to identify your competitors. Don't just think of your local competitors; also consider those in the region, the rest of the nation, and, depending on your areas of expertise, your global competitors. For example, practices that aim to attract patients from around the world to their country for orthopedic procedures, which are significantly cheaper than the same procedures performed in America, are establishing a medical tourism industry. They are making it possible for patients to obtain visas, book airline and hotel reservations before and after their surgery, and even arrange for doctors who will participate in their postoperative care once they return to their hometowns. This concept is branded to make it not only less expensive but also hassle-free for patients willing to undergo surgery in such a setting. How do you differentiate yourself from your competitors? What is it that makes you unique from those who offer the same services?

For example, a urology practice in New Orleans is branding itself to provide urologic oncology care for patients from South America, a form of "reverse tourism." They have Spanish-speaking doctors and staff; they meet patients at the airport and provide them with transportation to the medical center. They choreograph every aspect of the patient's care by providing outstanding patient services alongside clinical care. To make this work, you need to create a list of the unique benefits patients may experience from being in your practice.

As another example, an academic practice in Boston that specializes in the treatment of urinary incontinence can evaluate the patient in one visit by conducting a history and physical exam, performing diagnostic testing, providing a discussion on the treatment options, obtaining consent, and doing the pre- and postop teaching on the very first visit. This one-stop approach contrasts with the three or four trips that are typically required by many other urogynecologic practices, as they can't charge patients for diagnostic studies on the same day as the initial office visit when the E and M codes are generated. This Boston practice has branded itself as a "one-stop shop," which makes it attractive to patients, insurance companies, and payors.

During brainstorming sessions, to generate many ideas, it is important to avoid judging those who offer suggestions. You want to have as many unfiltered ideas and thoughts as possible to work from during this first brainstorming session. After this first brainstorming session, print your branding statement and share it with all your staff before your next meeting. Your next meeting will allow you to refine your responses to the questions that were generated during your first branding meeting. At the second meeting, fine-tune your branding statement, then use it to develop your strategy and tactics for implementing the branding message.

Displaying Your Brand

Look for opportunities to display your brand. If you have a website, take an objective look at it. Can you add your brand message? What about your business cards? You could have them redesigned to include your brand message. You can create signage for your office to set the tone or display your brand. Next, you can find ways to share your message through your words, attitude, and behavior. No matter what you display externally, it's who you are internally that defines your authentic brand.

Every successful business, including your medical practice, benefits from having a strong branding message. When you create your brand, please make sure it's a proclamation and a promise, not a pitch. Because what you're delivering is a promise, and that's what the branding buzz is all about.

Kaila's Story

Kaila's branding experience involved creating a website, with her multispecialty group's permission, that focused on nutrition and its role in maintaining good health, as well as its use to improve various medical conditions. Kaila also began a monthly blog highlighting the importance of good nutrition. Kaila prepared a newsletter and sent it to existing patients and referring physicians. The newsletter was sent to her target market every quarter. Kaila created a slogan, "Kaila loves kale," which she used on her website, stationery, and blogs. As a result, Kaila increased the number of patients she referred from existing patients and other primary care physicians. She soon found herself seeing patients with nutritional needs and using her skills as a nutritionist to address unmet needs in her community. She had a real sense that she was seeing the types of patients she wanted to see and felt that her practice was becoming a good fit for her skills and interests. This was a real branding success story.

Bottom Line

Branding is not just for soft drink companies, Amazon, and Nike shoes. Additionally, branding in healthcare is not exclusive to the Mayo Clinic or the Cleveland Clinic. Nearly every practice and hospital has the potential to create a brand or an area of expertise that sets it apart from others in the community or region. Einstein said, "If you can't explain it to a six-year-old, you don't understand it yourself." Look to what makes you unique and special—the essence of your practice—and distill it into a simple statement that guides your brand in every aspect of your practice. Be consistent and use that brand to define the visual image, verbal communication, and the patient experience in all patient encounters.

If you fail to uphold your brand's promise to the patient at any stage, the relationship and the implied trust will be at risk. Instead, create the best possible experience for your patients and establish a long-lasting brand that attracts new patients and fosters the loyalty of existing ones.

Key Takeaways

- A brand is an opportunity to distinguish your practice from your competitors.
- A brand demonstrates the unique features of your practice.
- Branding can improve a practice's online presence and visibility, making it easier for potential patients to discover and choose the practice.
- Branding also enhances your search engine optimization and may help you land on the first page of Google search results.
- Branding is only effective if you keep the promise of your message.

Resources

Baum L. Healthcare Professionals, Consider Yourself Creative – Go Digital, Harvard Business Review, December 2011

Marketing and branding for private practices. Nov 15, 2023. https://www.ama-assn.org/practice-management/private-practices/marketing-and-branding-private-practices

Physicians Practice. (2017, May 30). 5 tips for developing a strong medical practice brand. https://www.physicianspractice.com/practice-management/5-tips-developing-strong-medical-practice-brand

Marlowe, D. (2017). Branding Your Medical Practice: A Guide to Successful Branding for Physicians. Amazon.

11 Legal Considerations in Hiring and Firing of Healthcare Staff

Case Study: Rochelle
Rochelle is working with a small group practice and has recognized the need for a medical assistant. Rochelle's partners agreed with her request and suggested that she conduct the necessary screening and evaluation to find a suitable medical assistant. How should Rochelle proceed?

Finding the Match Made in Heaven

For the health and ultimate success of your practice, you must have high-quality, efficient, and dedicated staff. Someone not suited to your practice can create a negative impression among your patients and cause a decline in the morale of your staff.

With today's tight healthcare labor market in many metropolitan communities, and competition from large hospitals and other industries offering higher salaries and more benefits, individual practices, which are often akin to small businesses, usually struggle to compete with larger employers. The challenge of finding the right person for the job is made even more difficult. Does this mean that you should settle for a less-than-qualified employee? Certainly not!

Despite other opportunities, job seekers still find the idea of working at a medical practice attractive. A position with a private practice offers status as well as the gratification and enjoyment that come from helping others. By offering fair salaries and challenging working conditions, you can attract and retain a top-notch staff.

Finding and hiring the right person to fill a staff position requires time and patience.

Hiring staff members is a delicate process that you will improve as you and your practice mature. Hiring someone hastily to fill a vacancy and making the wrong decision leads to costly turnover.

Studies show that the average cost of turnover, whether you are correcting a hiring mistake or replacing a long-time employee, is two and a half times the salary of the worker you are losing. But turnover also brings hidden costs beyond compensation and benefits. The time to interview, the overtime you pay others to pick up the slack, and the impact on morale of your existing staff can wreak havoc with your practice.

The most effective way to find candidates is through word of mouth. Consider utilizing job-listing services offered by local schools, universities, and professional organizations. Today, there are websites where you can post job opportunities. A popular job-listing site is Craigslist,

N. Baum, M. J. Kahn, *Business Basics for your Healthcare Practice*,
https://doi.org/10.1007/978-3-032-25241-8_11

<name of your city>. craigslist.org. This website features job postings, classified ads, etc. It is a networking tool for the younger generation of job seekers. Other online employment websites include Indeed.com, Monster.com, and ZipRecruiter.com.

Screening Applicants

Request that applicants submit their electronic resumes to your email address. Ask your office manager to screen the resumes and then call the applicants to schedule an interview. Your office manager or human resources department should speak to each applicant when they call your office. This phone call is too important to be screened by your receptionist. The office manager should specify the time of day when they can receive calls from applicants or set a time to return calls to the applicants. After the office manager has screened applicants and narrowed down the choices, the doctor interviews the finalists.

Talking with an applicant allows you to evaluate

- The applicant's telephone manners.
- The applicant's curiosity about you and your practice.

You want a vibrant individual who conveys enthusiasm. If you do not sense vitality and enthusiasm in a phone conversation with the applicant, your patients will not either.

Ask the applicant to send a handwritten letter, along with their resume and application. Suggest a topic for the letter. For example, you might suggest that the letter explain why the applicant wants the job, why the applicant is qualified for the job, or how the applicant could enhance your practice. You might also suggest that the letter address a nonmedical topic, such as the applicant's hobbies or last vacation. Suggest that the letter be emailed, faxed, snail-mailed, or hand-delivered to the office.

This letter serves several functions:

- It allows you to see how quickly the applicant responds. In most medical practices, a prompt response to patients and other healthcare professionals is crucial.
- It allows you to analyze the applicant's writing and spelling skills. (You do not want to hire someone who cannot spell correctly or whose handwriting is more illegible than yours!) If the applicant is emailing the letter, this also allows you to evaluate their "email etiquette"—an important feature these days, when too many people fail to proofread or edit before they hit the send button!
- Finally, a written letter will frequently reveal something about the applicant that is not available in their resume.

The Interview Process

Encourage preparation. The interview will be more productive if you allow applicants to prepare. Before an interview, send the applicant a job description and information about you and your practice. Please provide information about your practice, including the types of patients you see and the typical situations that someone working in your office might encounter. If you are a specialist, send the applicant information on the nature of your specialty or some educational material that you give to patients about the various diseases, illnesses, and conditions you treat. It is impressive when an applicant has read this information or has visited the practice's website and asks questions about anything they don't understand.

Make the most of each interviewing session. You can do this in several ways: The first few minutes of the interview can be used to break the ice. For example, introduce yourself, your practice, and the job description to the candidate.

Next, consider providing the candidate with a written list of questions at the time of their visit, which you will ask the applicant (Fig. 11.1).

Fig. 11.1 List of questions to ask job applicants

Name

1. What are your strengths?
2. What are your weaknesses?
3. Why are you interested in changing jobs?
4. What was your best job? Your worst?
5. Tell me about your best boss.
6. Tell me about your worst boss.
7. What do you think your references will say when I call to inquire about your past employment?
8. What do you want to be doing one year for now? Five years from now?

Using a written list encourages candidates to do the talking.

Try to interview promising applicants more than once. First impressions are important, but most couples don't get engaged on their first date. Many applicants will be eliminated after the phone call or the first interview. Those still in the running typically require a second, third, or even fourth interview before a job offer is extended.

Consider asking "curveball" questions. At least once during the interview process, ask the candidate a difficult question. Circumstances will arise that require the staff to think and respond quickly. Failure to react quickly can adversely affect patient health and may even lead to litigation. Suppose the candidate has worked in a medical office or has healthcare experience. In that case, you might ask a question such as, "What would you do if a patient called with a medical emergency and the physician couldn't be reached or located immediately?" Fig. 11.2 contains additional examples of curveball questions to ask.

After the first interview, give a potential applicant a "homework assignment." In addition to the curveball questions, which require immediate answers, present each applicant with a more complex problem that allows them time to respond after the interview is over. For example, you may ask the applicant to propose a solution to a common problem in practice. How quickly the applicant responds to this "homework assignment" tells you a lot about the applicant's creative problem-solving abilities as well as the strength of the applicant's desire to get the job.

Encourage the applicants to ask questions. This allows you to evaluate their level of interest in and curiosity about the job. Suppose an applicant fails to ask any questions. In that case, this suggests that the applicant is intimidated by the interview process or is not very curious. If either is the case, you are learning something important. You want to hire people who are both inquisitive and not easily intimidated. For instance, if an applicant's only question is about the salary or vacation pay, that would be a clue to their priorities. Suppose an applicant asked about furthering skills through seminars or attending night school. In that case, this might be an indication to consider putting this applicant on the short list.

1. If I did a procedure that did not have a CPT code, how would you attempt to obtain insurance coverage from a third-party payer?
2. How would you handle it if a patient began arguing with you in front of other patients about the cost of his visit?
3. If a patient called on the telephone and demanded that he be seen the same day as he called, and you knew that the problem was not an emergency, what would you tell him?
4. What would you say to a patient who requested that his records be sent to another physician?
5. Suppose that you saw a patient in the grocery store and you were with your spouse or significant other. How would you introduce them?

Fig. 11.2 List of curve ball questions to ask job applicants

Advice on Requesting References

There's an unwritten rule regarding references: do not give out references, but do not hire without them.

Many employers will make the mistake of calling the previous employer without any introduction and expect the former employer to discuss the applicant and their employment history. Accept that the information you receive will likely not be complete and should not be the determining factor in whether you hire the individual. You can obtain information on an applicant through a background check (with proper authorization from the applicant). Still, you should wait to conduct a criminal background check until you make a conditional offer of employment.

Many employers only give out a name, job title, and dates of employment. Still, they will not provide specific information on performance and the applicant's termination because they are fearful of a lawsuit. [1] This situation can be avoided by asking the applicant to sign a release-of-information letter (see Fig. 11.3) and emailing or faxing it to their previous employers before your call. This avoids your cold calling a reference and not receiving any useful information.

Applicants will often not give you names of references unless they expect the references to respond favorably. To get around this, ask applicants for additional references during follow-up interviews. The length of time it takes them to respond reveals the quality of the references.

Have your existing staff members conduct interviews with each applicant. They will let you know whether that person will be a good team player and a good fit with the existing staff.

Pay attention to the applicant's follow-up. Did the applicants return your phone calls in a timely manner? Did they send you a thank-you note after their interviews? Remember that the way they handle the business of looking for work today is how they will handle the business of working for you tomorrow. More importantly, the courtesies and manners they extend to you will be a barometer of how they will treat your patients.

Release Form

I am an applicant for employment with Dr. Baum. I am submitting a signed release form that provides you with permission to speak with Dr. Baum or one of his representatives regarding my previous employment and experience with you. I have read all the information the attached request concerning your experiences with me as an employee. I am in agreement with the content on the form and give you permission to release the information to Dr. Baum. I hold you harmless for any information you furnish regardless of the outcome of my application for employment.

Date:

Signature:

Notary Seal and Date

Fig. 11.3 Release-of-information letter

Rochelle's Story

Rochelle's search for a medical assistant. Rochelle got the word out in the medical community that she was looking for a medical assistant. She also posted a job description on Craigslist. Still, her best candidate came from one of her patients, who had a daughter who was a trained medical assistant looking to change jobs due to the great distance she had to travel from her home to her office. After thorough vetting and a paid day to shadow Rochelle, she was hired, and both Rochelle and the medical assistant were happy with the decision.

Bottom Line on Hiring

Although the hiring process is time-consuming and stressful, it is essential for creating an excellent practice where both the doctor and staff provide outstanding service. The cost of taking the time to hire the right employee is less than the costs of employee turnover.

Ready, Aim, Fire! Tactfully Terminating an Employee

The remainder of this chapter will discuss the legal process of terminating an employee and how to avoid violating labor laws, which could lead to a lawsuit if the termination is not conducted properly.

Case of Terminating Theresa

Theresa served as an office manager for a small group oncology practice for 20 years. She has been with the practice for over two decades, as it merged with two other oncology groups in the community. Although Theresa was an excellent employee and was highly respected by the staff and doctors, her skill level was insufficient for managing a large, multimillion-dollar group of oncologists. It became apparent that Theresa would have to be terminated. How does the practice terminate a long-serving employee?

Termination of Employees—Dot Your *I's* and Cross Your *T's*

Most medical practices, 95%, are non-unionized. The laws and guidelines that apply to unionized employees will apply to those without a union affiliation. Unionized employers, those that have contracts with unions covering wages, hours, and working conditions of their employees, are generally required by the contract to show that they had "just cause" to terminate an employee. This situation develops when an employee has been terminated and files a grievance with the union, which ultimately goes to arbitration. Arbitrators typically rule that the employer has the burden to prove cause by a preponderance of the evidence, which is a high standard. Arbitrators often send terminated employees back to work even though the employer felt it had good reason to terminate the person.

Why do we discuss unions when union contracts do not cover most clinics and medical practices? (In fact, most private employers in the United States are nonunion—93.5%). Since the enactment of the National Labor Relations Act of 1935, 29 U.S.C. §§ 151–169, and the Taft Hartley Act of 1947, 29 U.S.C. §§ 141–197, there have been significant changes in the laws affecting employment such that employees no longer need the help of a union to challenge their termination. Those laws include

- **Title VII of the Civil Rights Act of 1964 (Title VII)** (42 U.S.C. §§ 2000e-2000e-17), prohibiting discrimination based on race, color, sex (including amendments by the **Pregnancy Discrimination Act** and the Civil Rights Act of 1991), national origin, and religion.
- **Age Discrimination in Employment Act (ADEA)** (29 U.S.C. §§ 621–634), prohibiting discrimination based on age (40 and over).
- **Title I and Title V of the Americans with Disabilities Act (ADA)** (42 U.S.C. §§ 12,101–12,117), prohibiting discrimination based on disability (including amendments by the Civil Rights Act of 1991 and the **Americans with Disabilities Act Amendments Act (ADAAA)**.
- **Genetic Information Nondiscrimination Act (GINA)** (24 U.S.C. §§ 2000ff-2000ff-11), prohibiting discrimination on the basis of genetic information.
- **Uniformed Services Employment and Reemployment Rights Act (USERRA)** (38 U.S.C. § 43), prohibiting discrimination based on past, current, or prospective military service. This protects the civilian job rights and benefits of veterans and military personnel.
- **Section 1981 of the Civil Rights Act of 1866 (Section 1981)**, prohibiting discrimination based on race, color, and ethnicity in the area of contracts.
- Most states and some municipalities have their own laws that mirror many of the federal regulations, and some states protect other groups, such as those of LGBT status.
- **The Family and Medical Leave Act (FMLA)** (29 U.S.C. §§ 2601–2654) protects employee rights to take up to 12 weeks of leave for medical and family care purposes.
- **Workers' compensation laws** prohibit retaliation against employees for making workers' compensation claims.
- **National Labor Relations Act (NLRA)** (29 U.S.C. §§ 151–169), prohibiting termination because of an employee's protected and concerted activity on behalf of a group or for organizing or union activity.
- **Fair Labor Standards Act (FLSA)** 29 U.S.C. §§ 201–219), prohibiting termination for exercising wage and hour rights.

How do these laws affect your decisions to terminate employees? Let's consider the Bones Are Our Business Orthopedic Clinic, a clinic that has been in practice for 5 years and has five doctors and a support staff of 20. The clinic has been experiencing a decline in patient numbers, as well as the retirement of its head. To meet these financial demands, as well as to deal with certain personnel issues, the clinic has taken the following actions:

1. Martha, an X-ray technician, is pregnant and has been restricted to lifting no more than 50 pounds. The clinic advised her that she needed to go home, have the baby, and come back within 12 weeks. Walter, a 61-year-old maintenance worker, had a heart attack and was restricted from lifting over 40 pounds. The clinic assigned Henry to help Walter when lifting was needed. Martha heard about this and quit threatening to sue.
2. Horace, an African-American male technician, had five instances when he arrived late for work and two unexcused absences within the past 3 months. Sharon, a white female nurse, was late for work on 5 days and had three absences within the same time period. The clinic terminates Horace but does not terminate Sharon because it deems her an essential employee.
3. William, a physician's assistant, went on active duty with his reserve unit 6 months ago and is now seeking to return to work. The clinic eliminated his position while he was absent.
4. A patient complains that she does not want to be treated by Willie, a transgender male nurse, and she threatens to leave the clinic and take her large family, who are also patients, with her. The clinic terminates Willie to comply with the patient's request.
5. The clinic holds clinic-wide meetings for all employees and doctors every Friday morning. At one of the meetings, Jerry, an X-ray technician, complains that he and the rest of the staff are not treated fairly because they are not allowed to leave the clinic during their 45-minute lunch break, for which they are not paid. Dr. Arthur, the head of the clinic, tells him that these are the rules, and if he doesn't like it, he can leave. Jerry responds that the clinic doesn't care about the employees, and he urges the rest of the staff to protest. Dr. Arthur terminates Jerry immediately.
6. Abdul, a Muslim physician's assistant, tells you he must pray five times a day. You tell him this would be too disruptive to the workplace and patient care at the clinic, and he should look for other work.

What problems do you see with the above actions, and what laws do you think might apply?[1]

So, how can a doctor or a clinic avoid termination problems, such as those that befell Bones Are Our Business Orthopedic Clinic? The following steps are recommended:

1. Be familiar with the laws that may apply to your employees.
2. Develop appropriate policies covering termination as a part of your employee handbook and/or personnel manual.
3. Educate the staff, especially the doctors and supervisors, as to the policies and legal ramifications covering employment termination.
4. Have the employees acknowledge in writing receipt of the policies and agreement to comply with them.
5. Consistently apply policies and procedures to all employees without any exceptions.
6. Evaluations—be honest—don't sugarcoat the employee's performance deficiencies—this can well come back to haunt you when you are considering termination. Train your evaluators to be objective.
7. Consider placing a problem employee on an improvement plan, for example, 60 or 90 days, to achieve satisfactory performance. Review performance every 30 days and document any improvement or lack thereof.
8. Document disciplinary actions as they occur and make sure that you have sufficient documentation to support a termination.
9. Ensure that the decision to terminate is based upon objective criteria and does not involve personal feelings.
10. Before deciding to terminate, conduct an impartial internal investigation and adequately document the results of the investigation.

[1] Martha—Title VII violation—making an accommodation for Walter, but not for Martha

Horace—Title VII and Section 1981 violation—different treatment based on race.
William—USERRA.
Willie—Title VII—sex.
Jerry—National Labor Relations Act—protected activity.
Abdul—Title VII—religion.

11. Determine if any employees have engaged in similar conduct and what disciplinary action was taken.
12. Analyze whether termination of the employee will have an adverse impact based on race, sex, age, or any protected category.
13. Where circumstances call for termination, act; do not delay.
14. Delivering the message to the employee:
    (a) Have a witness with you.
    (b) Arrange for the meeting with the employee to be private.
    (c) Collect and review the employee's personnel file with particular attention to disciplinary write-ups.
    (d) Be prepared and rehearse for the meeting.
    (e) Discuss any employment agreements with the employee.
    (f) Present the termination decision directly and avoid arguing with the employee.
    (g) Have the employee's final pay and benefits prepared and pay him. Decide beforehand whether the employee will receive severance and whether a waiver and release will be required. For this action, you may need the advice of a labor or employment lawyer.
    (h) Be sensitive to the termination and recognize that this will be an emotional situation for the employee.
    (i) Allow the employee to speak, but do not argue with him or allow him to go on at length. If possible, refrain from interrupting the employee while they are speaking.
    (j) Document the termination and have the witness also sign off on the document.
    (k) Obtain all clinic property from the employee, such as the computer, parking pass, and keys to the office.
    (l) Disable electronic resources the employee had, including email, voice mail, passwords, and logins.
    (m) Remind the employee of any continuing obligations, including non-competition and non-solicitation agreements, and protection of confidential information and trade secrets.
    (n) Escort the employee to his desk, allow him to gather his belongings, and politely escort him from the premises. If you anticipate resistance or violence, consider requesting a security officer from the hospital to accompany you and the employee.
    (o) Advise the remaining employees of the termination either directly by the person who handled the termination or through other supervisors or managers.
    (p) Decide how to inform patients of the action.
15. Determine what information will be provided to inquiries or references concerning the employee's employment and termination. You can't go wrong if you give the dates and titles of the work the employee performed in the practice.

Following these guidelines will help you make the right decision and defend it if you are challenged by a discharged employee seeking damages for wrongful termination.

Importance of Documentation

Your word may be good, but not when it comes to "he says, she says" discussions from each of the employee's memories and the firing doctor's or office manager's account, especially if litigation is involved. A weak pen on paper rather than a strong memory is more likely to avoid costly litigation. Meticulous documentation avoids a confrontation with an employee who remembers something different than the doctor or the office manager. All discussions should be in writing or, at a minimum, documented via email, and the discussion should be acknowledged by the employee by having them sign the document. This documentation should be placed in the employee's personnel file. If you didn't document the discussion with the employee, then you are setting the stage for expensive litigation or a costly settlement. Avoid saying anything to a departing employee that could be used against the practice in a wrongful termination lawsuit. That is why the history leading to the termination is documented.

Usually, less is better. The more discussion that takes place with a departing employee, the greater the risk of saying something that could be used by the employee to file a wrongful termination lawsuit. Provide the employee with the reason for their termination. Employment lawyers suggest avoiding dumping a litany of previous mistakes the departing employee has made during the termination discussion. By doing so, you allow the employee to refute each point or mistake. State with unequivocal certainty that the employee is being terminated and bring the discussion to a prompt close. If you have decided to terminate the employee, don't leave any "wiggle room" or make the discussion another warning. Also, avoid stating that you are going to give the employee one more chance to improve their performance or behavior. If firing an employee is inevitable, sever the connection between the employee and the practice promptly and without delay.

Inform the employee that if a future employer contacts you for references, you will only provide the position held by the employee, the date the employee started, and the date the employee left the practice. Reassure the employee that no mention will be made of the termination or any discussion of the employee's performance in the practice.

Following the termination discussion, ask the employee to return their keys and computer badges. Walk the employee to their desk or workstation and allow them to retrieve all their personal belongings. Then, escort them out of the office. This approach may seem cold and heartless; you avoid the departing employee from interacting with the remaining staff and cause a deterioration in staff morale.

Final message on firing an employee: good documentation will protect your practice. If you didn't document it, you didn't do it or say it!

Follow Up on the Termination of Theresa

Theresa was an excellent employee, and the doctors and the staff appreciated her service over many years. However, her skills were outdated and would not be able to handle the complexity and new technology, including AI, of managing a large group practice. She was given 4 months' severance pay and a 6-month payment of her health insurance. A glowing letter of recommendation was provided, which she could use if she decided to look for new employment. She was reassured that she could use the practice as a reference for any new job, and a retirement party was held on her last day of work.

Bottom Line on Hiring and Firing

Hiring and firing an employee is not an easy task. Doctors don't receive any training in medical school or residency to learn the skills necessary to perform these functions without incurring any legal risk to the practice.

You may find the hiring process time-consuming and stressful, but that does not come close to comparing with the time and stress it will cost you if the candidate you hire is not a good "fit" with your practice. Follow the suggestions in this chapter, and you are much more likely to hire right the first time!

Circumstances surrounding hiring and firing are a source of stress among doctors, office managers, and human resources in the healthcare setting. It is imperative that the practice develop skills and techniques to find the right person for various positions in the practice. Hiring takes time and energy, and mistakes can be very costly to the practice. Having the wrong employee in a position can significantly impact the efficiency and productivity of the practice. When an employee is not working out and fitting in with the practice, the difficult process of terminating the employee ensues. Termination can result in deterioration of morale and can be very costly to find a replacement. Additionally, there is concern about the potential risk of liability for wrongful termination if the termination process isn't followed as we have shared with you in this chapter. This process of hiring and firing should not be minimized or delegated to a doctor or manager who lacks the skills to find the right person or the necessary knowledge to terminate an employee.

Key Takeaways

- There's an art to the practice of medicine and as well as an art to the hiring and firing of staff.
- You can control the turnover rate by hiring the right person; however, this takes time and requires careful vetting of applicants.
- Terminating an employee is never a comfortable task, which requires careful documentation and sensitivity to the departing employee.

Resources

"Hiring, Firing, and Managing Healthcare Employees: Legal Pitfalls and Best Practices" by Michael J. Sacopulos: This book provides healthcare managers and human resource professionals with practical guidance on hiring, firing, and managing employees while navigating the legal landscape of healthcare employment.

Websites/Articles:

American Medical Association (AMA): The AMA offers a wealth of resources on various healthcare topics, including employment and management issues. Visit their website for articles and guides on hiring and firing best practices: https://www.ama-assn.org/

Healthcare Finance: This website features articles on various aspects of healthcare management, including hiring and firing employees. Browse their site for relevant content: https://www.healthcarefinancenews.com/

Society for Human Resource Management (SHRM): SHRM is an excellent resource for HR professionals in any industry, including healthcare. Their website offers articles, templates, and tools to help organizations manage their workforce effectively: https://www.shrm.org/

Legal Services/Consulting Firms:

Jackson Lewis P.C.: This law firm specializes in employment and labor law and offers services to help healthcare organizations navigate hiring, firing, and other employment-related matters. Visit their website for more information: https://www.jacksonlewis.com/

Ogletree Deakins: Another law firm focusing on labor and employment law, Ogletree Deakins provides resources and services for healthcare organizations. Their website offers valuable insights into various employment-related topics: https://www.ogletree.com/

Reference

1. Many states, including Louisiana, have adopted legislation protecting an employer from civil liability in providing accurate information about a current or former employee's job performance or reason for separation. The statute also protects employers who rely on such information in hiring from civil liability. See La. R.S. 23:291.

12 Malpractice: What You Need to Know to Stay Out of Trouble

> **Case Study: Tomika and the Tail**
> Tomika is completing her training as an internist and plans to join a large group practice in the same community where she trained. She is married, her husband is finishing his training, and they plan to move closer to their families in 2 years. Tomika knows she will be employed in her current position for only 2 years. Her contract stipulates that she has a claims-made policy and that there is no tail coverage after she and her husband leave the community. What are Tomika's options?

If you are faced with a lawsuit, know that you are not alone. The likelihood of a physician facing a medical malpractice suit during their career is high, with one study finding that approximately one-third of physicians will be sued at some point during their career, and the risk increases significantly with more years in practice [1]. Factors like physician specialty, with obstetrics and gynecology and general surgery having higher risks, and gender, with men facing higher odds than women, also influence this likelihood.

Most malpractice policies cover the expenses incurred while defending and settling a malpractice suit. These include attorney fees, damages, arbitration, settlement costs, court costs, and punitive and compensatory damages. These are subject to the limits of the policy.

Types of Malpractice Insurance

There are two categories of malpractice insurance: (1) claims-made and (2) occurrence. A claims-made policy provides coverage only if the policy was in effect when the incident occurred and a lawsuit was filed. Occurrence policies cover any claim for an event that takes place during the period the policy was in effect, even if the claim is filed after the policy lapses. Because a claim can be filed years after an event and after a claims-made policy expires, these policies often include a "tail" that extends coverage for a specified number of years beyond the expiration date of the malpractice policy. Tail coverage can be purchased separately if it's not part of the original policy.

For example, suppose a physician has a malpractice claims-made policy and receives a malpractice lawsuit during their employment. In that case, the doctor will be covered under a claims-made policy. If the doctor has an occurrence policy and is sued *after* they leave the practice, but the policy was in effect while the doctor was practicing, the doctor will be covered and protected by the policy.

N. Baum, M. J. Kahn, *Business Basics for your Healthcare Practice*,
https://doi.org/10.1007/978-3-032-25241-8_12

Tail coverage offers protection when a physician is changing jobs or retiring. Sometimes the cost of tail coverage will be covered by a previous employer to protect itself, or it can be negotiated with a new employer. Occurrence policies generally don't require tail coverage, but occurrence policies are only available in some states.

If you or your employer is buying a claims-made policy, ensure the beginning date for coverage is accurate and matches the expiration date on the prior policy to avoid any coverage gaps between policies.

The required coverage amount can vary by state, specialty, and arrangements with hospitals or your employer. Some states require doctors to have minimum coverage, but you can request additional coverage depending on your specialty.

Usual malpractice insurance limits are expressed as two numbers, such as "$1,000,000/$3,000,000," where the first number is the maximum payout per claim and the second is the maximum payout for all claims in the policy period. While limits vary by state, specialty, and risk, common ranges are $100,000/$300,000 to $1,000,000/$3,000,000, though higher limits are available and sometimes required by hospitals or state laws. $1,000,000/$3,000,000 is the most common and widely recommended limit, especially with increasing "mega verdicts."

The proper limits depend on your personal assets, the risk of your specialty, and local regulations, as you are personally responsible for any amount exceeding your policy's limits.

Generally, standard coverage limits are $1 million per claim and $3 million aggregate, which is the most the policy will pay in a year for all claims. However, specific states require different limits based on medical malpractice caps on damages. States with more litigious climates might need additional coverage.

Suppose a lawsuit is filed and found to be credible or legitimate. In that case, malpractice insurance will cover the injured patient's costs up to a limit set by the policy. Some states have patient compensation or catastrophe loss funds, which provide an additional layer of coverage over the primary policy limits. Doctors must pay into these state-run funds through a surcharge on medical malpractice insurance premiums. In such cases, when a lawsuit is filed and found to be credible or legitimate, malpractice insurance will cover the injured patient's damages up to a limit set by the policy. The state's fund pays the rest.

Finding a Malpractice Carrier

We emphasize that price certainly is one factor, but it shouldn't be the only one in selecting a malpractice carrier. Most states have a few carriers licensed to sell insurance in the state. If you focus only on price, you might be hiring an unreliable or financially precarious carrier.

Ensure that the policy includes a consent-to-settle clause. This clause prevents the insurer from settling a claim without the doctor's permission. Sometimes, insurance companies find it cheaper to pay a claim than to defend it. However, the doctor's reputation is at stake, and doctors are reticent to settle a claim if there is no evidence of malpractice.

The very best malpractice carriers will act as resources for their physician clients. They will offer advice on how to avoid claims and will guide the doctor through any litigation.

A few suggestions for screening potential carriers include

- Ask colleagues in your area where you plan to buy insurance about the malpractice carrier's reputation.
- You want to know their experience of settling claims.
- Go to AM Best (www.ambest.com) and check the carrier's financial position. AM Best provides the financial stability of the carriers and rates each carrier. Using this service, you can compare apples to apples.
- Check how long the carrier has been in business.
- Does the carrier specialize in specific medical fields such as obstetrics, neurosurgery, or anesthesia?

- Do they want to have a relationship with you and meet you personally, or is it only through the Internet that they communicate with their clients/doctors? Depending on your personality and preferences, you may be comfortable with internet communication, or you may prefer more personable face-to-face interactions.
- You will want to know if the carrier encourages or mandates that you settle a claim made against you. Paying a claim is often in the best interest and less expensive for the malpractice carrier than the expense of defending a claim. Settling a claim, especially if you feel you have not deviated from the standard of care, may not be in your best interest and may place you in the National Practitioner Data Bank, which can negatively impact your reputation. The National Practitioner Data Bank (NPDB) is a confidential, web-based federal repository for reports on medical malpractice payments and adverse actions against healthcare practitioners, providers, and suppliers, established to promote quality healthcare and deter fraud.

To Broker or Not to Broker

A broker possesses the depth of knowledge and experience to determine the coverage a doctor or practice requires and identify the best insurers to provide it.

A malpractice insurance broker helps keep us informed of what our needs are and what changes must be made. For example, if a practice bought a general insurance policy 10 years ago, there was probably no provision for cyber insurance in case of a hack and loss of your data. A good broker will contact the doctor/practice and suggest that cyber insurance be added to the policy. Other insurance coverage risks include regulatory requirements such as compliance with the Health Insurance Portability and Accountability Act (HIPAA).

We suggest you contact your broker every periodically to ensure you are up to date and adequately covered, and to check for new developments since the policy was purchased. Examples of a need for evaluation and changes in the policy include

- Adding a new provider.
- Starting a new business, joint venture, or adding ancillary services.
- Forming a new entity, that is, sale of the practice to a hospital or merger with another practice.
- Adding new services or equipment.

Our take-home message is that if you can find a knowledgeable broker, it's much easier to hire them to do the heavy lifting, get the quotes, and inform you or the office manager of any legal issues that may affect your malpractice coverage.

Tomika's Story

Tomika approached her employer and asked about tail coverage. The large group practice said they couldn't make any exceptions regarding tail coverage for her. Tomika contacted a broker who found a tail-only policy at a reasonable premium that would be in effect for 5 years after she left the practice. Tomika purchased this policy and received additional compensation from the large group by offering her a "moving allowance" to help defray the extra cost of the tail insurance. Lesson learned: You can always get your own way if you have more than one way to do it!

Bottom Line

Malpractice insurance is required in every state. Most hospitals, ambulatory treatment centers, or outpatient surgery centers will require a malpractice policy to practice. For most employed physicians, medical liability coverage is typically provided as part of their employment contract by the hospital or health system. It is essential to check your contract and make sure you have coverage if you leave the practice for any reason. The old CYA is now CYT or "cover your tail!"

Key Takeaways

- If you practice long enough, you will likely be involved in a lawsuit.
- An occurrence policy is desirable, which will provide coverage even after you leave the practice or retire from practice.
- If you have a claims-made policy, we suggest that you purchase tail coverage if you are changing practices or retiring.

Resources

Liang, B. A., Maroulis, J., & Mackey, T. K. (2023). Understanding medical malpractice lawsuits. *Stroke*, *54*(3), e95-e99.

Hyman, D. A., Lerner, J., Magid, D. J., & Black, B. (2023, February). Association of past and future paid medical malpractice claims. In *JAMA Health Forum* (Vol. 4, No. 2, pp. e225436-e225436). American Medical Association.

Aaron, D. G., Robertson, C. T., King, L. P., & Sage, W. M. (2025). A new legal standard for medical malpractice. *JAMA*, *333*(13), 1161-1165.

Smith, H. (2025). Self-Defense in Medical Malpractice: How to Derail a Frivolous Malpractice Lawsuit. *Physician Leadership Journal*, *12*(2).

Reference

1. American Medical Association. Medical liability claim frequency among US physicians. Philadelphia: American Medical Association; 2020.

13 Mid-Level Providers and Use of Scribes to Improve Efficiency and Productivity

Case Study: Cassandra
Cassandra is a recent medical school graduate who worked for 3 years in a primary care medical practice. She found that she was soon overwhelmed and was required to see more patients than she was comfortable with. As a result, she and the staff had to work overtime, which the office manager informed her was increasing the practice's overhead. What were some solutions to her dilemma?

Who will provide medical care to millions of newly insured and aging patients? When Massachusetts made health insurance mandatory, physician practices were overwhelmed by the increased demand. Many doctors stopped taking new patients, and those who continued to accept new patients saw waiting times for appointments lengthen significantly [4].

One of the solutions to this dire situation is to use mid-level providers (MLPs). This is an area that is receiving recognition from both the medical profession and patients. However, it is an area of controversy. The controversial issue has been settled—mid-level providers are in our offices and in our hospitals, and the numbers are increasing rapidly. There is no going back, and MLPs are gaining momentum.

Who Are the Mid-Level Providers?

There's confusion among the medical profession and, of course, the public, about the names and titles associated with MLPs. Other terms that include MLPs include limited providers, nonphysician providers, allied health providers, midwives, advanced practice providers, and even medical assistants.

Where Are MLPs Working?

Today, 385,000 NPs and 145,000 PAs work in a variety of settings around the country. They have traditionally provided care in rural and underserved settings, where they work under the supervision of a physician who may or may not be in the same office or community. In these settings, mid-level providers diagnose and treat a broad range of routine medical conditions, referring the more complicated cases to the supervising physician. In our modern healthcare marketplace, clinics located in pharmacies and other retail locations are often staffed with MLPs.

Over the last 30 years, the role of MLP has expanded well beyond the primary care environment [5]. Today, mid-level providers work in hospitals, emergency departments, inpatient and outpatient surgical facilities, and in specialty practices such as cardiology and oncol-

N. Baum, M. J. Kahn, *Business Basics for your Healthcare Practice*,
https://doi.org/10.1007/978-3-032-25241-8_13

ogy, as part of the team that serves patients receiving ongoing treatment. It is often a mid-level provider who monitors fragile diabetics, sees cancer patients between treatments, reduces bone fractures in the emergency department, or closes the surgical incision for the doctor at the end of surgery.

MLPs include two distinct groups, physician assistants (PAs) and nurse practitioners (NPs). Their educational requirements and training are quite different. PAs receive three times more clinical hours in training than NPs. On the flipside, NPs usually have more clinical work experience, which frequently balances out their lack of clinical training hours and, perhaps levels the playing field.

The difference between PAs and NPs lies less in training and ability, and more in a cultural difference, or a difference in practice expectations. Depending on the state where MLPs practice, NPs increasingly are free of the requirements of physician supervision. In contrast, PAs appear to have a career goal that takes them along a path to work dependently with practicing physicians. The cultural and clinical training and competencies of the two groups and the difference between NPs and PAs are subtle, often nuanced.

Training aside, it is important to understand that for lower acuity patients, beyond the diagnostic work, most of the tasks (and time) to manage these patients do not require the skill sets of a physician. These tasks involve data-gathering, reviewing past medical history, EMR data entry, documenting the patient encounter, tracking, and reviewing lab and imaging results, writing prescriptions, and other routine patient management tasks.

The job of the physician working with PAs and NPs is to engage in the critical portions of the patient encounter, including diagnostic decision-making, management, and treatment planning. By offloading the perfunctory work, physicians gain leverage in productivity, at the same time providing that critically important contribution to quality of patient care. This is the direction we should be adopting regardless of whether the mid-level provider is a PA or an NP. Since the real deliverable of medicinal care is often time-critical, time-sensitive care, the MLP allows physicians to be more productive, more available, and more responsive with improved access of our patients to care. This results in improved quality of care, and from the patient's perspective, enhances the patient's experience and satisfaction with their care, and will probably decrease healthcare costs. MLPs work throughout the entirety of healthcare, from health promotion and disease prevention to diagnosis that prevents and limits disability [6].

Compensation for MLPs

Clearly, it is important to understand the productivity and workflow advantages generated through the employment of MLPs. The average range of a mid-level provider in 2023 is $103,000–$158,000 per year [7]. That's 25–35% of a physician's salary. The average productivity of an MLP in the office setting is 1.6 patients per hour, or about 80% of the productivity of a physician in the same environment. Adjusting the cost of an MLP for this variance in productivity generates at a minimum a 50% improvement in the cost of care for this lower acuity subset of patients. That's a significant improvement in financial margins. Theoretically, if we reinvest those margins, we could significantly increase the number of providers available to evaluate patients, thereby reducing wait times and improving both patient safety and patient satisfaction. This is where this workforce strategy begins to solve our demand management dilemma, balancing cost, and service.

MLPs in surgical and other medical subspecialties are paid 5–15% more than the NPs and PAs working in primary care practices [8]. Even so, salaries for MLPs are far lower than those of physicians. This suggests that mid-level providers may represent an option for increasing the capacity of physician specialty practices without significantly increasing payroll costs.

Some bean counters would argue with the ROI of MLPs by pointing to increased costs associated with their higher utilization of tests and labs. However, there is little data to support this argument. This does not mean that over-utilization of resources is not an issue for physicians and practices who decide to utilize MLPs. What is important is that oversight and appropriate supervision allow the physician to reduce this risk. The best advice is to have "rules of engagement" for the MLPs that flag both complicated patients requiring complex workups and/or monitor high-cost procedures, triggering physician engagement and oversight.

Outcomes and Liability of MLPs

Malpractice costs for mid-level providers are 10–20% of the cost of physicians' malpractice insurance. There is no evidence in the literature supporting increased litigation or larger malpractice claims related to independent MLPs in medical offices. In fact, the overall incidence of malpractice claims per provider is similar between mid-level providers and physicians. Payments for claims involving MLPs are lower than payments for claims against physicians. Also, the data suggest that patient outcomes for MLPs are comparable to those of physicians [9].

It is necessary in some states to have physician oversight. While many MLPs have their own schedules and see patients autonomously, it is important to remember that physician oversight is necessary. State regulations dictate what degree of physician oversight is needed for MLPs, so it is essential to be knowledgeable of these requirements.

Credentialing an MLP

Checking any medical professional's credentialing is essential, and MLPs are no different. Most states require that MLPs be certified to practice. State regulation requirements can vary considerably, so it is important to verify what your individual state's regulations require for licensing. National Certifications can be verified at

- American Academy of Nurse Practitioners National Certification Board
- National Commission on Certification of Physician Assistants (NCCPA)

Where Do MLPs Come from

Hospitals and medical practices can recruit mid-level providers directly from the medical schools and nursing schools or can identify candidates from their own staff and offer them the additional training they need to step into the role.

Several recruiting organizations locate MLPs for your practice. An example is iHireAdvanced Practitioners (https://www.ihireadvancedpractitioners.com/).

Do You Need an MLP?

Soon, the medical community will be expected to serve more patients because there will be fewer physicians. This reality will require a redesign in the way medical care is delivered, and MLPs will likely play a bigger role than they do today. Practices that are going to consider hiring an MLP should ask several questions:

- Does your practice have a backlog and an inability to accommodate new patients? If a practice can't see a new patient for 4–6 weeks, this may be ego-gratifying for the doctors, but this situation may result in patients seeking their healthcare elsewhere.

- Is the practice paying costly overtime to see patients at the end of the day?
- Are there signs of burnout among the physicians and the staff?
- Are there delays seeing patients for more than 20 min? (Twenty minutes is considered by patients as the upper limit of a reasonable wait time. Longer wait times to see the doctor result in deterioration in patient satisfaction and poor online reviews.)
- Where will your practice find MLPs to see an influx of new patients?
- Will MLPs be part of the solution to physician shortages in your practice?

- What strategies will you adopt to recruit and retain the MLPs you need?
- How will your organization compensate physicians for supervising mid-level providers?

The way your hospital or practice answers these questions will determine your need for an MLP.

Benefits of MLPs

Physician assistants have become increasingly popular over the last three decades, quickly becoming valued members in many medical hospitals and medical practices.

Patient satisfaction is one of the greatest benefits of MLPs. Patients frequently report high satisfaction levels when it comes to visiting with an MLP [9]. Many patients report that MLPs are more empathetic, and MLPs have more time for them during the visit when compared to physicians. These benefits of MLPs may be a result of taking more time per patient on health education and answering questions than other medical providers.

A significant advantage associated with hiring MLPs is that they can boost the practice's revenue. If you compare an MLP's salary versus their revenue, they can produce 3–4 times their salary for a practice, depending on the specialty. Hiring MLPs can also have the benefit of freeing up physician time. This free time allows physicians to be more focused on higher-grossing procedures and services.

Hiring an MLP can help expand your organization's services. For example, MLPs can be a part of a walk-in clinic, provide specialty procedures, or offer patient educational services. Their clinical flexibility also allows them to adapt to a variety of medical specialties without the need for additional certifications. Many MLPs moonlight in specialties that are different than their primary employment and provide care for pediatric, adult, and geriatric patients.

Hiring MLPs can help augment clinical coverage for overextended physicians on holiday, or if the physician is delayed in surgery or has a backlog of patients in the clinic. It is reassuring to know you will have backup coverage when you need it most.

There are reasons to consider expanding the roles of MLPs in both hospitals and physician practices. The timeframe for educating mid-level providers is much shorter than the timeframe for educating physicians, making it easier to increase their presence in the workplace quickly.

MLPs are cost-effective in primary care settings, where they can relieve physicians of providing routine care. This approach enriches the work experience for physicians and enhances patient retention. MLPs are cost-effective in specialty practice settings, allowing physicians to focus more attention on the complex issues that make the best use of their knowledge and experience.

Including MLPs on the clinical staff can enhance scheduling flexibility and make it easier to offer part-time jobs without compromising quality of care. This may help attract and retain physicians beyond normal retirement age and women physicians who may be reluctant to commit to full-time schedules.

As MLPs take on expanded roles like those of physicians, there will need to be incentive plans that become a standard component of pay. Like physicians, we expect mid-level providers to receive incentive awards for productivity, patient satisfaction, adherence to quality standards, and achievement of other organizational goals. The design of compensation programs for mid-level providers will also influence the design of programs for the physicians who supervise them.

MLP-Lite or Using a Scribe to Improve Efficiency and Productivity.

One of the challenges that is impacting nearly every physician is the need to improve the efficiency of our practices. In the past, we had the luxury of low patient volumes and fat, juicy profit margins. Today, it is the reverse: large patient volumes and razor-thin profit margins. As a result, to maintain our incomes, we are motivated to improve the efficiency of our practices.

A frequent complaint by physicians pertains to the increased amount of nonclinical administrative tasks they are asked to perform. Many physicians think that using an EMR distracts them from patient care. By utilizing scribes, physicians can concentrate on patient care and reduce the administrative burden. Employing scribes has also been shown to improve physician satisfaction and productivity, while decreasing burnout [10].

How Does the Scribe Work?

The scribe interacts with a new patient after the doctor introduces themselves to the patient. The scribe then takes the history of the present illness (HOPI), records the past medical history, and reviews the systems. The scribe then presents the HOPI to the physician and then accompanies the physician into the room. The physician may ask a few additional questions or probe any aspects of the HOPI that are not clear or require further clarification. The doctor conducts the physical exam, and the scribe records the positive findings in the chart or the EMR. At this juncture, the doctor can have a discussion with the patient regarding the diagnosis and the plan of management, and the scribe records the doctor's plan of action. The doctor can then answer any questions, and the scribe can give the chart or the computer to the nurse who will make the necessary arrangements for any lab tests, studies, or surgeries, provide the patient with sample medications and written instructions for the use of the medications, provide pertinent educational materials, and make the follow-up appointments. While the nurse is taking care of one patient, the scribe has moved to the next patient, staying one patient ahead of the physician.

The scribe improves the efficiency of the practice. You are now able to make eyeball-to-eyeball contact with the patient and focus on communicating with the patient instead of entering data into the EMR. Physicians can see 5–6 additional patients each full day in the office.

Scribes who aspire to be physicians can be found in the gap year between undergraduate school and medical school. The scribe does not need to have a medical background. You are looking for someone with people skills and the ability to communicate with patients sensitively and compassionately. The cost of a scribe is roughly $20–25/h [11]. Consider starting at the lower end and move up as they become trained and comfortable in the scribe position.

The disadvantages of having a scribe are cost, time to train the scribe, and the changing of habits from the physician writing in the chart or entering data into the computers to allowing someone else to do it for you. In the beginning, this can be frustrating, but when you see how efficient you become, you will enjoy the luxury of having a scribe. As a matter of fact, when the scribe is absent or on vacation and you have to use the computer, you will realize how invaluable they are and how effective the technique is to enhance your practice.

Getting Started Using a Scribe.

First, decide if you need a scribe. If patients need to wait more than 4–6 weeks to make an appointment for a routine visit, then you have a backlog of patients, and a scribe will help you reduce that backlog. Suppose your last patient is scheduled at 4 or 4:30 and you aren't finished with patients until 5:30 or 6:00 and your staff is working overtime. In that case, a scribe will help improve the efficiency of the practice. Finally, if you are considering a move to an EMR but are technophobic, then a scribe might be a natural segue to implementing the EMR.

The take-home message on scribes: few of us can increase reimbursements or make significant cuts in overhead without impacting quality of care and patient satisfaction. However, we all find ways to improve our efficiency and productivity. A scribe may be just what the doctor ordered.

The Economics of a Scribe

It is very easy to calculate the return on investment of a scribe. First, multiply the hours by the scribe's salary. For example, if the scribe's salary is $25/hr. And the scribe works 8 h, the cost of the scribe would be $200/day. Next, add the cost of benefits: insurance, parking, taxes, uniform, or about 25% of the salary. In this case, it would be $50, or $250/day.

Next, calculate the incremental increase in revenue by having a scribe.

This requires determining how many more patients the provider can see in each period with the help of a scribe. In most circumstances, the scribe makes it possible to see an additional 10 more established office patients a day and an additional 4 new patients/day. With an average reimbursement for an office follow-up patient of $150 and an average reimbursement of $250 for a new patient, the daily incremental revenue is $1500 for established patients plus $1000 for new patients, or a total of $2500/day. Subtract the cost of the scribe $250, and that is an ROI of $2250/day. This is perhaps the best investment you can make.

The economics of having a scribe is shown in Fig. 13.1. You can see that the breakeven for a scribe is an additional 1–2 patients a day. If the scribe can increase productivity beyond two patients a day, that added income will go right to the practice's bottom line.

The take-home message on using a scribe: There are advantages and disadvantages to the use of a scribe. Your adoption will depend on your comfort after weighing the pros and cons. There is no one right answer for everyone, and we encourage you to explore your options to maximize your practice efficiency.

Fig. 13.1 The economics of a scribe

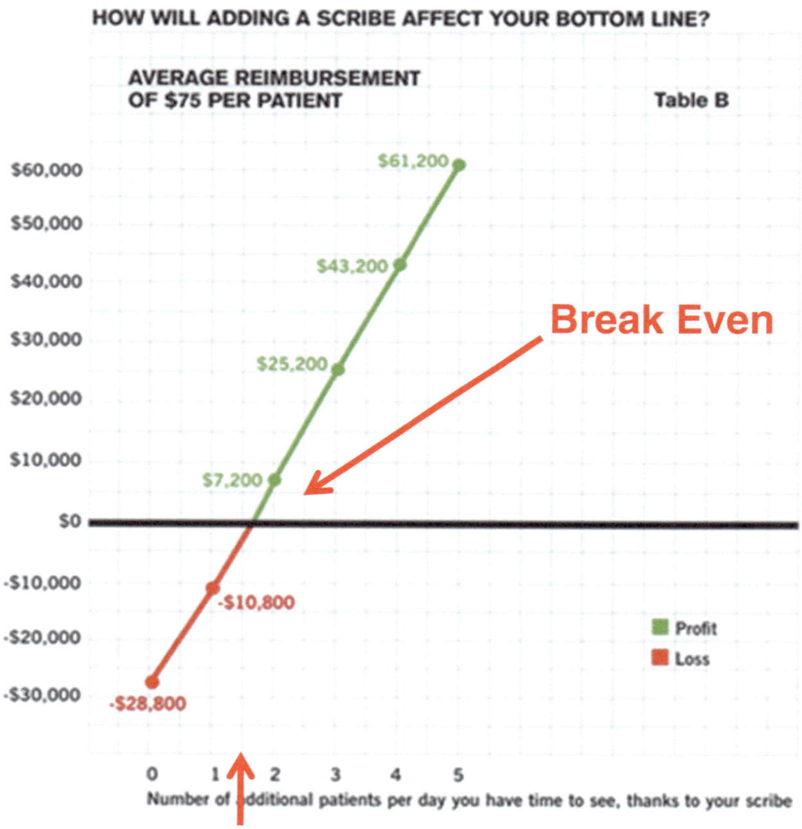

Case of Cassandra

Cassandra investigated bringing on an MLP. She ran the numbers and showed the office manager that it was in the economic interest of the practice to hire an MLP. She was able to show that she could see at least four additional patients each day and that any patients beyond the breakeven rate of two extra patients a day would make more money for the practice, increase access for patients in the practice, reduce overhead costs, put less stress on Cassandra and the staff, and would ultimately be a win-win-win for patients, staff, and Cassandra.

Bottom Line

Despite the issues and controversies surrounding the use of mid-level providers or scribes, this option is going to continue to grow. Hospitals and physician practices will need to change the way they deliver care as the healthcare environment continues to evolve. The aging of our population, looming shortages of physicians and nurses, and increasing access to health insurance all point to the need to care for more patients with fewer providers. Physician practices and hospitals will need to redesign work processes and introduce new technologies to increase efficiency, effectiveness, and employee satisfaction; retain employees and reduce employee turnover; and attract a new generation of employees, which will include MLPs.

Key Takeaways

- There's a significant shortage of primary care physicians, which is projected to worsen in the coming years, potentially affecting patient access to regular healthcare.
- Mid-level providers, such as nurse practitioners and physician assistants, can help fill the gap in primary care and improve patient outcomes.
- Implementing scribes in healthcare settings can enhance efficiency and productivity, allowing primary care providers to focus more on the patient rather than data entry into a computer.

References

1. Shepherd M. What proposed Medicaid cuts could mean for rural communities, hospital access. University of Michigan, School of Public Health. https://sph.umich.edu/news/2025posts/what-proposed-medicaid-cuts-could-mean-for-rural-communities-hospital-access.html#:~:text=Major%20cuts%20to%20Medicaid%20funding,these%20proposed%20changes%20could%20mean
2. Heimlich R. Baby boomers retire. Pew Research Center, December 29, 2010. https://www.pewresearch.org/short-reads/2010/12/29/baby-boomers-retire/#:~:text=By%20Russell%20Heimlich,Pew%20Research%20Center%20population%20projections
3. Physician Workforce Projections. 2022-2037. Data. HRSA.gov
4. Pande AH, et al. Effects of healthcare reforms on coverage, access, and disparities. Am J Prevent Med. 41(1):1–8.
5. O'Hare S. Mid-level providers in a changing healthcare workforce. Becker's Hosp Rev. 2010;
6. Institute of Medicine. The future of nursing: leading change, advancing health. Washington, DC: The National Academic Press; 2011.
7. How much do nurse practitioners make? Barton Associates, July 2023.
8. Top five factors impacting PA salaries. Comp Health, November 24, 2020.
9. Carranza AN, Munoz PJ, Nash AJ. Comparing quality of care in medical specialties between nurse practitioners and physicians. J Am Assoc Nurse Pract. 2020;33(3):184–93.
10. Henry TA. Scribes linked to 27% lower burnout rates in primary care. AMA. 2023; https://www.ama-assn.org/practice-management/physician-health/scribes-linked-27-lower-burnout-rate-primary-care#:~:text=Before%20being%20assigned%20a%20scribe,is%20going%20down%2C%E2%80%9D%20Dr
11. Medical Scribe salary in the United States. Salary.com. https://www.salary.com/research/salary/benchmark/medical-scribe-salary?utm=semsts?utm_source=google&utm_medium=Performance%20Max&utm_campaign=22209827665&gad_source=1&gad_campaignid=22738159154&gbraid=0AAAAABgNuZdC7cGPKjlCv3aPepoebOZPF&gclid=Cj0KCQjwqebEBhD9ARIsAFZMbfxzb8xtQLEUYUSE_zoMBY7DFRX_FvD79wXC8YTW_XXZPxDgtMRmI88aAvZeEALw_wcB

14 Team Building for Healthcare Practices

> **Case Study: Tania's Challenge on Team Building**
> *Tania is the office manager of a multispecialty group practice. She believes that there has been a decline in the morale of the doctors and staff. This situation has been compounded by physicians leaving the practice and several staff members requesting to work remotely following the COVID-19 pandemic. Tania monitors the online reputation of the doctors and has noted an increase in complaints from patients and referring physicians. She needs help rebuilding the staff's morale and improving the online reviews.*

Many medical practices and hospitals are experiencing openings that are going unfilled. As a result, this stresses the existing staff, which may impact patient care. This chapter offers practical suggestions to stem the exodus of skilled healthcare employees from the healthcare sector. This blog will cover the reasons employees are leaving the profession.

Approximately one in five healthcare workers has left the medical field since the pandemic began [1]. Employee turnover is one of the costliest challenges medical practices face today. It only threatens to become more problematic as the demand for care exceeds the available supply of healthcare workers. The cost of replacing a departing employee is approximately one year's salary. The obvious conclusion is that a hospital or practice that fails to prioritize employee retention will likely result in understaffing, financial instability, and a deterioration in patient care.

The Bureau of Labor Statistics estimates that the US healthcare sector has lost nearly 500,000 workers since February 2020. Eighteen percent of healthcare staff have quit since the pandemic began, while 12% have been laid off, according to survey research company Morning Consult. Of the remaining workers, 31% have thought about leaving their employer, according to Morning Consult [2].

In 2022, nearly 1.7 million people have quit their healthcare jobs—equivalent to almost 3% of the healthcare workforce each month, according to the U.S. Bureau of Labor Statistics [3].

It is not just nurses and allied health professionals leaving, but also physicians who have decided to leave their medical practices.

With the Great Resignation comes an increased workload on existing employees. Just imagine it is Monday morning, and a message has been left with the answering service stating that the receptionist and a medical assistant have called to say they will not be coming to work. Do you call a temp organization, and they send you someone who has never worked in a medical office and is unfamiliar with the scheduling process? Or will you try to make do with your exist-

N. Baum, M. J. Kahn, *Business Basics for your Healthcare Practice*,
https://doi.org/10.1007/978-3-032-25241-8_14

ing staff, which will undoubtedly disrupt your schedule? Do you call patients, reschedule several patients, and only see those deemed necessary and urgent? None of these options is desirable, and the situation is likely to cause stress on the existing staff. This could lead to problems with patient care. The best answer is to anticipate this situation if a suddenly absent employee(s) occur. Then cross-train your staff so that employees can work in multiple positions. By cross-training your team, you can maintain the full schedule without delays or disruptions. It is necessary to inform patients that there is a shortage of staff and that we appreciate their understanding of any delays that may occur.

All practices, especially small practices, benefit from cross-training. When staff members are prepared to work in multiple positions, physicians and managers can ensure that all employees have enough work to keep them busy while keeping staffing needs to a minimum.

Staffing shortages are not just a result of COVID. When there are not enough employees, it may mean that fewer workers will be required to care for more patients. Shortages and the additional workload may lead to burnout, personal illness, and costly turnover.

When there is not enough staff, sometimes mandatory overtime will be necessary for some employees. Working extra hours can affect sleep quality and performance, leading many employees to consider a different job.

The other major issue that impacts staff morale is burnout. Before the pandemic, between 35% and 54% of US nurses and physicians experienced one or more symptoms of burnout [4] (https://www.washingtonpost.com/health/2019/10/23/broken-health-care-system-is-causing-rampant-burnout-among-doctors-nurses/). Burnout has reached epidemic proportions, and more physicians, nurses, and healthcare employees are leaving the profession because burnout has resulted in mental and physical issues. A survey of 1000 healthcare professionals revealed that 28% had quit their jobs due to burnout [5].

The pandemic has created additional responsibilities and new workflows. The daily reality of potential virus exposure to doctors and staff has increased the stress and exhaustion already felt by many providers. Burnout, in turn, can lead to lower-quality care, medical errors, poor health outcomes, and patient dissatisfaction.

We are all aware that medicine can be a physically and emotionally demanding job. Often, there is a need for more staff to accommodate the number of patients, and the demand placed on providers has increased significantly in recent years. The patient volume and acuity of illnesses have increased, necessitating the need for more staff to meet that demand. Many healthcare staff are burnt out and leave the profession to regain their physical and mental health.

A few suggestions for enhancing morale and team building include the following.

Effective Staff Meetings

There are three types of staff meetings. There are formal or standard meetings that are scheduled monthly. Less formal meetings are held during lunch and may be sponsored by a pharmaceutical company or a vendor that calls on the practice. These meetings usually do not have an agenda. They provide an opportunity to have open discussions about the practice. The third type of staff meeting is very informal and usually lacks structure but is intended for staff to share issues that may affect patient care, as well as discuss nonmedical and nonclinical topics. Staff meetings can be scheduled more often if any problems or new programs are introduced into the practice.

When organizing staff meetings, keep the following points in mind:

1. Avoid meetings on Monday and Friday, as those days usually have added patients that must be worked into the schedule.
2. Meet in the morning when everyone is rested.
3. Limit the meeting to 30–40 min.
4. Avoid interruptions—turn off cell phones and have the answering service pick up calls.
5. Serve refreshments.
6. Have an agenda that is shared with the staff before the meeting starts.

Start Positive

Many positive events and circumstances happen to the staff. It is essential to share those positive comments with the team. At the beginning of a staff meeting, ask everyone to share a compliment or a positive event that has occurred since the last meeting. Such incidents might include

- Successfully dealing with a difficult patient.
- Getting new uniforms.
- An employee receives an accolade or award.

We suggest starting the meeting with these favorable comments, which create a positive atmosphere and help avoid the staff meeting from becoming a gripe session.

Another suggestion is to ask everyone to contribute one idea to improve the practice. Each suggestion is recorded in the meeting notes. Implemented ideas are rewarded verbally or monetarily, especially if the cost savings are significant. Remember to respect all the staff's suggestions. Failure to provide respect will stifle future creativity if you indicate that some ideas are ridiculous or useless. Creating a positive atmosphere is a prerequisite for generating ideas that will enhance the practice. Suppose your team is unhappy, not engaged, and feels negative about their work. In that case, your practice will not have the best results in patient care. A disgruntled staff also impacts patient satisfaction and your online reputation.

Stimulating Staff Involvement

Have you thought about how your patients feel and experience when interacting with your practice? Did you ever wonder what it feels like to grow old? What is it like when you have difficulty lifting your hand above your head? How does it feel when you're recovering from a heart attack? How embarrassing it is to wear a diaper? Looking through the lens of a patient can be very helpful in identifying the doctor–patient encounter from the patient's perspective.

Role-playing during a staff meeting is another technique for enhancing morale within the practice. For example, one staff member can assume the role of an angry patient calling to complain about a bill, while another staff member attempts to calm the patient and resolve their issue. The rest of the staff can critique the dialogue.

Another example is a senior citizen simulation designed for younger staff members to understand the limitations and challenges that older patients face when navigating a medical practice. The senior citizen simulation is accomplished in the following fashion:

A middle-aged team member is converted to a senior citizen by (1) making her hard of hearing by placing a cotton ball in each ear, (2) impairing her vision by giving her glasses that distort the reading material, and (3) making her arthritic by having her wear gloves and immobilizing one leg with a splint (see Fig. 14.1). Before the staff meeting, she is asked to go to the bank in the building, make a transaction, enter the office, sign in at the reception desk, take a seat, and review some of our patient education materials.

The team member then returns to the reality of a middle-aged woman. We started the staff meeting, and she explained that she had trouble reading materials at the bank and in our reception area. She also had difficulty getting into and out of the chairs in the reception area. She also had problems using the doorknobs to open doors in the restroom and the exam room. Finally, she had trouble hearing the receptionist in the office and the bank teller.

What did we learn? We learned that the font size, 12-point, on our print material in the reception area was too small. We knew that most of the chairs in our reception area and the exam rooms were not accessible to seniors. We learned that one of the staff members may need help with seniors'paperwork due to difficulty with fine motor skills, such as writing. We also added rubber door handle grips to assist seniors in opening doors (Fig. 14.2). Most of all, we increased the sensitivity of the entire staff to the unique concerns of older patients and how we might provide better care for them.

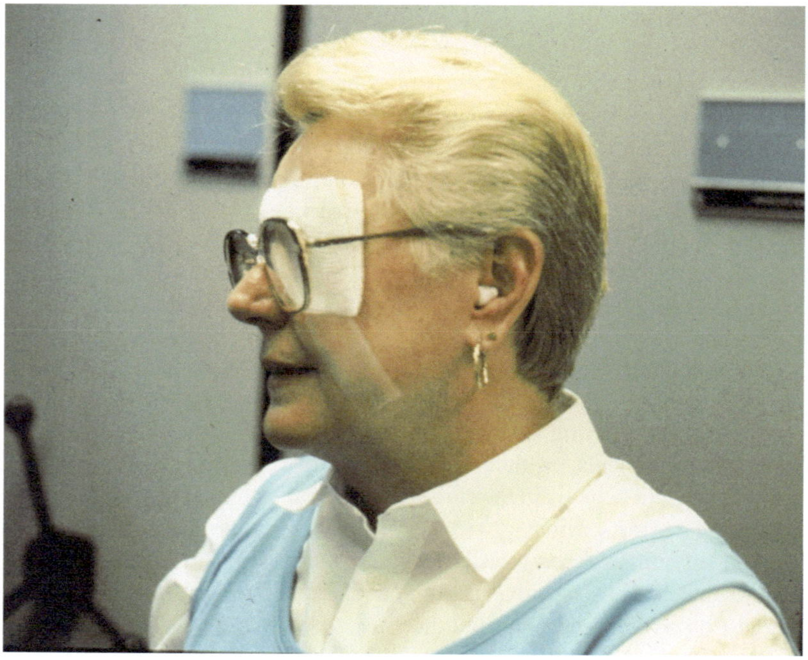

Fig. 14.1 Example of senior citizen simulation by using ear plugs and impairing her vision

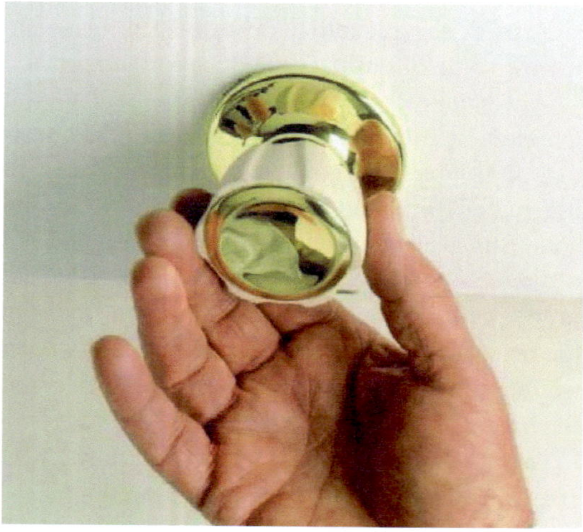

Fig. 14.2 Addition of rubber door handle covers

Create a "to-do" list for the next meeting. This list should be distributed to all the staff members, including those staff who could not attend the meeting. Every staff meeting should conclude with a summary of the accomplishments.

For a staff meeting to be effective, doctors and office managers must be good listeners and accept constructive criticism. Listening is one of the most challenging tasks for a doctor to perform during a staff meeting. If good ideas are suggested, implement them. Show your employees that the time spent participating in staff meetings is well spent.

The take-home message on staff meetings is the importance of making them fun, enjoyable, and positive. Adding a little sparkle can transform those meetings into a team-building experience that yields positive results for your practice.

The Morning Huddle

A huddle in football serves the purpose of the quarterback informing the rest of the team about the play and the role of each of the other 10 members of the offense. The same concept of the huddle can occur in your practice. This huddle takes place about 2–3 min each morning before we start seeing patients.

The doctor calls the staff together and tells everyone the game plan for the day. The morning huddle anticipates potential issues and problems that might occur during the day in the office.

The huddle can make your workflow go more smoothly. It is an opportunity to review the upcoming patients and schedule. You will identify space for work-ins, urgencies, and emergencies, or areas where you might fall behind due to slow or more challenging patients.

For example, the doctor can review the schedule and identify which patients require reports of blood work, pathology reports, or imaging studies, ensuring that the reports are available for discussion with the patients. If a patient has special needs, such as the requirement of a heater in the room, the huddle can serve as a reminder to have this available in the room before the patient is placed in the exam room. Every practice has some very important patients who require some extra time, and you want everyone on the staff to be aware that a VIP is on the schedule.

The morning huddle is used to motivate the staff to increase their commitment to ensuring that every patient has a positive experience with the practice. A comment in the huddle might be, "We have a great schedule today with wonderful patients. Let's make sure that we see them on time and give them a star-studded experience with our practice."

These meetings are held in the employee lounge, where there's a sign on the wall that says, "You are on stage. Now go out there and light up the room and give them a performance that will be like no other healthcare experience the patient has ever had."

Finally, another benefit of the morning huddle is that the meeting motivates the doctor to arrive just a few minutes *before* patients are placed in the exam rooms to start the day. Nothing can be more detrimental to a schedule than the doctor arriving more than 15 min late and trying to play catch-up, which is a game you almost always lose.

A huddle is an excellent method to get everyone on the same page before the day starts. It just might be the best 2–3 min you spend with your staff.

Practice Retreat [6]

The traditional in-person strategic retreat is making a comeback after being postponed during the 2020–2022 pandemic. The format is simple—the managing partner and/or practice manager hosts a strategic planning meeting for the physicians, typically off-site and often held over the weekend. The goal is for the team to return with a clear vision for the future and a renewed sense of teamwork among their fellow physicians.

Most medical practices manage problems like small wastebasket fires, which can be quickly extinguished with a fire extinguisher or resolved in the short term. Thus, the likelihood that the issue(s) persist is high.

Furthermore, staff and doctors are overwhelmed with additional, nonclinical tasks, such as excessive documentation and paperwork, which leads to a decrease in morale and increased burnout. When doctors/staff are continuously working in the "catch-up" mode, it is difficult or nearly impossible to create long-term goals or establish an action plan to achieve them.

It can be challenging to convince physicians to take a "time out" or give up their valuable time off to facilitate strategic retreats, despite many successful businesses touting the importance of such sessions. Therefore, the following outlines the benefits of these sessions in resetting priorities and creating a unified approach to growth, challenges, and opportunities.

Practice Retreat Goals and Objectives

A practice retreat addresses strategic or long-term issues and creates a roadmap toward future success. The intent is to free your doctors and administrative/executive staff from their day-to-day tasks, allowing them to consider the big picture rather than the minutiae and ongoing challenges of daily practice.

The four primary objectives for strategic planning retreats include.

1. **Increase engagement:** Invite practice leaders to contribute their ideas and make them feel like a part of the solution.
2. **Build camaraderie and teamwork**: Make time to build connections and create a more effective team, establishing further opportunities for practice leaders and retention.
3. **Develop a cohesive plan**: Create a roadmap for the future that highlights key opportunities for growth and development within the practice.
4. **Address issues**: Discuss ongoing challenges more thoughtfully than at a standard staff or board meeting.

To ensure participants see the benefit of these meetings, it is essential to ask them about their specific goals and expected outcomes for the retreat (potentially through a pre-retreat survey, as discussed below). Ideally, this feedback is received before or at the start of the retreat, allowing the session to address critical issues.

Retreat Preparation

Appropriate planning and preparation will ensure the retreat runs smoothly and yields greater results. Focus on identifying key themes or issues among stakeholders that can be addressed at the retreat and determining potential areas of contention or negativity to allow for an adequate response. We suggest distributing a survey before the retreat, creating an opportunity for attendee input, and establishing the foundation for retreat topics.

This survey can be a simple web-based form (there are many free and user-friendly options available online) (ref) that allows participants to share their opinions on potential topics while ensuring confidentiality and facilitating more effective data review. A few examples of questions applicable to physician groups include.

1. Do you feel the practice is moving in the right direction in this ever-changing healthcare environment?
2. What are the practice's three greatest strengths currently? What are its three most significant weaknesses?
3. What two actions should the group take to hold the physicians more accountable?
4. Communication is a two-way street. What two areas need the most improvement in communication?
5. Is there any area where you see the shareholders acting more from an individual perspective versus a group mindset?
6. What three objectives would you like to see accomplished from the upcoming retreat?

Additionally, this survey can be utilized for various administrative functions, such as determining attendance, gathering feedback on the food menu, assessing social interactions, or even selecting the location and date.

Additionally, we suggest sending a packet to all participants *before* the retreat, typically 1–2 weeks prior. This packet should include the initial goals and objectives of the retreat, specific topics for discussion, and clear expectations of the participants. This may include additional details on the retreat facilitator, an explicit agenda, and a summary of the pre-meeting survey results. Finally, the welcome package may also include recommended materials to read before the meeting (e.g., short articles on topics to be discussed during the retreat, intended to help establish a consistent baseline understanding among all attendees).

These items will set the tone of the retreat—an interactive, collaborative session with the expectation of physician involvement.

Practice Retreat Facilitation

A strategic planning retreat differs from an office meeting, with the latter used to enhance communication, solve minor problems, and address immediate crises (usually bonding over food provided by a pharmaceutical company). Alternatively, a retreat focuses on generating ideas, setting goals, and strengthening relationships.

The retreat should not consist of hours of PowerPoint presentations with talking heads, followed by brief discussions. That results in information flowing in one direction, leading to dissatisfaction with the outcomes and a lack of buy-in from the physicians. Instead, the retreat should aim to establish a clear vision for the future, supported by specific action items (as discussed further below), as identified and endorsed by the physicians.

While retreats often comprise most of a day, that is, 6–8 hours, it is important to remember that keeping participants engaged for an extended period is a challenge. Thus, facilitators should incorporate informal breaks throughout the day. Also, avoid using large-group didactic lecturing as the sole method of presentation/engagement. Utilize small group sessions to delve deeper into specific educational topics or develop singular initiatives. Give each small group a task-driven mission focused on outcomes, rather than just discussion, and assign them a time limit to complete their tasks. Ask them to report to the larger group at the end of the breakout session.

Organizations may also find that a role-play exercise is particularly effective during a retreat, truly engaging the audience and establishing a new way to solve problems. Participants are often more eager to challenge themselves in new and innovative ways in this atmosphere, rather than in a traditional discussion methodology.

Finally, we recommend that retreats include time for relaxation and socialization. For example, kick off the retreat with a group dinner and encourage participants to engage with peers they don't normally interact with as often in the office setting. This will further facilitate teamwork and more informal discussions before the retreat.

The retreat should yield a clear and shared vision for the future, with goals established for the practice over the coming months and years. Goals should be lofty yet achievable and quantifiable, encouraging physicians and staff to think creatively and drive meaningful change within the organization. For example, your goal is to improve the practice's profitability. In that case, the retreat should aim to establish specific goals, such as a 10% improvement within the first year and a 25% improvement within 2 years. Simply stating a goal of improved profitability will probably yield insignificant results. Still, a specific goal forces participants to come up with more creative ideas.

Practice Retreat Objectives

One of the most significant challenges of a retreat is maintaining the momentum. Therefore, before the retreat ends, the following should occur:

1. Goals should be clearly identified and prioritized (suggested topics for the retreat are shown in Table 14.1).
2. Each goal should receive a deadline and assigned check-in points to ensure progress throughout the year.

Individuals should be assigned to these goals, distributing the responsibility throughout the group, rather than simply assigning all tasks to the practice administrator.

If the retreat concludes without measurable items and deadlines, the goals are relegated to a wish list and will most likely not be realized.

Following the retreat, draft a written summary to document outcomes and agreements and foster accountability. That synopsis should include an overview of the retreat, a detailed listing of the conclusions and recommendations, and a list of action items as determined during the retreat (including specific timelines and assignments). The summary may be disseminated to physicians or relevant leaders who did not attend the retreat but are assigned specific responsibilities.

Once the retreat is over, participants should provide feedback on both the positive and negative aspects of the retreat, enabling the organization to identify areas for improvement for the following year. This is accomplished using a survey of all the attendees.

Table 14.1 A list of potential retreat topics

Provider recruitment and retention
Growth of the practice
Provider engagement and leadership
Operational and financial efficiency
Alignment opportunities and evaluation of potential strategic partners
Response to new payment models
Clinical quality initiatives
Implementation of AI

Several organizations specialize in medical retreats. We also recommend reading *The Ultimate Retreat Planning Guide* by Andy McClung [7].

Practice retreats help medical groups remain vibrant in today's changing healthcare industry. Even the most traditional and deeply rooted behaviors of large organizations can be innovated. Sometimes, a great strategy needs a bit of creativity, which can be fostered during an off-site retreat.

Tania, the Team Builder

Tania met with the doctors and expressed her concern about the loss of employees and the dismal online reviews. She made copies of comments from patients and shared them with the doctors. The most common complaints were that patients needed to be able to schedule appointments in a timely manner and that doctors seemed distracted, spending more time looking at their computers than at the patients. Tania arranged staff meetings to address these complaints and organized a practice retreat. These issues were presented to the physicians, and corrective action was taken. The practice now has nearly four-star ratings on multiple online review sites. Tania also organized a weekend retreat for the doctors and key staff members. As a result, everyone was on the same page. Patients were now complimenting the practice instead of complaining about the deterioration of care.

Bottom Line

Team-building efforts, such as dressing up for Halloween or doling out employee of the month certificates, will not be effective in creating a team-building atmosphere in today's healthcare environment. Finding time to set aside staff meetings and an office retreat can be time-consuming and effort intensive. However, clear communication with doctors and staff is essential for a successful practice where patient satisfaction is paramount, and online reputation must be addressed. Any loss of online review stars must be acknowledged and promptly addressed.

Key Takeaways

- Following the pandemic, there has been an increase in staff turnover and added stress on our existing employees.
- Regular staff meetings provide an opportunity for staff to communicate, address existing issues, and introduce new solutions to enhance the patient experience.
- A morning huddle is an effective way to start each day in the clinic.
- A practice retreat fosters a renewed sense of teamwork among fellow physicians.

References

1. Masson G. About 1 in 5 healthcare workers have left medicine since the pandemic started. Becker's Hospital, Review. 2021;
2. Yong E. The Atlantic, November 2021. Why healthcare workers are quitting in droves.
3. https://www.bls.gov/news.release/jolts.t04.htm#jolts_table4.f.2
4. Shah MK, Gandrakota N, Cimiotti JP, Ghose N, Moore M, Ali MK. Prevalence of and factors associated with nurse burnout in the US. JAMA Netw Open. 2021;4(2):e2036469.
5. Saha S, Saha SK, Jha A, Kumar S. Why do healthcare professionals quit their jobs? A bibliographic analysis. Int J Learn Intellect Cap. 2024;21(6):646–67.
6. Cowart T, Baum N. It's not obsolete to have a practice retreat. The Journal of Medical Practice Management: MPM. 2023;38(4):160–2.
7. McClung A. The ultimate retreat planning guide: a complete resource for anyone who wants to Plan Great Retreats & Camps with practical step by step instructions. Christian Camp Pro; 2016.

15 Effective and Ethical Marketing of Your Practice

Case Study: Sammy

Sammy joined a five-person orthopedic practice following residency. He holds an undergraduate degree in business, with extensive knowledge in computer science, having spent his younger years as an avid video game player and developer. The practice hired a high school student to convert the three-colored practice brochure into an electronic format. The student cut and pasted the document into the free WordPress.com *website builder in under an hour. Despite attempting to maintain a presence on social media, the site has remained inactive for over a year. What is Sammy's next action step regarding social media?*

Using Social Media

When Wayne Gretzky was asked about his great hockey skills, he said, "I skate to where the puck is going to be, not to where it has been." Suppose you ask a successful medical practice about where they place their marketing materials on social media. They will tell you they create and post where the patients and potential patients are hanging out, that is, on the Internet through social media. Practices need to be where the patients are. Having a presence on a social media site is like locating your office in a prime location with easy access to highways or mass transit. With a presence on Facebook, LinkedIn, and other sites, you create more opportunities for more people to learn about you and your medical practice.

Social media enables you and your practice to stay in touch with existing patients and provides a means to offer value to your current patients. You can reach potential patients with a social media presence, including your website. These potential patients can search for you on social media sites and review the recommendations of friends and family. You can also utilize social media to strengthen your professional relationships and partnerships by networking with colleagues and groups that focus on medical issues. Ultimately, social media enables you to enhance your professional stature.

By using social media, you generate more traffic to your website by providing links to it. You can expect that social media will increase your ranking in search engines, leading to more links and higher rankings in search engines such as Google. Also, your social media pages and the pages of people connected to you can all generate more traffic to your website and, ultimately, to your practice.

One of the best applications of social media is the opportunity for interaction with patients, such as answering questions, providing advice, and giving existing and potential patients a sense of what kind of physician you are. And it does not hurt to

N. Baum, M. J. Kahn, *Business Basics for your Healthcare Practice*,
https://doi.org/10.1007/978-3-032-25241-8_15

convey an appearance of being tech-savvy, especially if you are reaching out to a millennial audience. Finally, ratings from patients on social media sites can be an important way of supporting the all-important word-of-mouth that builds a medical practice. This is particularly important for young physicians who want to establish themselves in the community with a positive reputation.

Examples of Social Media and Ethical Marketing

LinkedIn

LinkedIn is considered the largest social media site devoted to the needs of educated professionals, including physicians. LinkedIn was launched in 2003 and now has over 1 billion members worldwide, spanning more than 200 countries [1]. More than 2 million companies, organizations, and practices have LinkedIn pages, and over one million LinkedIn Groups are dedicated to specific topics or professions [2].

LinkedIn is a great way to promote yourself and build a network, and it's particularly beneficial if you are searching for a job. However, LinkedIn is also used in other ways: to communicate and share insights with like-minded colleagues, conduct market research on new ideas, and foster collegial relationships.

It is easy to get started on LinkedIn: Set up your profile and invite other people in the LinkedIn network to connect with you (most often starting with people you know well). Dozens of medical practices have LinkedIn accounts. Prospective patients can search for you on LinkedIn, or they may seek you out because you share a mutual connection with another LinkedIn member. You can join a group of like-minded physicians on LinkedIn or form a group to share ideas and insights.

You can set up a free LinkedIn profile. The free version is a great way to get started. However, you then become an active LinkedIn user, regularly exchanging communications and links with other members and leading groups. In that case, consider one of the paid plans.

Because LinkedIn is designed for educated professionals, it is the social media site that most closely meets the needs of physicians. However, LinkedIn lacks the mass of users necessary to make it truly valuable as a form of patient outreach. For that, you need to look at Facebook.

Facebook

There are approximately 3.07 billion monthly active users on Facebook worldwide [3]. This makes it the largest global social media platform. Facebook is almost synonymous with social media. After gaining popularity among college students, Facebook entered the mainstream and is now the primary way many people stay connected with family and friends, sharing updates, posting photos, and arranging meetings.

With so many Facebook users spending hours on the platform every week, it was inevitable that medical practices would utilize Facebook to promote their products and services, provide customer support, test ideas, and keep patients and potential patients informed about their practice. Facebook accepts advertising, but more importantly, when a Facebook user declares that they "like" a product, they advertise that fact to all their friends and followers. For the medical profession, especially for new physicians who have traditionally relied primarily on word of mouth, Facebook can help build a practice.

Surveys have shown that well over half of all medical school graduates have a profile on Facebook. Organizations like the Mayo Clinic have given Facebook their approval. The American Medical Association and many medical specialty organizations all have Facebook pages.

Facebook offers numerous benefits to healthcare practitioners. A well-designed Facebook page becomes like another website. You can provide key information about your practice on Facebook, including your address, phone number, office hours, and services provided. The hundreds of millions of users and the hours they spend every month are a significant market potential for your practice. Many people now do their web searching on Facebook.

Posting new information on Facebook makes it easy to educate patients by providing engaging, accurate health information and advice. Additionally, there is potential for interactivity, including the ability to answer questions, schedule appointments, and refill prescriptions.

We caution against physicians "friending" their patients. The American Medical Association has taken a strong position, advising medical staff and medical students to reject any approaches by current and former patients to avoid the risk of blurring the boundaries of the doctor–patient relationship.

Due to these issues, the best approach to Facebook is to maintain a separate business or professional page from your personal page and closely monitor it. Another option is to look at a social media platform that offers more control, such as X.

X (Previously Twitter)

Every day, more than 500 million "tweets" (messages of up to 140 characters) are sent by more than 326 million active X users [4]. X was initially popular with politicians, celebrities, and sports figures who used it to stay in touch with their fans.

You can tweet messages about newsworthy issues and provide links to engaging content. Let people know of your involvement in events and activities, such as national meetings that you are attending. You can tweet about the new information presented. It is possible to tweet in real time while the meeting is taking place. What you do with X is limited only by your imagination.

Getting started is easy. Go to X.com and sign up. Choose a short, descriptive name and include a brief description of yourself under the "bio" section so people will know your background. Followers can differentiate you from marketing spammers. Registering as a "skin doctor," your X name becomes @skindoctor.

The best way to make the most of X is to first "follow" some people on the X platform. Numerous places provide lists of current X users, including lists of physicians. (Try twellow.com or twibes.com.) Additionally, once you start using Twitter, it can quickly become out of control. A free program like Tweetdeck or HootSuite helps organize your tweets.

Caveat: The same issues with patient privacy and the patient–doctor relationship that arise from Facebook also apply to X.

Blogging

A blog is an opportunity to share new content. There are easy-to-use blogging templates, and when you write your blog postings, you are not limited to a specific word count, as in the 140 characters of X.

The evolution of easy-to-use blogging software, such as WordPress, Movable Type, and Typepad, a popular blogging platform, makes it easy to create and manage content. It is estimated that over 164 million active public blogs exist today, with more than 1 million new posts added each day [5].

Blogs provide the opportunity to interact with your readers. When you write a blog, you encourage viewers to leave comments or to ask questions. A typical blog combines text, images, and links to other blogs, web pages, and social media platforms.

Of all the social media vehicles, blogs give you the greatest opportunity to establish your own voice and expertise. The ideal scenario is that your blog posts are perceived as valuable, so viewers share them with others, thereby promoting your practice. This also increases your rankings in search engines, attracting more patients, thereby making the investment of time worthwhile.

Getting Started

Before launching your social media presence, take a few minutes to read, listen to, and watch what others are writing and doing. Start by paying attention to what gets noticed by others (blog, posts, comments, and retweets) and what appeals to you, and identify your comfort zone. We recommend you participate in other people's conversations before starting your social media presence.

A social media caveat: take private conversations offline. Never mention a patient by name or allude to a patient in a way that could identify them in the content.

Utilizing social media tools incurs little to no cost. Allocating time to manage and stay current is your highest cost. Plan to allocate several hours a week to social media, including research and writing, to provide content for tweets, Facebook, and blogs.

You cannot maintain a social media presence by being absent on your social media sites. If you plan to be involved in social media, be prepared to contribute regularly. We recommend publishing content on your blog, Facebook page, or LinkedIn group at least once a week.

Keep the needs of your audience in mind. What do they want to know, and what do you want them to know about you and your practice? Remember, content is king. Your content must attract and hold the viewer. The word technophiles use is "sticky," and your goal is to attract and inform viewers, have them stick on your site, and eventually call your office for an appointment.

YouTube for Medical Practices

An excellent opportunity to showcase yourself and your practice is to create and share videos on YouTube. There are 2.7 billion viewers on YouTube each month. According to Google, people watched YouTube videos related to health conditions 110 billion times globally in 2024. And that number is increasing [6].

YouTube is a medium where people can upload and share their videos for free. Video is an increasingly important aspect of any Internet marketing campaign. Video attracts people to your website, engages them, and keeps them on your website longer.

Importance of Video

Video is a vital medium for showcasing your practice on the Internet. Along with your website, blog, and various forms of social media, your mission is to provide potential and existing patients with the best and most comprehensive information in a format that works best for them.

Just as people are inclined to understand and believe what they see on television, video on the Internet has the same effect. Allowing a potential patient to find a basic answer to a medical question, which will enable you to discuss it with them, is a compelling opportunity.

One of social media's primary goals is to appear on the first page of a Google search, and search engines tend to favor video content. At the time of writing this book, search engines are only able to catalog that a video exists on your website. Search engines can scan the audio of your video file for keywords. This will provide better search engine results for your videos. Adding your videos to YouTube will increase your visibility online.

Getting Started on YouTube

Smartphones, such as the iPhone, have a video camera that records high-definition videos. iPhones even feature the ability to upload directly to YouTube without saving the file to a computer.

We suggest purchasing a universal or flexible iPhone holder that contains a Bluetooth remote shutter. The cost is $10–20 (available from Amazon.com; https://www.amazon.com/flexible-phone-holder/s?k=flexible+phone+holder).

A few healthcare content ideas include

- Quick tips and patient-friendly advice.
- Showcasing physician and staff accomplishments.
- New technology used in the practice.
- Latest advances in diagnosis and treatments for conditions you treat.
- If possible, include patient testimonials.
- FAQs for common questions.
- Trends taking place in your areas of interest and expertise.
- Announcing events like speaking engagements, healthcare screenings.

Select a well-lit area of your home or office to create your videos. The microphone on your computer is usually of good quality for videos. Avoid any distractions or outside noise. Silence your office telephones and your mobile devices.

Editing a video is easy; most computers come with software to simplify the process. With your computer's software, you can add a title frame, text subtitle, and images.

Once your video is edited, you are ready to upload to YouTube by creating an account on www.YouTube.com.

Ensure your videos are accessible to the public. This way, they are cataloged by search engines and are viewable by prospective patients.

Aside from posting your videos on YouTube, to increase visibility for your patients and potential patients, consider including the videos on your website, in a blog post, or on Facebook.

We suggest that the video also be loaded onto your EMR to show patients while they are in the exam room, preparing for the doctor–patient encounter. Finally, we encourage your front office or receptionist to direct patients to your YouTube site to watch videos on various medical topics before their office visit.

Like anything in medicine, there is a learning curve, and you will find the first foray into video production will be time-consuming and may take several hours. After making just a few videos, you'll see how easy it is to create a 5–7-min video that can send new patients to your office.

Our take-home message: Trust, clarity, and connection are essential in the healthcare industry, making video a strategic imperative. Suppose your healthcare social media content strategy doesn't include video. In that case, you're missing out on brand visibility, patient engagement, and revenue growth.

Video Cornerstone of Today's Healthcare Social Strategy

Social media is more than just a marketing opportunity. It's a lever for growth, patient engagement, and reputation management.

If your practice isn't competing with trust-building video content across your social media channels, you're already behind. Why? Patients are researching care options, checking reviews, and watching videos before booking an appointment.

Position your brand as a trusted resource and engage patients interactively and compellingly through compelling healthcare content creation and video content for social media.

Using a Hook on Social Media to Attract and Hold Viewers' Attention

Just like a billboard on the highway, you have 3 s to grab your viewers' attention. Put your hook front and center to keep your viewer engaged. Examples of powerful hooks include

- A bold statement.
- An interesting statistic.
- An intriguing question.
- A visual that evokes emotion.

TikTok

TikTok is the fastest-growing social media platform ever created. It has created over a billion users in a matter of seconds. The concept is primarily embraced by users aged 16–29. TikTok reached over 2 billion downloads worldwide as of April 2021. Over 850 million unique users log in to the video platform every month. It currently has more than 30 million active users in the United States alone and was the most downloaded social media app in the first quarter of this year. All of this means it's something your practice should consider [7].

TikTok is a popular app that delivers engaging and unique special effects, enabling users to create short, attention-grabbing videos with the potential to go viral. It is a homemade application developed in China. This free app provides 15–20-s opportunities to build creative ultrashort videos for a broad audience of viewers.

The significant advantage of TikTok is that it provides an excellent opportunity to entertain your patients. The program is suitable for people aged 12 and older. This app enables every doctor to create engaging videos and gain instant publicity.

In addition to being free, one unique feature is that TikTok doesn't require specialized equipment. Everything can be accomplished with a mobile device with a video recorder.

For healthcare professionals, the primary purpose may be patient and community education. TikTok is available in over 75 languages. This video app offers a straightforward interface, featuring audio and video editing options for ease of use.

TikTok does not require any skill set or previous video experience. TikTok has the potential to make learning about health fun, so if a doctor comes up with a unique way of giving you a few facts in a few seconds, it sticks.

Currently, few medical practices and physicians have adopted TikTok as a social medium for communicating with existing and potential new patients. It's also an opportunity to attract and educate a younger population.

Doximity

Doximity is designed to connect colleagues and classmates on a HIPAA-secure platform.

It is estimated that 70% of US physicians are on Doximity, and that 90% of fourth-year med students are now members [8]. (https://press.doximity.com/articles/doximity-reaches-70-percent-of-all-us-doctors.)

Doctors and medical students can upload their CVs, listing their areas of interest and expertise, education, board certifications, and publications. Doximity also offers data on compensation trends in nearly every specialty and geographic location. The site also contains a job board and tools to earn and track CME credits. It includes a personalized medical news and research feed, and its collaboration with the University of Pittsburgh Medical Center allows physicians to earn Category 1 continuing medical education credits by reading medical journals.

The Doximity app is free and HIPAA-compliant. Users have unlimited access to pages and are allowed to sign, edit, and annotate documents, such as lab tests and imaging study results.

Instagram

Doctors and practices can use Instagram for publishing informative content to keep their followers updated; tell patient success stories; introduce new doctors and the medical staff; promote events, contributions and fundraising; answer frequently asked questions; publish procedural information; share news about events and visitors; welcome patients; educate patients on procedures and treatments; provide simple "how to" directions; participate in awareness day events; announce new products, services, new equipment and technology. This widely used platform helps practices generate conversations, and those who utilize Instagram in **their marketing** will have a competitive advantage.

QR Codes

QR codes, or quick response codes, offer a dynamic way to engage patients and direct them to your website and online content. They can be used to provide instant access to information, facilitate appointment scheduling, and enhance communication between patients and physicians.

QR codes can link to specific pages on a practice's website. QR codes link to videos, articles, FAQs, or educational guides related to particular health conditions, preventive measures, or treatment options.

QR codes enable patients to book or reschedule appointments directly from their smartphones.

For practices that engage patients through virtual platforms, QR codes can be used to link to telehealth platforms for remote consultations.

If a practice doesn't have access to a patient portal, in that case, the QR codes can offer secure and convenient access to patient records, provided the patient's permission is obtained.

This technology offers an option to gather feedback on patient experiences through surveys or by completing survey forms linked to QR codes.

Benefits of Using QR Codes

QR codes enable patients to access information and interact with their physicians and practices easily. This technology reduces paperwork and saves time for both patients and staff.

This technology is cost-effective, as printing costs are reduced and it eliminates the expensive costs associated with using traditional marketing materials, such as brochures and newsletters [9].

Sammy's Experience with Social Media

Sammy quickly recognized that he lacked the time, energy, or skills to develop a website and a social media presence. He contacted a marketing company that had extensive experience in medical websites and social media. He then divided the responsibility of creating content for the website and social media among two younger doctors in his practice. He committed to making one YouTube video a month.

Within a few months, his practice had risen to the top of Google's first page. More importantly, he received 2–3 calls or responses daily from the website and from online viewers requesting appointments.

Key Takeaways

The days of Dr. Marcus Welby have disappeared. Today's physicians have more in common with Mark Zuckerberg and Bill Gates than with the fictional character Marcus Welby. The advent of technology has differentiated the doctors of today from those of decades ago. We have grown comfortable with computers in diagnosing and treating diseases; now, we must become comfortable using computers and social media to help communicate with patients.

Every doctor's challenge is to see and care for an increasing number of patients within the same amount of time, educate them, and maintain the quality of care that patients are accustomed to, while also avoiding the ever-present threat of litigation. The Internet and social media offer solutions to some of the problems impacting physicians today.

There is good news. All the statistics suggest that the doctor–patient relationship is changing, and patients will likely receive a different kind of care than that offered by Dr. Welby. Doctors will have to embrace the digital age, which includes social media, and think creatively about communicating with patients, educating them, and teaching them wellness rather than just treating illness. Doctors will need to utilize new digital solutions to foster a complementary relationship between the doctor and the patient.

References

1. Behrend TS, Ravid DM, Thapa S. Implications of social media for a changing work landscape. Annu Rev Organ Psych Organ Behav. 2024;11(1):337–61.
2. Leo C, Halloran T, Valdez C, Martinou I, Connell L, Morin J. The LinkedIn effect: building personal brands, enhancing self-esteem and job search behaviors for the next generation. Mark Educ Rev. 2024;34(2):107–20.
3. Rishi B, Bandyopadhyay S. Social Media Marketing: Trends and challenges. In: Contemporary issues in social media marketing; 2025. p. 1–14. Gunter J. For better or maybe, worse, patients are judging your care online. 2011, Obg Management 23(3), 47–51.
4. Bastos MT. So long twitter, and thanks for all the tweets. Available at SSRN 5206365; 2025.
5. Kaye BK. It's a blog, blog, blog world: users and uses of weblogs. Atlantic J Commun. 2005;13(2):73–95.
6. Hollenbeck S. 35 YouTube stats to know in 2025. https://www.rev.com/blog/youtube-statistics.
7. Jia J. IT business model: case study of TikTok. J Mod Soc Sci. 2024;1(2):269–76.
8. Ventola CL. Social media and health care professionals: benefits. Risks, and Best Practices Pharmacy and Therapeutics. 2014;39(7):491–9. https://press.doximity.com/articles/doximity-reaches-70-percent-of-all-us-doctors
9. Joshi P, Sawant S. The impact and potential of quick response (QR) codes in healthcare: a comprehensive review. In: Proceedings of the human factors and ergonomics society annual meeting, vol. 68 (1). Los Angeles, CA: SAGE; 2024. p. 1153–8.

One-Page Marketing Plan 16

"A goal without a plan is just a wish."—Antoine de Saint-Exupéry

Case Study: Dr. Mendoza
Doctor Mendoza is the managing partner of a multispecialty group practice. The practice has a website cobbled together from its original tricolor, threefold brochure, created years ago. Doctor Mendoza recognizes the importance of medical marketing but is unsure how to proceed. He received several marketing proposals from marketing firms, but his next steps remain unclear.

Today, marketing in medical practices is ubiquitous. Who would've ever thought that renowned medical institutions such as Mayo Clinic, Cleveland Clinic, and Kaiser Permanente would embark on marketing strategies for their institutions? Marketing consists of attracting new patients to the practice, providing them with a stellar patient experience, and then implementing a system to keep them within the practice and turn them into raving fans. This can be accomplished with a one-page marketing plan.

Every profession, including healthcare, has a well-thought-out plan that is created, distributed to the staff, and followed meticulously. This is true in the airline industry, where pilots follow a flight plan, and in the military, where soldiers follow an operational plan. Marketing is not a subject taught in medical school, and most physicians and office managers are unfamiliar with marketing and practice promotions. We have seen many practices hire a marketing consultant who provides a comprehensive business plan, identifying the practice's needs and wants for marketing. Consultants prepare an expensive, multipage plan that is put on a shelf, never looked at, and more importantly, never implemented. The result is a waste of precious marketing dollars that doesn't work for the practice.

We suggest creating a one-page marketing plan that encourages action, and you are likely to see more patients enter the practice as a result.

The Circus and Marketing

Historically, physicians have believed that marketing is merely advertising and requires a significant financial outlay. Let's think of marketing as preparing for the circus coming to town. If the circus is coming to town and there is a sign saying, "Circus Coming to the Showground on Saturday," that is advertising. If the sign is on the back of an elephant that strolls into town, that's promotion. If the elephant walks through the

N. Baum, M. J. Kahn, *Business Basics for your Healthcare Practice*,
https://doi.org/10.1007/978-3-032-25241-8_16

town's flower bed in front of city hall and the newspaper writes a story about the debacle, that's publicity. However, if the mayor offers his observation of the elephant and laughs about the elephant, that's public relations. Now, if the town's citizens show up at the circus and buy a ticket to see the show, that's sales!

The one-page marketing plan consists of nine elements, which are divided into three phases. (Fig. 16.1, use Figure 32.1 from The Business of Building and Managing a Healthcare Practice, Baum, Kahn, Daigrepont, Springer, 2003.) There are three phases of every marketing plan: (1) identifying a target market and follow-up on any

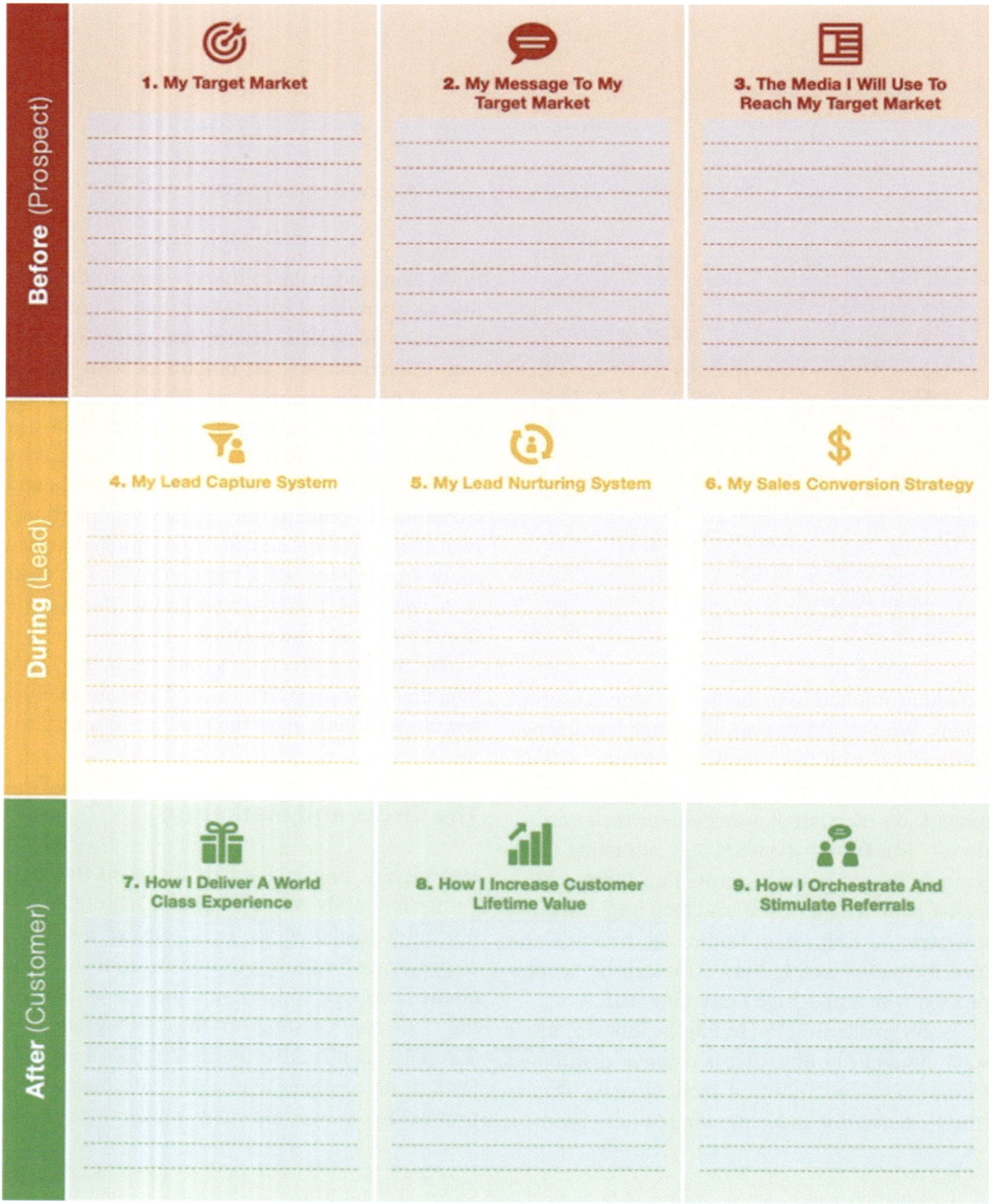
Before (Prospect)
1. My Target Market
2. My Message To My Target Market
3. The Media I Will Use To Reach My Target Market
During (Lead)
4. My Lead Capture System
5. My Lead Nurturing System
6. My Sales Conversion Strategy
After (Customer)
7. How I Deliver A World Class Experience
8. How I Increase Customer Lifetime Value
9. How I Orchestrate And Stimulate Referrals

Fig. 16.1 Three components of the 1-Page Marketing Plan

potential patients needing the services of the practice, (2) providing the patient with educational materials before they enter the practice and the patient is given an outstanding experience, and (3) after the patient leaves the practice they continue to return regularly, and, more importantly, become raving fans who tell others about the wonderful experience they had with the doctors and the practice.

Phase Number 1: Before the Patient Enters the Service Cycle.

It is at this stage that the future patient knows nothing about you or your practice. If you can raise awareness of your practice, you have accomplished the first and most important part of the patient cycle. This phase serves as a magnet or hook that entices the patient to provide information about themselves and encourages them to take advantage of phase 2, when they become part of your practice.

Phase Number 2: During this phase, the patient becomes a patient and has an experience with the practice. If that experience is positive, the patient is likely to remain in the practice and will segue to phase 3.

Phase Number 3: After you and your practice have participated in the patient's care and the patient has had a positive experience, you will want them to share that experience with others. The patient has interacted with your staff from the time they made the phone call to the practice until the moment you ended the doctor–patient relationship, when they paid their bill, left with educational materials, and had all their questions answered. Your marketing has promised access to the practice, timely follow-up, and the resolution of all the patient's questions at the time of the visit. Now the patient has a favorable relationship with the doctor and the staff and is very likely to refer others to the practice.

You will notice in Fig. 16.1 that each phase of the one-page marketing plan consists of three components. Let's look at the three components of the first phase with practical examples of each element that will hopefully lead not only to adding more patients to your practice but will also maintain the loyalty of those patients who are already in your practice.

First Component of the before Phase of the One-Page Marketing Plan

The goal of this component is to enable your patients to become familiar with you and your practice. When you create a message to prospective patients and have demonstrated even a modicum of interest, you must continue to connect with them to motivate them to enter the practice.

This usually begins by identifying your target market. Let's be very honest: it is nearly impossible, or unreasonable, to target everyone with what you do and how you do it so that everyone enters your practice. Phase 1 also means avoiding a mass-marketing or scatter-shot plan, such as TV, radio, or newspaper ads with bland comments about your outstanding services or about being the first in the area to offer such a service or treatment.

The "PVP" approach is used to identify your ideal patient. This consists of "personal" enjoyment, "value" to the marketplace, and "profitability."

Personal enjoyment is the pleasure you derive from providing care for a specific type of patient. For example, if you are a primary care doctor, do you enjoy helping patients achieve their ideal weight and support their diet, nutrition, and supplement use? If you are an orthopedic surgeon, you may be interested in sports medicine and helping weekend warriors overcome injuries common among middle-aged and older adults who engage in sports. Another example is the urologist who offers treatment for middle-aged men with difficulty with urination and erectile dysfunction.

The value to the marketplace is the benefit of your service to your target market. If your target market is women with problems achieving pregnancy, you can be sure that this is a very high value to the couple who are trying desperately to become pregnant.

Finally, you must determine the profitability of providing care and services for your target market. You want to avoid any target where the fees you charge are not worth the effort or the expense of your marketing programs. You want to avoid at all costs having a target market that is not profitable.

1. NAME____________________ D.O.B.______________________

2. TELEPHONE NUMBER (W)__________ (H)____________ FAX:_______________ EMAIL:_________________

3. ADDRESS (W)_____________________ (H)__________________________

4. EDUCATION:____

5. SPECIAL AREAS OF INTEREST:____________________________________

6. HOBBIES AND RECREATIONAL ACTIVITIES:_________________________

7. MARITAL STATUS:_________________ PARTNER:_____________________

8. CHILDREN:____

9. CONVERSATIONAL INTERESTS: ___________________________________

10. DINING PREFERENCES:____

11. ADDITIONAL NOTES:____

Fig. 16.2 Important information on referring physicians and other referral sources

Next, you want to learn as much as possible about your target market. Suppose you have a medical practice that relies on referrals from other physicians. In that case, you want to know as much as possible about how to target your marketing efforts to physicians.

A simple worksheet for the purpose of identifying the hot buttons of referring physicians is shown in Fig. 16.2. (Use Figure 32.2 shown below, but also in The Business of Building and Managing a Healthcare Practice, Baum, Kahn, Daigrepont, Springer, 2003.) This brief survey of your existing and potential referring physicians can provide valuable insights into their practices and personal lives.

Second Component of the Before Phase of the One-Page Marketing Plan

This second component consists of crafting your message. Most marketing messages are boring, like all other messages, and ineffective. Most medical marketing fails to address the needs and wants of the target market, instead offering platitudes that fail to attract patients. The practice logo and a laundry list of the diseases and conditions treated, along with the procedures performed, are ineffective. We refer to this as "me too" marketing, which is likely the same as all the other practices in the community. So why are you wasting your precious time and dollars?

We recommend that you develop a unique service proposition (USP). What is it that makes you different and special, and that distinguishes you from others who are also trying to attract the same kind of patients that you are reaching for?

Let's consider the example of water—one of the most abundant commodities on earth. In contrast to many areas of the world, in our country, most tap water is free and safe to drink. Yet millions of Americans pay $2.00–4.00 or more for a liter of bottled water, such as Evian, Fiji, or SmartWater. The price of bottled water is 20% more than the same volume of Budweiser beer, 40% more than the same volume of milk, and three times the cost of gasoline! Now that's the power of your USP: motivating people to pay more for water than what is available for free at the tap. What is your USP to become the Evian of healthcare?

Most of the choices we make—from the coffee shop we frequent for our jolt of java to the company that provides the medical supplies for our medical office—are based on having a USP. Doctors may not even be aware of it, because subliminal suggestions, social media, and word-of-mouth marketing can be as contagious as a multimillion-dollar advertising campaign.

A medical practice is a business and needs brand recognition. In fact, if a practice doesn't take the time to build a unique brand, patients will seek care elsewhere. They may form opinions of the doctors and the practice that may not align with what the doctors or the practice intended. Perhaps the practice has had the unfortunate situation of just one "negative online review" giving the practice a one-star rating, or the practice may have a label or reputation that can't be erased or prevented, such as long wait times, an unfriendly front desk, and can't get through by phone because of the phone tree, are some examples. As in other businesses, the most successful hospitals and practices usually have a strong USP that clearly differentiates them from competitors who provide similar services.

We recommend that you identify your USP and craft your message for your target market, emphasizing what makes your practice unique. The goal of your USP is to answer the question, "Why would a potential patient prefer to become a patient in your practice than a similar practice in the area?" It is a fact that most patients discover your USP after becoming part of your practice. We emphasize that your USP should be used to attract patients before they enter your practice.

Third Component of Phase 1: Reaching Potential Patients Using Social Media

John Wanamaker, a media mogul, once said, "Half the money I spend on advertising (practice promotion) is wasted; the trouble is I don't know which half." That comment was made over 100 years ago, when tracking of marketing efforts was in its infancy. Today, technology is readily available to track our marketing effectiveness quickly, inexpensively, and easily.

For the most part, this cannot be accomplished in-house, especially in small- to medium-sized practices that don't have a marketing expert on board. To determine the success of your marketing using the website and social media analytics, you will probably need to hire an expert who specializes in medical marketing and is familiar with your target market and the media that you use to reach that market, whether it is print advertising, direct mail, the Internet, or social media. To be successful in marketing and promoting your practice, you will want to achieve a return on your marketing expenditures.

An example of measuring the return on your marketing investment is assuming you use a direct mail campaign and send out 100 letters. The cost of printing and mailing your 100 letters to potential patients is $300. Your response to those 100 letters resulted in 10 potential patients, or a 10% response rate. Of the 10 who responded, only 2 requested an appointment, resulting in a 20% closure rate. Based on the calculation, you acquired two new patients at $300 each or $150 each from the marketing effort. If each new patient received medical services for $200, you made $50 per patient. Suppose you are in primary care and the patient stays with you for 10 or more years. In that case, the return on your investment will be substantial, especially if the patient has a positive experience and shares it with others about you and your practice.

The take-home message is more than just getting your name out or using word-of-mouth promotion; it's about focusing on getting potential patients to become actual patients in your practice.

The second phase of the one-page marketing plan involves understanding what happens when you receive leads from your marketing efforts. You will need to develop a system for follow-up and maintaining contact with potential new patients. In prehistoric times (probably during the Paleolithic age), a man (most likely a male member of the clan or tribe) woke up every morning, collected his primitive weapons, and headed out to hunt for food for his clan or family. On a successful day, he would return with a deer or antelope, and the family would be able to eat. However, I am sure there were days when he returned empty-handed, and the family might go hungry. There was pressure every single day to hunt successfully, as the clan's survival depended on it.

Compare the daily life of the hunter with that of the farmer, or with that of hunter-gatherers who became involved in agriculture. The farmer planted seeds, and the clan would wait weeks or months before the wheat, barley, or corn was ready for harvest. From planting to harvesting, the plot of land needed to be watered, weeds removed, and the crops tended to regularly.

What does the hunter-farmer story, which is perhaps the most significant single development in human history, have to do with one-page medical marketing? Our observation regarding practice marketing is that most physicians behave more like hunters rather than farmers. They take their trifold brochure, electronically convert the content, and then hire a high school student to paste it into a website template, declaring, "Our practice has a website." Another example is the practice hires a marketing firm that has little or no experience in medical marketing to create a logo and write a newsletter and add some meaningless slogan like "state-of-the-art technology" and then claiming to be a leader or expert in the area and send it out for a few months but without any follow-up to any potential patients who contact the practice for more information and are disappointed and state, "Marketing doesn't work." Merely "getting the word out" or "getting the practice name out there" will be futile and a waste of time and money.

Most medical practices are clueless about the purpose behind practice promotion and effective marketing. These practices and doctors believe that marketing primarily consists of getting the word out, getting recognized, or creating a buzz about the doctors or the practice. Suppose you ask doctors about the goal of their marketing. In that case, they will state that they are interested in attracting more patients and/or performing more procedures. This hunting approach is akin to flushing water down the toilet. Successful medical practices that truly understand practice promotion describe marketing as both retaining existing patients and attracting new patients who are interested in your area of expertise or specialty. This kind of marketing is a long-haul, farming approach, rather than the instant, hunting approach to practice promotion.

The successful practice identifies potential patients and enters them into a database, and then follows up with additional educational material regularly or provides useful products that are a constant reminder of the practice, so that when "the time is right" and the patient needs to avail themselves of your services, your practice will be remembered. They will call for an appointment and become members of your practice. Now, your practice is building value that will serve as a magnet to attract new patients and keep your existing patients within your practice.

Humanity made progress by moving from hunter-gatherers to farmers. However, farming did require regular care and attention to the crops. The same applies to your practice promotion and marketing efforts. You can't create just one newsletter, one blog post, or one social media post and have the phone ring off the hook. It requires frequent, consistent offerings so that when the time comes for a potential patient to need your services, your practice and your name will be easily recalled. You will have captured a new patient from your marketing efforts.

The next step in your one-page marketing plan is to create a database system for organized follow-up to any potential patients. For example, make a presentation to a lay audience and collect their names, addresses, and email addresses. You must have a process for connecting with everyone in your audience. The likelihood of giving a single talk to a church group or a service club is that a significant number of those in the audience will eventually become patients.

Let's apply some numbers to having a database system. For example, you have a monthly support group for a medical condition that is in your repertoire or in your strike zone of medical care. On average, 3% of those attending the program may be highly motivated and ready to schedule an appointment. An additional 7% are very amenable to becoming patients. Then there may be another 30% who are interested in your services but not at this time. Then there are 30% who are not at all interested. Finally, the reality is that 30% of attendees come to the meeting solely for the coffee and cookies and are never interested in becoming patients, even if you wouldn't charge them. Suppose you measure your marketing by the number of new patients who contact your practice immediately after the program, the 3%. In that case, you are missing out on the other 97%. You must be a farmer and continue to take care of your field, or of those who may eventually need your services. You need a system to continue reaching out to those you can identify as potential patients. Now, by increasing the number of participants from the 3% who are immediately interested to nearly 40%, you are multiplying the effectiveness of conducting a support group by 1233%. Now that's what we call a real return on your investment (ROI).

Therefore, it is essential to track your potential patients using a customer relationship management (CRM) system. You will want all your potential patient leads entered in your CRM. (Fig. 16.3 is a list of software programs for healthcare practices that offer CRM.)

Next comes nurturing your leads. Most medical practices have an attitude of "one and done."

Zendesk (Zendesk.com)

Salesforce (Salesforce.com)

Monday.com (Monday.com)

Scoro (Scoro.com)

Hubspot (Hubspot.com)

NetSuite (NetSuite.com)

Nutshell (Nutshell.com)

Qucikbase (Quickbase)

Freshworks (Freshworks)

Fig. 16.3 Customer Relationship Management systems

They write a blog, add an article to their website, or send out a newsletter. Nothing happens after one or two attempts, and the statistics on the success of nurturing your leads in all areas of marketing and practice promotion are that 50% of practices will give up after one contact with a potential patient; 65% give up after two, and 80% give up after three attempts [1].

With each interaction with the patient, you have an opportunity to create a negative impression, a neutral impression, or a mind-blowing, knock-your-socks-off impression. Most practices accept the negative or neutral impression. The successful practices employ a shock-and-awe approach, ensuring that whenever a patient needs the services they offer, they will be quickly remembered and make the call to become a patient at the practice.

A shock-and-awe approach is most effective when a physical package is mailed to the potential patient. This provides information or surprises so unique that the recipient cannot forget where they came from or who the sender was.

Examples of a shock-and-awe package include a book on a medical topic. This is even more meaningful if you have written the book. One of the authors (NHB) gives a program on impotence/erectile dysfunction. In that case, I distribute a sign-in sheet and inform the audience that if they sign the sheet with their name, home address, and email address, I will send them a copy of a book I have written on the topic. Of course, I could save on postage if I gave out copies to audience members right after the program; however, it is better to send the book a few days later. Almost every member of the audience provides this information to receive a copy of the book. This creates a shock-and-awe impact, and I have the names and contact information of potential patients.

Another "present" in the shock and awe package is a DVD or CD that introduces the doctors in the practice, a tour of the office, and testimonials from a few patients.

If you have articles that appeared in the local or national media, send copies to the patients, as this enhances your credibility. It's also effective to send papers or articles that you have written, which appeared in professional journals, which adds credibility to your expertise.

The least effective way to create shock-and-awe is to give out scratch pads, pens, magnetic refrigerator calendars, or mouse pads with the practice's name, contact information, and logo. These are typically given out by other practices, usually at the point of service, and your trinkets will not stand out among the "tchotchkes"* from other practices.

The best shock-and-awe packages include a handwritten or personalized note from the doctor, expressing interest in the potential patient and offering to be available to answer any questions.

In summary, a shock and awe package should (1) give potential patients a fantastic surprise that is valued by the recipient, (2) demonstrate your expertise in a particular medical area and that you are a trusted authority in your field, and (3) move the potential patient closer to picking up the phone and making a call to your office if they need your services. Our message is that a shock-and-awe package provides you with a competitive advantage. It's ethical, it's easy, and it's effective.

It is common for those not skilled at marketing to dip their toe in the water before fully immersing themselves in the river. They will often send out one or two practice newsletters but fail to attract new patients through their efforts, then cease all marketing endeavors. Our take-home message is that an attitude of "if you build it, they will come" may apply to baseball fields but not to marketing and practice promotion. A newsletter, like all others, is screaming "me too," and you may be left with competing on price, which is a losing marketing plan.

***Tchotchkes**: (pronounced *chahch-kê* or *chotch-kee*) This is a Yiddish word, derived from Slavic languages, meaning an inexpensive souvenir, trinket, or ornamental knickknack.

A true story about virtuoso violinist Joshua Bell highlights the importance of context.

Joshua Bell is one of the world's most renowned concert violinists. As an experiment sponsored by *The Washington Post*, Mr. Bell wore a baseball cap and sunglasses. He played for 45 minutes on a 300-year-old Stradivarius violin worth $3.5 million at a Washington, D.C., subway station during rush hour on January 12, 2007. Over a thousand people passed by Bell; however, only seven stopped to listen to him play, and only one person recognized him. Just a few nights before his performance in the subway station, he had played at the Kennedy Center, and the cost of each ticket was $100. He had a hat placed conspicuously to collect tips and received a grand total of $32. Here was a virtuoso who would receive $1000 per minute to play in front of a sold-out audience.

This is no surprise; the social context in which a behavior occurs affects how it is interpreted. The very same talented musician, playing the same music on the same violin, earns $32 an hour in one instance and $60,000 per hour in another. What made the dramatic difference? It was positioning.

If you are a professional musician and think of yourself as a subway performer, your audience/patients will pay you accordingly. On the other hand, if you position yourself as a professional concert performer, you attract a totally different customer, client, or patient and get paid accordingly. Our key takeaway is that the public will accept you at your own self-appraisal.

If you provide superior service, you can position yourself at a significantly higher level. You can charge a much higher price and attract a higher-quality patient. Don't try to compete on price, because there will always be someone who charges less than you do. Then you may be forced to reduce your price even further, and ultimately, the quality of your service will deteriorate.

Think in terms of providing value to your patients. Offer useful material that educates potential patients and enhances the trust that potential patients will have in you and your practice. It is essential to consider the pain points patients are experiencing and how you can provide solutions to address them. If you are a primary care physician focused on being an obesity expert who can help patients lose weight—and, more importantly, keep the weight off—then offer that information regularly to potential patients. If you are an orthopedic surgeon specializing in sports medicine, provide information on injuries incurred by weekend warriors and focus on the prevention of soft tissue injuries. If you are a urologist and your area of interest and expertise is erectile dysfunction, speak to your patients about nonmedical, nonsurgical solutions to this common problem impacting millions of middle-aged men.

The road to conversion is paved with expertise and education. You must see yourself as a virtuoso violin player playing on one of the world's finest violins. In this context, you are a creator of great value—a resource for good health—that will positively change the lives of patients who become part of your practice.

The third phase of the one-page marketing plan is creating raving fans who will promote your practice to others. If you define tribe, you will find that it is a group of people connected to one another by a leader who serves as the connector. Outstanding practices lead tribes of raving fans. If your practice has raving fans, you have patients who are special—they are promoters and cheerleaders for your practice. Your raving fans will amplify your marketing message and elevate your reputation beyond what you can do alone.

To create these raving fans, it is essential to consistently deliver exceptional services that continually impress your patients. Practices with raving fans strive to foster a lifelong relationship with their patients. These practices that attract raving fans will make it a slam dunk for them to interact with the doctors and the practice. These practices have a system in place that enables them to consistently deliver a stellar experience. It is essential to have a strategy for building a following of raving fans and to make every effort to take exceptional care of them. You must consider that each raving fan generates exponential results, because each patient doesn't generate revenue on their first visit; instead, it's the recurring revenue that comes from this patient serving as a magnifier, creating new business for your practice.

Delivering a World-Class Patient Experience

There's an advantage to being small, flexible, and able to make decisions quickly.

Large practices and groups are hindered by their bloated bureaucracy, which features layers and hierarchies of people who must approve every decision. Smaller practices have the advantage of being agile. They can respond to patients' needs and make decisions more quickly and efficiently than large organizations. More importantly, small practices can micromanage the doctor–patient relationship. As a result, the patient doesn't feel adrift among other patients, and the practice has an opportunity to offer a personal and customized interaction that is conducive to creating a raving fan.

The first step in creating a raving fan is to find out what your patient wants. It is imperative to think about not only what the patient wants, but also what the patient needs. For example, in an IVF practice, the woman wants to become pregnant and have a baby. Every woman who enters the practice wants that result. How can you give her what she wants, but if not, what she needs? It is necessary to understand both needs and wants. Needs and wants may overlap, but they are often distinct. Our challenge is to motivate patients to take the steps required to achieve the results they want and need. This is the topic of compliance, which can often be challenging to achieve. The take-home message is that we want our patients to achieve the results both the doctors and the patients want. The benefit of reaching this goal is that patients who achieve it will spread the word to others who are likely to become patients in your practice. We've found that the best way to encourage compliance is to divide the process into bite-sized chunks, making it less daunting.

In this era of technology, you can make healthcare more seamless. For example, make it easy for patients to make an online appointment. This is particularly important and attractive to Millennials. Another friction point is the process of paying for services. When this can be made easy and quick, your practice will be appealing to patients. Another way to reduce payment friction is to set prices for your services. There should be no secret about the cost of visits and procedures that you offer, and they should be readily available to patients. Receptionists should be able to quickly quote the cost of each service the patient is likely to encounter. These prices should also be posted on the website. As of 2021, the government will require hospitals to disclose the prices they negotiate with insurers [2]. The purpose of any new technology implemented in your practice should be to eliminate friction.

Increasing Patient Lifetime Value

First, it is essential to understand the lifetime value (LTV) of a patient to your practice. The LTV calculation is the average value of an appointment multiplied by the average number of appointments per year, multiplied by the average number of years a patient is likely to remain in your practice.

The calculation of the lifetime value = V × N × Y, where,

V = average value of appointment.
N = average number of appointments each year.
Y = average number of years they visit your practice.

For example, if you are a middle-aged otolaryngologist and your average patient is seen three times a year, with each visit worth approximately $150, and patients stay within your practice for 6 years. Then, the average lifetime value of your patients would be 3 × $150 × 6, or $2700.

A classic story is Russell Conwell's Acres of Diamonds (available online at https://www.google.com/books/edition/Acres_of_Diamonds/O44DAAAAYAAJ?hl=en&gbpv=1&printsec=frontcover). The story is about a farmer living between the Tigris and Euphrates rivers who wanted to find diamonds so badly that he sold his farm, left his family, and went off on a search that took him all over the world to search for diamonds. His search was futile and ultimately led to extreme poverty, including the loss of his family. The new owner of the farm discovered a mother lode of diamonds on the property he had purchased from the original owner.

The moral of this story is to dig first on your own property when seeking a treasure, or more succinctly, look first at what you already have. If you apply that to your marketing efforts, look at your existing patients and ensure they have a stellar experience before reaching out to new patients.

Numerous studies have shown that it is far easier to satisfy an existing patient than the time, money, and energy required to attract new ones. Those studies indicate that a person is 21 times more likely to buy from a business or practice they've already used compared to one they have never visited [3]. There can be plenty of productivity from your existing or past patients, and there are diamonds right in your own practice.

Nearly every practice has dozens and perhaps hundreds of patients who have fallen through the cracks and have missed appointments for follow-up examinations. In this pandemic era, there are large numbers of patients who have been fearful of coming to the doctor and have skipped follow-up appointments.

More than a third of adults report they've delayed or forgone healthcare either due to fear of COVID-19 infection or their physician offering limited services during the pandemic [4]. An even larger portion (40.7%) of respondents with one or more chronic conditions reported they've delayed or forgone care, while 56.3% of respondents with both a physical and a mental health condition have failed to follow up with their doctor [5].

Black adults were more likely (39.7%) to report forgoing or delaying care than Hispanic (35.5%) or White (34.3%) adults, and more likely to report forgoing or delaying multiple types of care, with 28.5% compared to 22.3% and 21.1%, respectively [5]. The most common types of medical care delayed or forgone were visits to a primary care physician or specialist (20.6%) and preventive health screenings or medical tests (15.5%) [6].

Respondents with one or more chronic health conditions, like hypertension, diabetes, respiratory illness, heart disease, cancer, kidney disease, and mental health disorders, made up the vast majority (76%) of those who have delayed or forgone healthcare [6].

Delaying and forgoing care isn't without its dangers, as 32.6% of respondents say that doing so has worsened one or more of their health conditions or limited their ability to work or do other daily activities, according to the report [6].

This would be a perfect time to institute telemedicine for those patients who have missed appointments (See Chap. 22 on telemedicine.) A primary care doctor likely has numerous patients who require follow-up cholesterol testing and blood pressure monitoring. A urologist has patients with low-grade bladder cancer who need follow-up office cystoscopies. Men who are using testosterone for hypoandrogenism require monitoring of the hemoglobin/hematocrit and PSA levels.

How can we keep these existing patients informed and within the practice? We suggest sending the patients reminders by email, SMS, or even snail mail. With modern technology, it is possible to send automatic reminders to patients who are likely to need follow-up appointments.

You can make your practice user-friendly by making it accessible. Inform existing patients that they can schedule same-day or next-day appointments. Another convenience is to offer early morning, late afternoon, evening, or weekend appointments. If you are delivering extra value that your competitors do not provide, your existing patients will continue to remain loyal members of your practice.

Consider developing a reactivation campaign. This involves reviewing your patient database to identify patients who need to return to the practice. You need to give them a strong reason to return to the practice. An example would be type 2 diabetic patients who need to monitor their blood glucose levels several times a day. We suggest using one of the small wearable devices that transmit glucose readings to their mobile phones.

When the electronic contact method fails, consider calling patients to ask why they haven't returned. Let the patient know you care about them and their health. Inform them that you want them to return to the practice and make it as convenient as possible for them to re-enter. Ideally, a reactivation should not be necessary. However, situations such as pandemics, hurricanes, floods, and other natural disasters will make it difficult for patients to return to the practice. However, a reactivation campaign can be your ace in the hole, significantly increasing the lifetime value of your existing patients.

The basics of conducting a reactivation campaign begin with looking at your patient database and retrieving the names of patients who haven't returned for follow-up. Next, create a compelling offer to entice them to return. In most healthcare practices, returning is beneficial for their health, and failure to return may lead to deterioration in their health and well-being. Finally, when they call to schedule a follow-up appointment, send them a note indicating that you look forward to seeing them.

It is essential to stay in touch with patients who haven't followed up. Let them know that you are concerned about them, that you're available, and you will find that they will handsomely reward you by reactivating you in the practice. On the other hand, if you don't reach out to them, then they will forget you, and their health may deteriorate.

Repetition will lead to repeat visits and patient loyalty. One contact is unlikely to remember both your name and your practice name for recall when patients may need your services. By sending patients regular reminders, newsletters, and emails, you become a familiar name, and they are more likely to call for an appointment when they need your services. Reaching out to patients in your database can be easily automated with current technology, allowing it to do the heavy lifting. This technology enables you to easily stay in touch and continue developing and maintaining relationships through your customer relationship management (CRM) system. Maintaining that connection can be as simple as a monthly postcard or text message.

Orchestrating and Stimulating Referrals

Several decades ago, the concept of marketing and spreading the word was relegated to "word of mouth," or what we call "hopeium," where the doctor and the practice "hope" that patients who have had a favorable experience will walk out of the practice and tell others about it. That's a "sit-

and-wait" approach to building and maintaining a practice. That approach may have worked a few decades ago, but it's passive. You may wait a very long time for it to yield results, while others take a more active approach, creating raving fans who do the marketing and practice promotion on your behalf.

The attitude of asking for referrals is often considered beneath us and akin to begging for business. It is possible to initiate the process by asking patients whom you have delivered outstanding care and have had a favorable result to share that experience with others, including their primary care doctor. However, you need to provide them with the tools they need to be your publicist.

For example, a patient returns for a follow-up semen analysis after a vasectomy, and he is sterile with the outcome he and his partner desired. A follow-up letter mentioning that you would appreciate it if they would share their experience with other men who need the procedure. You might include several packets that provide educational material on vasectomy and offer their friends a free consultation if they would consider having the male sterilization procedure. These satisfied patients will be able to inform others in a similar situation who need family planning. They will very likely share their vasectomy experience.

Remember, it is human nature to be drawn to people with similar interests, likes, and situations. Also, no man is looking to have a vasectomy. However, he is seeking a solution to a specific problem: having no more children. The practical approach is to identify the problem and offer a solution that addresses it.

This process acknowledges them and appeals to their ego, as nearly everyone likes being acknowledged. Rather than appearing to ask for a favor, consider offering something of value that they can share with their family and friends. This process is far more effective, taking an extra dose of "hopeium"!

Case of Dr. Mendoza

Dr. Mendoza developed a comprehensive marketing plan using this one-page format for his practice and found it beneficial.

Key Takeaways

The one-page marketing plan is not a sprint but a marathon. Outcomes and gratification are deferred, but it all begins with a plan of action. The one-page marketing plan is a practical approach to medical marketing that is well within the reach of every medical practice, regardless of size, location, and current level of marketing and practice promotion.

There's a popular Chinese proverb that says, "The best time to plant a tree was 20 years ago. The second-best time is now." This means that if you want success and growth tomorrow, the best time to act is now. So, consider starting to plant your one-page marketing page today!

References

1. Contrera J. Violinist bell to play metro again. The Washington Post; 2014.
2. Wheeler C, Taylor R. New year, new CMS price transparency rule for hospitals. Health Affairs; 2021. *Forefront*-healthaffairs.org
3. Gallo A. The value of keeping the right customers. Harv Bus Rev. 2014;29(10):304–9.
4. Czeisler MÉ. Delay or avoidance of medical care because of COVID-19–related concerns—United States, June 2020. MMWR. Morbidity and mortality weekly report. 2020;69:1250.
5. Claxton G, Damico A, Rae M, Young G, McDermott D, Whitmore H. Health benefits in 2020: premiums in employer-sponsored plans grow 4 percent; employers consider responses to pandemic: the annual Kaiser Family Foundation employer health benefits survey of the cost and coverage of US employer-sponsored health benefits. Health Aff. 2020;39(11):2018–28.
6. Gonzalez D, Zuckerman S, Kenney GM, Karpman M. Almost half of adults in families losing work during the pandemic avoided health care because of costs or COVID-19 concerns. Washington, DC: Urban Institute; 2020. p. 11.

17 Crisis Management

> **Case Study: Ben**
> Ben had been the dean at a southern medical school for 2 years when a Category 4 hurricane struck his city. The storm led to massive destruction of his city's infrastructure, and the resulting flooding damaged many of the facilities on his campus. Ben evacuated to a city 350 miles from home and was trying to plan for the future of his school. Unfortunately, the storm had disrupted major communication systems, including cell phone service and email. The easiest course of action might be to suspend his school for a semester, an idea favored by the president of his university. Still, Ben was concerned that this course of action might have dire consequences as faculty and students may choose to go elsewhere, costing the school a loss of tuition, grants, and clinical dollars. How should Ben proceed?

The first step in managing a crisis is to identify your leadership team. In his book, *Good to Great*, James Collins describes this process as "getting the right people on the bus." Identifying specific job descriptions for the leadership team at the beginning of a crisis is often less important because the right team will usually effectively solve problems. Recovery from a crisis is not achieved through the micromanagement of a single leader but through creating an empowered team that can make decisions, solve problems, and think outside of the box.

When Tulane University School of Medicine was recovering from the devastation of Hurricane Katrina, a group of leaders was assembled in Houston, Texas, to plan to reopen the medical school. The small group worked closely, and each was empowered to make decisions consistent with the overall goal of reopening the school. Although the dean had the final say on decisions, the success of the recovery was closely linked to teamwork and cooperation [1, 2].

Once your team is identified, the next step is quickly establishing a recovery plan with clear objectives. This involves setting a single thematic goal that is clear, concise, and consistent throughout the organization. The public, your employees, and your patients want to feel that the situation is controlled and managed adeptly.

Although crisis management is complex, raising the tendency to have multiple goals, a thematic goal should identify the single top priority. If everything is important, then nothing is important. In the Tulane example, the overriding goal was to get the school back in business.

A thematic goal requires a definable action and a time frame for results. The thematic goal should dictate the organization's steps during the recovery and the time frame in which milestones are expected to be reached. Suppose the thematic

N. Baum, M. J. Kahn, *Business Basics for your Healthcare Practice*,
https://doi.org/10.1007/978-3-032-25241-8_17

goal is to open a new clinic to recover market share by a particular date. In that case, the business strategy should center around this goal. The thematic goal becomes the defining rationale for strategic planning.

Any change in operation that is inconsistent with or irrelevant to the goal should be questioned and dismissed. In crises, management needs to be coordinated, iterative, and precise. Since time is of the essence, efficiency and agility are essential in the planning process.

A crisis requires quick action. After establishing a thematic goal, the team needs to set measurable objectives. Having measurable outcomes ensures accountability for all management decisions at all levels.

Establishing an effective and comprehensive communication plan is almost as important as selecting the crisis team and identifying a plan with goals. In any crisis, stakeholders must know that the leadership team has everyone's best interests. To properly communicate during a crisis, identify a spokesperson, preferably someone with training in communicating with the media, and communicate often. In medical practice, your stakeholders include your patients, your employees, the hospitals where you work, other referring physicians, your community, and the public. Think broadly. Are there other stakeholders who may feel left out if not directly contacted?

In 2017, Adidas sent an email to all finishers of the Boston Marathon stating, "you survived" [3]. This email was sent 4 years after three people were killed and several hundred injured by an explosion near the finish line. Adidas recognized its mistake and quickly apologized for its perceived lack of sensitivity. Their quick response and apology prevented a worse public relations disaster.

In the aftermath of Hurricane Katrina, leaders at Tulane University School of Medicine created a "war room" where the team would meet to discuss each objective (obtaining housing for the students, bringing faculty to Houston, providing financial resources for students in need) and where they were in the process of accomplishing this objective. Frequent communication kept the team on task and helped them feel accountable for the overall thematic goal of getting the school back into operation. During the time of crisis, frequent status updates are imperative.

Niccolò Machiavelli is credited with first saying, "Never let a good crisis go to waste." This sentiment has been echoed by Winston Churchill during post-World War II Europe and Rahm Emanuel when describing the 2008 financial crisis. Certainly, nothing is better at breaking down silos than a crisis. Silos are bad in business because they lead to distrust, conflicting goals, and turf wars where people on the same team can work against each other. Nearly every silo can be attributed to leaders who have not fostered interdependence between different units of an organization. The silver lining of a crisis is that it brings people together toward a common goal. When a country goes to war, a president's popularity typically increases due to a sense of loyalty. To break down silos, identify key objectives, gather consensus, and involve as many constituents as possible.

During a crisis, honesty is essential. Successful recovery depends on the ability of leaders to communicate recovery plans and to have people trust their decisions. Many of us remember, during the first Iraq war in 2003, Iraqi Information Minister Mohammed Saeed al-Sahaf, nicknamed "Baghdad Bob." He appeared on TV daily to predict an Iraqi victory and deny the American Baghdad invasion even when US tanks were seen on the screen behind him. Al-Sahaf did not waver from his story until Baghdad fell. American forces captured and interrogated him and ended up in Abu Dhabi, where he dropped into obscurity. The term "Baghdad Bob" is now used colloquially to refer to a leader who confidently attests to something everyone else sees as false.

If you are a leader in a time of crisis, lead by example. Be honest, show integrity, and take charge. The mayhem imparted by a crisis requires people to act quickly and follow through with plans. You need to be the first to volunteer and the last to go home. It is also important to show emotion and empathy when appropriate. No one wants a leader who appears detached from their organization. Some crises are emotion-driven by their very nature. For example, physician suicide is an unfortunate reality that confronts practices, medical staff, and medical schools. Suicide produces feelings of guilt, sadness, and anger among survivors. A good leader in this type of crisis does not appear detached but one who is warm, consoling, and emotionally involved in such a time of sorrow.

An example of not showing leadership and understanding occurred in May 2010 when the British Petroleum Deep Water Horizon rig exploded in the Gulf of Mexico, killing several roustabouts on the rig. During the crisis, the CEO of British Petroleum, Tony Hayward, opted to take time off to sail with his son instead of dealing with the Gulf of Mexico oil spill. This was an example of a leader "missing in action" just when his company, the families of the men who were killed, and those who were injured in the explosion needed to see a leader demonstrate ethical principles of responsibility, accountability, and humanistic care. The case of the BP oil spill in 2010 provides an important example for understanding how these principles are valued by public opinion in a crisis situation and how the communication actions by a corporation in this type of circumstance might have a long-term effect on the image of the organization.

This is a textbook example of how not to conduct a crisis management resolution. (By the way, Tony Hayward was relieved of his CEO position a few months later.)

Finally, with any crisis, plan for next time. What will you do the next time your competitor opens an office down the street from you? What will you do with the next market crash? The next product recall? The next drug shortage? In his book, *The Black Swan*, Nassim Taleb describes a black swan as an unpredictable event with significant impact. After the event, the facts are interpreted such that the event appears less random. The term "black swan" comes from the assumption that they represent a rare species mutation, yet they are reasonably common. The danger of black swans is that the human brain uses black swans to create the illusion that we know more than we actually know. The human brain is programmed to focus on specifics rather than generalities. For example, following 9/11, every airport has instituted a rigorous screening process assuming that airplanes as weapons would be used in future attacks on American soil. Unfortunately, the specific is not important. In fact, the next terrorist attack is probably less likely to be via a weaponized airplane than a mass poisoning of our water supply. Preventing such an attack was the goal of airport security and remains today. But we do not focus on generalities, such as making our world safer for everyone. Do not assume it to be a black swan when planning for the next crisis. In New Orleans, the next hurricane is not likely to be complicated by levee breaches. A narrow focus will not make the next crisis easier.

In healthcare, the next epidemic will not be AIDS, so to assume that efforts to reduce the spread of HIV will be effective for a future epidemic is foolhardy. Plan ahead with a general approach. This includes planning for personnel changes, financial stresses, and changes in hospital management through mergers and acquisitions. Do not plan for specifics such as planning for the subsequent merger with a for-profit or planning for a shortage of one particular medication.

The next crisis might be a cyberattack. Crowdsource indicates that in 2024, more than half of the world's cyber intrusions occurred in North America [4]. These intrusions can affect damage in under 4 min! Many of these attacks start out as "vishing," or voice phishing, a cyberattack where scammers use fraudulent phone calls to get employees to divulge sensitive information about the company including log-in credentials, banking information, or even protected health information. In fact, healthcare cyberattacks are on the rise. Because of the sensitive nature of health information, it is not uncommon for a bad actor to enter into a system like an electronic health record, corrupt it, and demand a ransom to return the data to its original form. There were nearly 500 such ransomware attacks affecting healthcare enterprises in 2024. Such ransomware attacks are not only financially costly, but also are a potential threat to life. Many of the bad actors are from oversees, especially from hostile nations.

The best way to deal with an attack on cybersecurity is to prevent it in the first place. Simple methods such as requiring multifactor security to enter systems, and to restrict information to those most in need can go a long way to preventing a successful cyberattack. Training employees on cyber security practices and performing periodic risk assessments are key. Installing firewalls and compartmentalizing data can limit exposure in the case of a successful attack. Finally, using an effective data encryption program can limit the ability of others to intrude into your systems. Finally, many companies offer insurance for cyber damage. Although costly, these should be considered to mitigate financial loss due to interruption of a medical or hospital practice.

Back to Ben and the Hurricane

Ben decided that he would not suspend school operations for the semester. Realizing that his city would not be ready for a medical school for at least 6 months to 12 months, Ben moved the medical school to a city 350 miles away. Ben gathered a management team, including his associate deans, key chains, key faculty, and key students. His management team communicated with students, faculty, and staff, assembled a curriculum, organized housing, and created an alliance with other medical schools in the new location to train clinical students and residents. The school remained in the new city for the entire academic year and even recruited a new medical school class from their new location.

Key Takeaways

- Crises happen and, by their very nature, are unexpected.
- Crisis management involves deliberative steps, including identifying your leadership team, articulating a recovery plan, communicating effectively and often, breaking down silos, being honest, leading by example, and planning ahead for the next crisis.
- In planning ahead, do not be deceived by black swans; the next crisis will never be identical to the last one.

References

1. Kahn MJ, Sachs BP. Crises and turnaround management: lessons learned from recovery of New Orleans and Tulane University following hurricane Katrina. Rambam Maimonides Med J. 2018;9(4):e0031.
2. Krane NK, Kahn MJ, Markert RJ, Whelton PK, et al. Surviving hurricane Katrina; reconstructing the educational enterprise of Tulane University School of Medicine. Acad Med. 2007;82(8):757–62.
3. Calfas J. Adidas apologizes after sending "You survived" email to Boston Marathon finishers. Time, Inc. April 18, 2017. https://time.com/4745066/adidas-boston-marathon-email/
4. Crowdstrike 2025 Global Threat Report. https://go.crowdstrike.com/2025-global-threat-report-thank-you.html

18 Managing Burnout

Case Study: Lancelot
Lancelot is the youngest member of a five-person neurologic practice. One of the senior members, Arthur, appears to be detached from the practice and his patients. Arthur is consistently late to start his clinic and has been delinquent in completing his medical records, leading to payment delays that are adversely affecting the practice. Arthur is receiving negative comments on his lack of compassion and caring on online review sites. Arthur was recently involved in a lawsuit involving a patient who contends that he missed the diagnosis of a brain tumor. Lancelot worries that Arthur may be depressed. What is Lancelot, the young doctor in the practice, to do?

Physician burnout is reaching epidemic proportions. That is the bad news. The good news is that burnout is easily recognized, and there are effective solutions to this common problem.

Most articles report a prevalence of burnout among physicians of approximately 50%. As a result of physician burnout, our profession is witnessing a trend of young doctors choosing alternative career pathways in technology, consulting, and healthcare policy rather than pursuing a career in clinical medicine. Also, we are seeing a rise in online communities of dissatisfied and disaffected doctors looking to change careers and even form their own "club." The Drop Out Club and Physicians Nonclinical Career Hunters (www.docjobs.com and www.nonclinicaldoctors.com) are two such examples [1].

Additionally, burnout is more common among physicians than among other US workers and other nonmedical professionals [1]. We have a crisis on our hands as physicians are becoming disillusioned, depressed, and because of burnout, our profession has a very high rate of suicide. The burnout rate is emblematic of the problems facing our profession. We want to emphasize that burnout isn't just affecting older or near-retiring physicians. More than 50% of medical students, residents, fellows, and early-career physicians are already experiencing burnout [2].

Definition of Burnout

Burnout is characterized by a state of emotional, mental, and physical exhaustion caused by excessive and prolonged stress. Although burnout can occur in any profession and any field of work, it occurs most frequently among people in the caring professions of medicine, nursing, social work, counseling, and teaching.

N. Baum, M. J. Kahn, *Business Basics for your Healthcare Practice*,
https://doi.org/10.1007/978-3-032-25241-8_18

Causes of Burnout

Physician burnout is most often attributed to external factors such as workload, loss of autonomy, increased paperwork, and navigating the electronic medical record. For the most part, physicians can manage difficult situations, especially in the clinical arena. However, external factors perceived as beyond a physician's control increase the stress physicians regularly face [3]. In the not-too-distant past, it was common in medical education to emphasize the concept of high touch with physicians in training. Many entered medicine to spend time talking with and providing counsel to patients. Today, the concept of high touch has been replaced by high tech. Young physicians today are being micromanaged by many external forces, leading them to feel a loss of control and less valued.

Autonomy is the basic ability of physicians to exercise their judgment about how to allocate their time, attention, and resources. In the past, doctors were in control of many decisions, including when to see each patient, how much time to spend with each patient, what questions to ask patients, when to see the patient next, what kinds of tests to perform, what medications to prescribe, and what types of treatments to recommend, without asking for permission or obtaining authorization. Today, control and autonomy no longer exist. The current methods of medical reimbursement and technological advances are constantly mandating that physicians spend less time with each patient, more time looking at a computer than at the patient, more time complying with voluminous regulations and compliance guidelines, and large amounts of information to process on behalf of our patients. Doctors become discouraged when caring for patients requires focusing on the monitor rather than on the actual patient. Most physicians complain of the tsunami of electronic paperwork. Filling out paperwork is not the reason anyone decided to become a doctor. Most physicians remain altruistic and have a mission to treat patients and change the world—not to check boxes on paper or an electronic record. We often hear doctors say they feel they are treating a computer, not a patient.

Young physicians experience sticker shock when their training teaches them to focus on the patient. Then there is a transition to the real world of private practice, which requires an adjustment to a new environment and the learning of the facts of business life, including rules from government, insurance companies, and hospitals that limit the time physicians can spend with patients. Those rules also require that the patient's visit comply with the Health Information Portability and Accountability Act (HIPAA).

If we had to select one significant cause of burnout today, it would be the electronic health record (EHR). Physicians who had to transition from paper charts to electronic records often describe the computer shackles or handcuffs and that every "additional click of the mouse inflicts a nick on physicians' morale" [4].

For many physicians, the EHR has become the final straw. Although intended to overcome the flaws inherent in a paper-based system, the EHR has produced its own set of problems; the most significant impact is a loss of eye contact with the patient. An article in JAMA tells it all [5]. It is a drawing made by a pediatric patient of her experience with her doctor. In this narrative medical essay, a primary care physician describes a drawing by a 7-year-old patient who is sitting on an examination table with her mother cradling her baby sister, with the physician's back to the patient and her mother as he enters data in the computer as an example of a system that is sacrificing human contact for electronics. This drawing shows that the patient recognizes the doctor is paying more attention to the computer than to her or her mother.

Another complaint of young doctors is the time required to complete the electronic record, long after the encounter with the patient is over. One study involved ambulatory care in four specialties (family medicine, internal medicine, cardiology, and orthopedics) in four states (Illinois, New Hampshire, Virginia, and Washington). For every hour the physicians spent facing their patients, they spent nearly two additional hours facing the computer, entering data. They also spent 1–2 h working at home each night to keep up with their paperwork [6].

What a sad commentary on our profession, which prides itself on high touch in addition to high tech, at the cost of losing interaction with our greatest commodity: our patients. The electronic record requires the doctor to be a government data collector and to focus on processes of care rather than outcomes. This is compounded by the fact that most electronic medical records are built primarily for billing, not for patient care. It is not surprising that the technology intended to improve healthcare—the EHR—is causing burnout and is among the most common reasons doctors decide to leave the practice of medicine.

Symptoms of Burnout

Burnout is reasonably easy to recognize. Usually, it is not possible to see it in yourself, but others can easily identify doctors who are experiencing burnout, which can lead them to help.

In the early stages of burnout, doctors appear anxious, worried, and sad. Uncontrolled anxiety may become so severe that it interferes with the doctor's ability to work productively and may cause problems in their personal life.

Partners and colleagues of the burned-out doctor may notice irritability between the doctor and staff, and between the doctor and their patients. The burned-out doctor has a short fuse, and unexplained outbursts may occur. If anger reaches the point where it turns to thoughts or acts of violence toward family or coworkers, then this is a sign that professional help is needed.

Burned-out doctors will often complain of chronic fatigue. They may note a lack of energy and feel tired and lethargic on most days. If burnout goes untreated, the doctor may feel a sense of fear and anxiety and be unable to function in the office or hospital setting.

Another symptom of burnout is insomnia. The doctor often reports trouble falling and staying asleep. As a result, the doctor is exhausted upon awakening in the morning.

The burned-out doctor will complain of difficulty concentrating and forgetfulness. It is common for those doctors who are experiencing burnout to forget to attend meetings, to be chronically late for clinic, to have marked delays reporting for surgery, and to miss significant events in their personal lives.

When burnout is untreated, doctors may experience physical symptoms such as chest pain, palpitations, shortness of breath, vague abdominal pain, and headaches. These are often confused with medical illness.

Even in its earliest stages, burnout is often accompanied by a loss of appetite. As a result, unexplained weight loss occurs.

In the early stages, the burned-out doctor may feel mildly sad, occasionally hopeless, and may experience feelings of guilt and worthlessness. In later stages, the doctor may experience frank depression and hopelessness, which puts those who suffer from depression at risk for suicide. The depressed doctor needs to obtain professional help as soon as possible.

The colleagues and partners of a burned-out doctor will notice a decline in the doctor's productivity. The burned-out doctor is not able to complete projects on time. Burned-out doctors are those with incomplete medical records in the office and at the hospital. The burned-out doctor does not complete charge sheets, resulting in delays in receiving compensation. The doctor will have a litany of excuses but never seems to "climb out from under the pile" of work or responsibilities.

Solutions for Burnout

Patrick Lencioni's book, *The Three Signs of a Miserable Job* [7], discusses job satisfaction from a management perspective. Lencioni identifies three characteristics that make a job untenable: anonymity, irrelevance, and a term he coined, "immeasurement." Anonymity among employees leads to feelings of frustration and isolation. Irrelevance leads to a loss of sense of meaning with work. Immeasurement, defined as the lack of accountability standards and metrics, leads to a lack of clarity about how one is doing their job and a lack of fulfillment. All three of these—anonymity, irrelevance, and immeasurement—lead directly to physician burnout.

When seeking solutions to physician burnout, each of the three signs of a miserable job must be addressed. To protect anonymity, we suggest joining organized medicine (see Chap. 6). This can be done on the local, regional, or national level. We recommend starting by joining hospital committees. Become the "go-to" person for questions of quality, credentialing, or pharmaceutical approval. At the regional or national level, get involved with your specialty or sub-specialty societies. Develop a reputation. Develop specific expertise.

Become relevant. Create a situation where you have decision-making capacity, either as part of a committee that writes guidelines for medical conditions at your hospital, or as someone who helps decide strategy by allocating funds for projects. Many hospitals and healthcare systems now employ a Chief Wellness Officer. Perhaps aspiring to be this person or at least to be on a wellness team can increase your sense of value. Teaching medical students, residents, fellows, or mid-level providers can provide a sense of job satisfaction and can help you keep up to date with your specialty. Additionally, psychosocial theorists suggest that we all seek to gain mastery over internal and external forces to establish a sense of wellness. Teaching allows us to feel competent, confirming our sense of worth.

Finally, insist on measurement. Ask your supervisor or your group, "What is expected of me in the upcoming year?" Develop a 1-, 5-, and 10-year plan with milestones and keep yourself on schedule. Demand feedback. Work on improving those things in which you are deficient and work on being even better at those things you do well.

As for other solutions to the burnout crisis, investigators have recently found that exposure to the arts and humanities is associated with decreased burnout among medical students.8 The authors of this study speculate that the humanities stimulate part of the brain that is associated with pleasure, which in turn improves the quality of life. Interestingly, in this study, there was no difference between active participation in the arts (playing an instrument, writing a play, painting a picture) and passive participation (listening to music, going to see a play, going to an art museum). We do not suggest that the entire problem of physician burnout can be solved with a single rock concert, but personal wellness is undoubtedly part of the solution.

Finally, create safe places for physicians to talk. Like a battlefield, the hospital workplace can be demoralizing and difficult to control. Feeling part of a team or connected can relieve feelings of isolation and talking with others experiencing the same problems can provide support. Narratives are powerful communication tools, and people typically feel good about talking about themselves. Sometimes talking about an operational inefficiency can give a sense of control, even when control is not present.

Of course, the best solutions to physician burnout are to create systems, including the process of entering data into the electronic health record, that are efficient in terms of time and effort. Limiting work hours, providing time off, and promoting work–life balance are also important strategies. Sharing decision-making among hospital leaders and physicians also helps to create a sense of control. The burnout issue among physicians is complex, and there is no one-size-fits-all solution. Addressing physician burnout is a priority for all of us—physicians, hospitals, and health systems—to provide the best care for our patients.

Back to the Case: Lancelot

It was clear to Lancelot that he was dealing with a burned-out doctor. Since Lancelot was the youngest doctor in the practice, he was uncomfortable confronting Arthur about Arthur's burnout. Lancelot approached two of the other older physicians in the practice and made sure they were aware of Lancelot's observations. The older doctors appreciated Lancelot's observation and met with Arthur, who strongly recommended that he receive professional help. Arthur saw a psychiatrist who specializes in substance abuse and burnout in physicians. Arthur received treatment and took a recommended 2-month leave of absence. His partners were very supportive, and

Arthur was able to return to practice and remained very appreciative of Lancelot's recognition of the reality of the situation.

Key Takeaways

Burnout is not a condition we can ignore. Nearly 50% of doctors, including medical students, residents, fellows, and young doctors, are experiencing the signs and symptoms of burnout [8]. The causes are a feeling of powerlessness, a loss of autonomy, and the intrusion of technology intended to improve healthcare that detracts from the care we provide our patients. The signs and symptoms are easily recognized, and treatment is available for the impaired physician.

- Burnout among physicians is reaching epidemic proportions.
- Fifty percent of physicians experience one or more symptoms of burnout.
- Burnout impacts nearly 50% of medical students, residents, fellows, and early-career physicians.
- It is important to recognize burnout in ourselves and our colleagues and seek help to be a competent and caring physician.

References

1. Shanafelt TD, Boone S, Tan L, Dyrbye LN, et al. Burnout and satisfaction with work-life balance among US physicians relative to the general US population. Arch Intern Med. 2012;172(18):1377–85.
2. Dyrbye LN, West CP, Satele D, Boone S, Tan L, Sloan J, Shanafelt TD. Burnout among U.S. medical students, residents, and early career physicians relative to the general U.S. population. Acad Med. 2014;89(3):443–51.
3. Fred HL, Scheid MS. Physician burnout: causes, consequences, and cures. Tex Heart Inst J. 2018;45(4):198–202.
4. Zulman DM, Shah NH, Verghese A. Evolutionary pressures on the electronic health record: caring for complexity. JAMA. 2016;316(9):923–4.
5. Tool E. The cost of technology. JAMA. 2020;323(17):1661–2. https://doi.org/10.1001/jama.2020.2752.
6. Sinsky C, Colligan L, Li L, Prgomet M, Reynolds S, Goeders L, et al. Allocation of physician time in ambulatory practice: a time and motion study in 4 specialties. Ann Intern Med. 2016;165(11):753–60.
7. Lencioni P. The three signs of a miserable job. San Francisco: Jossey-Bass; 2007.
8. Mangione S, Chakraborti C, Staltari G, et al. Medical students' exposure to the humanities correlates with positive personal qualities and reduced burnout: a multi-institutional study. J Gen Intern Med. 2018;33(5):628–34.

19 Practice Divorce: Painless Separation from Your Partners

Phillipe is a nephrologist who joined a practice in a rural community in the Midwest 2 years ago. He had an income guarantee for 2 years and was very productive, receiving a bonus in his third year of practice. However, his wife, a social worker, was unhappy in the community and could only find part-time work, feeling unfulfilled. As a result, Phillipe considered terminating his relationship with the practice. He was unaware of the process of terminating his contract.

Physicians are under tremendous pressure in today's healthcare environment, as costs escalate, reimbursement declines, and the malpractice crisis persists. Everyday workplace stresses are exacerbated by longer hours, lower pay, and increased tolerance for error, which can lead to dissatisfaction and ultimately the decision to leave a practice.

Reasons for a medical divorce or employment agreements fall into two categories: "for cause" and "without cause." For-cause termination generally means that a party to the contract can terminate the agreement, often immediately, if the other party breaches or violates the agreement in some way. The employment agreement should clearly spell out each of the causes for which the employment can be terminated. The causes for termination should be objective and reasonably within the employed physician's control, but not so restrictive as to leave the employer without recourse if some unexpected behavioral or performance issue arises.

Common causes for termination may include loss or suspension of a medical license, loss of medical staff privileges at the hospital, failure to obtain or maintain insurance participation, failure to obtain or maintain board certification, conviction of a crime or felony, patient safety-related issues, or use of illegal drugs or abuse of controlled substances. For certain types of causes, a physician may negotiate a provision requiring the employer to provide advance written notice of the complaint that, if uncorrected, will lead to termination, thus allowing the physician adequate time either to change the objectionable behavior or to find new employment.

Typically, physician employment agreements can also be terminated without cause, meaning either party can terminate the contract at any time. Without cause usually requires a notice of a certain number of days, without the need to identify any specific reason for the termination. It is common for these contracts to stipulate that either party may terminate without cause following a specified period of advance written notice, which is typically 90 or 180 days.

This type of termination provision can offer protection for both parties, as in the absence of a "without cause" provision, each party is obligated to abide by the terms of the initial agreement for the entire term unless they can find a valid reason for termination or are willing to breach the contract. If a departing physician

N. Baum, M. J. Kahn, *Business Basics for your Healthcare Practice*,
https://doi.org/10.1007/978-3-032-25241-8_19

chooses the latter option, this may result in a lawsuit for breaching the contract.

If you plan to terminate your relationship with your employer, we recommend following these steps to make the process as smooth as possible [1].

Before notifying your employer of your decision to depart, review all documents, especially the contract you have signed. This will most likely include an employment agreement, a shareholders' agreement (if the practice is a corporation) or an operating agreement (if the practice is a limited liability company), and, in some cases, a deferred compensation arrangement. During your review, pay careful attention to information about advance notice provisions, retirement plan details, and noncompete restrictive covenants, which are the key components of your contracts.

You must understand and adhere to the commitments you have made, and the promises made to you through these contractual agreements.

Review the practice's established policies. In addition to reviewing any documents you have signed, you should review any of the practice's policies applicable to employment and departures. Some employment agreements indicate that the practice's general policies and procedures may be applicable even if they are contrary to the physician's employment agreement.

Next, review the practice's policies. In addition to reviewing any documents you have signed, you should review any of the practice's policies applicable to employment and departures. Some employment agreements indicate that the practice's general policies and procedures may be applicable even if they are contrary to the physician's employment agreement.

One of the most important aspects of your departure is to develop a plan for notifying your patients of your departure. Many states have a requirement that all patients be notified when a physician is departing a practice. Some states even require or suggest 30 days prior notice before departure so that patients will have sufficient time to transfer their records if they desire to change physicians. If you are not familiar with your state's requirements, consider consulting a healthcare attorney in your area for guidance.

In addition to sending letters, carefully consider how you will address this topic when speaking with patients. For example, you would never want to be in a situation where you felt compelled to lie to a patient. Often, practices and departing physicians will agree on what to tell patients who inquire about the tenure of the departing physician. Some practices display placards in the reception area informing patients of a physician's departure. Voice mail systems can also be modified to provide new contact information after the physician has departed.

Think about patients first. When scheduling your departure from the practice, take reasonable steps to ensure that you are not leaving any patients in a bind. For example, if you are an obstetrician, you would not want to plan your departure during a week in which you are anticipating five deliveries. The key is to prevent patients from falling through the cracks because of tensions between the departing physician and the practice. You and the practice have an obligation to provide proper care for your patients. The key takeaway is to prioritize the patient's well-being and avoid actions that could compromise their health.

High-risk patients should be sent a letter by certified mail, with a return receipt requested to confirm their receipt of the notification. High-risk patients are those who are more likely to experience adverse outcomes and feel that they have been abandoned if their departing physician is unavailable for ongoing care. Examples include recent post-op patients and those currently being followed for serious or chronic conditions. Keep a copy of the notification letter and certification material in the patient's record.

Active patients who aren't high risk should be sent a letter by regular post. Examples of active patients include those seen within the last 12–18 months. Again, we suggest that you keep a copy of the notification letter in the patient's record.

Finally, notify other patients who won't be receiving a letter by placing a notice in the local newspaper with the most extensive local circulation. We also recommend posting a sign in the reception area to inform patients about the departing physician.

The practice should also provide a script for receptionists on what to say. This should include information on how to contact the departing physician.

Suppose the departing physician won't be available for ongoing care due to moving out of the area. In that case, the letter should explain this and state that care is available at the same location as other physicians within the practice. You should tell those patients who choose to seek care elsewhere that, upon their written authorization, a copy of their medical record will be forwarded to their new provider.

If the departing physician will be available for ongoing care, explain to patients that the physician is leaving the practice but is available in the area. Inform patients that they have the option to stay with the practice or continue seeing the same physician in their new location. Instruct patients who choose to follow the physician that, upon their written authorization, a copy of their medical record will be forwarded to the physician at their new location.

To expedite the transfer of records, consider including an authorization form with the notification letter. If your practice is going to charge the patient for photocopying costs, you should inform the patient of the fee. Any material related to patient care should be considered part of the medical record and provided to the new physician. Both the practice and the new physician should keep a copy of the medical records.

For patients who stay within the practice, the patient should be notified about any changes in their provider. The patient's preferences should be honored to either remain in the practice or continue care with the departing physician.

If another practitioner will provide the care with the same scope of practice as the departing physician, inform the patient of the new provider's name. However, if a practitioner will provide the care with a different subspecialty, you should verify that the new provider can safely meet the patient's clinical needs.

Figure 19.1 is a sample of a letter you might consider sending to your patients announcing your departure.

Review advance notice provisions. Your contract may require you to provide your practice with advance written notice of your departure. If you fail to provide notice, the practice may claim breach of contract, and you could be held legally responsible for their cost of hiring a locum tenens physician or recruiting a new physician to fulfill the remainder of your term. Furthermore, many deferred-compensation arrangements are tied to the amount of notice provided. Some require an extraordinarily long notice period (such as 1 year) before the physician can qualify for deferred compensation payments.

Review your retirement plans. This will ensure that your departure date does not result in unnecessary forfeitures. For example, some retirement plans require an employee to work the entire year before becoming eligible. While it may be convenient to resign shortly before Christmas so that you can spend the holidays at home, it could be a monumental mistake if it results in losing nearly 1 year of retirement benefits. Further, many retirement plans have vesting schedules that depend on the number of years you have worked with the employer to receive your deserved retirement compensation. You and your attorney should review the details of your plan so that you do not unwittingly forfeit significant amounts of retirement money.

CYT or cover your tail! Many practices obtain "claims made" malpractice insurance policies that insure you for claims made during your term of employment. This means that if a malpractice event occurs while you were employed, but no one filed a claim until after you left the practice, the malpractice insurer will not cover the claim because it was not made during your employment. To prevent this, you need to procure a supplemental policy, commonly referred to as "tail coverage," which insures you for claims made after your employment terminates. While some employers will contractually agree to pay tail insurance in certain events, a thorough review of your employment agreement will determine who is responsible for procuring tail coverage.

Sample letter to patients informing of leaving the practice

Dear (patient's name):

It is with mixed emotion that I am [announcing my retirement from active practice; relocating my practice; etc.] as of [date]. This decision has not been made lightly, as I have enjoyed working at ______________________.

As of [date], Dr. ______________ will be taking over my practice. [Describe the new physician's background in 1-2 sentences]. Dr. ______________ can be contacted at the address below:

[Name of Physician and/or Clinic] [Address]
[Telephone number]
[E-mail]

If you prefer, you may obtain the services of another physician. If you choose to do so, I would recommend proceeding as soon as possible to ensure a smooth transition for your health care. The local Health Region keeps a list of physicians who are accepting new patients.

Your medical records are confidential, and a copy can be sent to another physician or released to you or another person only through your consent. I will be pleased to provide a summary of my care while you have been my patient, and with your consent, will arrange to have a copy of your file transferred to your new physician's office. Please sign the enclosed authorization form and return it to our office as soon as possible before (date) so that we may make the appropriate arrangements concerning your file.

It has been my great pleasure to have provided you with health services in the past, and I am grateful to have had the opportunity to meet some wonderful people throughout my years in practice. Best wishes for a healthy future.

Sincerely,

Dr. ___________ [title]

Fig. 19.1 Notice of leaving practice to send to colleagues, professional associations, payors

Whether the practice pays for tail coverage often depends on the type of termination. For example, practices usually agree to pay for tail coverage if employment is terminated by the practice without cause, meaning there was no violation on your part. For example, if the practice was sold or merged with another group, the malpractice might not cover you in the event of a claim after the practice is sold or merged. Likewise, physicians often agree in their initial contract to pay for tail coverage if they terminate their employment without cause.

This tail coverage can be significant, especially for obstetricians. Thus, regardless of who is responsible for procuring tail coverage, that party should provide a certificate of insurance to the other party. Do not be seduced into foregoing the purchase of tail coverage. The cost of successfully defending a medical malpractice action is lifestyle-altering, and you don't want to bear this expense on your own.

While you can purchase tail coverage that has no end date, many malpractice carriers offer 1-year, 3-year, 5-year, or 7-year tail coverage policies. These finite tail coverage policies, as opposed to lifetime coverage, are generally less expensive. If you live in a state with a strong statute of limitations on medical malpractice insurance claims, these finite tail coverage policies can save you money without leaving your tail exposed.

If you are responsible for tail coverage, you can negotiate with your new practice to provide you with sufficient funds to purchase it. Or, in limited circumstances, the new practice may provide coverage through a new policy with a retroactive endorsement date. This is referred to as "nose" coverage. Our take-home message is to check out both your tail and your nose so that you are covered in the event of a malpractice suit after you leave a practice.

- Several companies offer free quotes for tail coverage
- https://www.cunninghamgroupins.com/request-a-free-quote/ or 866-213-3035) or The Doctors Insurance Agency, for a blog on the cost of the tail, www.doctorsagency.com or 800-553-9293

Parting with the patients' charts. Be aware that patient lists, patient charts, and other patient demographic information are the property of the practice, not the departing physician. Employment contracts usually reinforce this stipulation in the contract. Rarely do practices agree that patient charts are the property of the departing physician. These assets belong to the practice and cannot be removed by the physician without the practice's consent. You should note, however, that most states allow the patient to request that their chart be forwarded to a departing physician, in which case the physician can, at that time, receive the chart from the practice. Usually, the practice will charge the patient a fee for copying the chart, and the departing physician cannot request that a copy of the chart be sent to them in their new practice.

Taking employees with you is a no-no. Your contract may contain provisions prohibiting you from soliciting the employment of existing employees of the practice. Even without these prohibitions, you should not actively solicit the employment of existing employees, especially before your departure. Some states would consider this behavior an egregious act, and courts would find favor with the employer if a physician were to "raid" the practice for employees. It is, however, not uncommon for employees to solicit the departing physician before their departure. This creates a quandary because, although you may need new employees, you do not want to appear to be soliciting from the existing practice. Before making any decisions, review your employment contract and your state's laws regarding the issue. This is where a healthcare attorney can be very helpful.

Review noncompetition covenants. A noncompete covenant may prohibit you from practicing within a specific geographic radius of your current practice for a designated period of time, often 2 years. Your practice's location typically determines the radius, which can range from five miles in a suburban area to 50 miles or more in a rural area. Many departing physicians believe that these covenants will not be enforced; however, courts in most states will uphold them if they are reasonable. For this reason, you should review the covenant as if it were enforceable. Litigating a covenant, either from the employer's or the departing physician's perspective, is expensive. Don't hesitate to contact an attorney if you have any questions.

Even when leaving a position under less-than-ideal circumstances, the departing physicians should leave adequate forwarding information. Patients may need to contact the physician who is departing. Payors may also need to contact them, especially regarding audits and adjustments that are the responsibility of the departing physician. If the practice doesn't know where the departing physician is located, complaints to the medical board will likely occur. A physician also doesn't want a complaint when they are trying to obtain a license in another state or secure hospital privileges at another institution.

Dependent upon the provisions of contracts and state law, both the departing physician and the practice may need to notify various third parties:

1. The malpractice insurance carrier needs to know of any changes to ensure coverage of the care rendered in both the prior and future practice settings.
2. Managed care companies with whom you have contracts.
3. The medical staff committee of hospitals where the departing physician has privileges. If they are on-call at the hospital, notify the emergency department as well.
4. The state board of medicine (if required by state law).

5. Legal counsel for assistance as needed in contract provisions and employment law.

Figure 19.1 is a letter you might consider using to notify colleagues of your departure from a practice.

Advice on securing the counsel of a healthcare attorney. Just as the words "cure," "remission," and "no evidence of disease" are pleasant to the ears of the treating physician and their team, "divorce" is a pleasant word for healthcare attorneys. Although physicians are transitioning from volume to value, attorneys still are reimbursed by the volume of cases they have, and they'll be just delighted to help you through a potentially expensive experience. That is why we suggest seeking the counsel of an attorney with healthcare experience and one who has experience in managing medical terminations on behalf of an employed doctor. We also recommend that you ask your attorney that you are considering for an estimate of the charges for managing your case. You can't hold their feet to the fire, but they should provide you with a ballpark estimate of the cost of managing your case. If the attorney comes back with a response that they "log in their hours" and then give you an hourly fee, we suggest you consider walking to the next healthcare attorney, as many are available who will provide you with an estimate of the fees you will likely be paying.

Phillipe's Case

Phillipe contacted his employer and explained the situation with his family and his desire to leave the practice. Phillipe made a point that he was happy with the group and wished to leave on good terms, but that he had to think about the happiness of his family first. Phillipe sought the counsel of a healthcare attorney, wrote a letter to all of his patients several months before his departure date, and then ensured that he had tail coverage in the event of any lawsuit after he left the practice. As a result, Phillipe had a reasonably amicable separation from the practice, moved to a large community where his wife was able to obtain full-time employment, and they lived happily ever after!

Bottom Line Most young physicians lack the knowledge and skills required to depart from a practice. It is for this reason that we suggest consulting a healthcare attorney who has experience with medical contracts before deciding to leave a practice. Leaving a practice can be a stressful time in any physician's career. A clean departure will save you headaches and possibly dollars in both the immediate and long-term future. Your careful attention to these details will ensure a smooth transition to a new practice.

Key Takeaways

- Develop an exit strategy to minimize disruption to your patients and the practice. This includes providing adequate notice, ensuring a smooth transition of care to another physician, and maintaining professionalism during the process.
- Consult legal and financial advisors to ensure your rights are safeguarded, particularly regarding employment contracts, noncompete clauses, and any financial obligations.
- This will help you complete the divorce and protect you in future employments

References

1. Wall JD. A must-do list for the departing physician. Fam Pract Manag. 2005;12(9):54–6.

Resources

2. Physician Employment Contract Guide by American College of Physicians, 2017. https://www.acponline.org/system/files/documents/running_practice/practice_management/human_resources/employment_contracts.pdf
3. Little KS. The Exit: Terminating Physician Employment Agreements. Healthcare Law Blog; 2017. https://www.healthcarelaw-blog.com/exit-terminating-physician-employment-agreements/
4. Leaving practice-A guide for physicians and surgeons. October 2017. http://www.cps.sk.ca/iMIS/Documents/Brochures/Leaving_Practice-guide.pdf

20 Telemedicine

Case of Roberto

Roberto, a primary care physician, was receiving inquiries from patients about whether he would consider using telemedicine for follow-up visits. He knew that other primary care practices in his community were offering telemedicine visits for established patients. He was fearful of losing patients unless he implemented telemedicine services for his patients. Roberto is interested in this concept but didn't know how to proceed using this new technology.

Telemedicine offers an opportunity to enhance communication between physicians and patients, meeting the needs of patients who prefer to receive care through telemedicine technology. Telemedicine saves patients the time and effort of coming to the office. A telemedicine visit provides a detailed record of the interaction, leading to improved healthcare outcomes. Many patients can receive medical care without the need for an in-person visit. There is even the potential to provide post-operative care via telemedicine safely. This chapter discusses integrating telemedicine into practice with minimal time, energy, and expense.

Practices typically use telemedicine platforms to manage one or both of the following types of encounters: (1) walk-in visits through the practice's website. Patients accessing a practice through the website tend not to care which physicians they see. Their priority is usually the first available provider, and (2) appointment-based consultations, where patients schedule video chats in advance of an in-office visit, or for a quick follow-up with a provider.

Although incorporating telemedicine into practice may seem overwhelming, it requires minimal additional equipment and interfaces easily with a practice's website and electronic medical record (EMR) system, increasing productivity and improving workflow. And patients generally appreciate the option of not having to travel to the office for an appointment.

Most patients and physicians are already comfortable with mobile phones, tablets, social media, and wearable technology, such as Fitbits. Telemedicine is a logical next step.

Getting Started

Physicians, their colleagues, and staff need to become comfortable with telemedicine technology. Physicians can begin by using video communication for other purposes, such as conducting staff meetings. They should practice starting and ending calls, as well as adjusting audio volume and video quality, to ensure good reception for both the doctor and the patient.

N. Baum, M. J. Kahn, *Business Basics for your Healthcare Practice*,
https://doi.org/10.1007/978-3-032-25241-8_20

Selecting a Video Platform

Table 20.1 provides a list of the most popular video providers, along with their advantages and disadvantages. Table 20.2 lists free video chat apps. Apps are available that can:

- Share lab tests, images, and other medical documents.
- Securely send documents over a Health Insurance Portability and Accountability Act (HIPAA)-compliant video.
- Stream digital device images live while maintaining a view of the patient's face.

Physicians should ensure their implementation team has the necessary equipment, including webcams, microphones, and speakers. They should research and test several programs before selecting one for their practice. Consider appointing a telemedicine point person who is knowledgeable about technology and who can patiently explain it to others. Keep in mind that video chatting requires a fast, robust Internet connection with sufficient bandwidth to transport a large amount of data. If your practice experiences connectivity issues, consider consulting an information technology (IT) expert.

Table 20.1 Telemedicine video conferencing programs

Products	Pros	Cons
Google+	Free	No screen sharing
Secure/ video	HIPAA compliant	
Skype	Leader voice and video	No screen sharing Requires ample bandwidth Not HIPAA compliant
Tango	Both Android and iPhone	No screen sharing
WebEx	Excellent for presentations and webinars	Decreased video performance
Zoom	Both Android and iPhone free for <40 minutes	Minimal fee for meetings >40 minutes

Table 20.2 Telemedicine apps

Amwell
HealthTap
MDLive
SimplePractice
Iotum
ClinicTracker
Klara
PracticeSuite

Testing It Out and Obtaining Feedback

Once a practice is comfortable using video, it is time to test it out with a few patients and a few payers. Most patients are eager to start using video for their medical encounters. Even senior patients are often willing to try consultations via video. According to a recent survey, 64% of patients want to see a physician over video [1].

Among those who were comfortable accepting an invitation to participate in a video encounter, increasing age was associated with a higher likelihood of accepting an invitation.

Physician colleagues, medical assistants, and nurse practitioners will need some basic telemedicine skills, and physicians and staff should be prepared to make video connections seamless for patients. Usually, patients need guidance and encouragement, such as checking their spam folder for invitations if they fail to arrive in their email inbox, adjusting audio settings, or setting up a webcam. Fortunately, most computers come equipped with built-in video cameras, which greatly facilitate the use of virtual appointments. In the beginning, physicians should make sure they build in plenty of buffer time for the unexpected, as there will undoubtedly be some "bugs" that need to be worked out.

Physicians should encourage and collect patient feedback on such questions as:

- What types of devices (e.g., laptops, mobile phones) do your patients prefer to use?
- What kind of networks are they using (5G, corporate, home)?
- What features do they like? What features do they have a hard time finding?

- What do they like or not like about the video experience?
- Keep track of the types of questions patients ask and be patient as patients become acclimated to the video consultation experience.

Streaming Online Workflow

After receiving feedback from your patients, it is time to streamline the online workflow. Most physicians want to manage video visits similarly to how they manage face-to-face visits with patients. This may mean experimenting with a virtual waiting room. A virtual waiting room is a simple web page or link that can be sent to patients before their virtual visit. Patients sign in with minimal demographic information on that page and then select one of the available time slots. Typically, these programs are designed to alert the physicians and staff when patients enter the virtual waiting room. Patients have access to the online patient queue and can start a chat or video call when both parties are ready. Such a waiting room model serves as a stepping-stone for new practices to familiarize themselves with video conferencing. This approach is also perfect for practices with a practice management system that wants to add a video component.

Influences on Practice Workflow

With good time management, telemedicine can improve the efficiency and productivity of your practice. Your daily schedule and patient management will require some minor adjustments, but significant changes to your existing schedule and workflow are generally unnecessary. One of the advantages of telemedicine is the convenience of prompt care, and the easy access patients have to your practice. This easy access decreases the need for visits to the emergency department and urgent care centers. This not only reduces the cost of care but can also benefit any value-based contracts that the practice may have.

One piece of advice: consider scheduling telemedicine appointments at the end of the day when your staff has left the office, as no staff members are necessary for a telemedicine visit. Ideally, you should offer a set time to communicate with patients, as this avoids making multiple calls to reach a patient.

Another advantage of telemedicine is that it allows for care to be provided in the evenings and on weekends. Previously, you may have been fielding calls from patients during these times without compensation. With telemedicine, you can conduct virtual visits from any location using a computer or mobile phone and receive remuneration for your care.

Telemedicine and the Coronavirus

The COVID-19 healthcare crisis led to the widespread adoption and implementation of telemedicine by healthcare providers. Patients with COVID-19 can be helped safely in the comfort of their own homes without endangering others. In fact, whether infected with COVID-19 or any other virus, patients who are febrile or experiencing respiratory symptoms can continue to utilize virtual visits. Similarly, doctors concerned about infecting others with COVID-19, the common cold, or other minor illnesses can safely consult with patients through a telemedicine network.

There are several misconceptions about telemedicine. Physicians often assume that patients prefer face-to-face visits when, in fact, many may prefer the convenience of virtual visits. More than 80% of surveyed patients report that their experience with telemedicine has helped improve their relationship with their providers [2].

Telemedicine has grown exponentially during the COVID-19 pandemic to the point where many patients now *expect* their healthcare providers to be able to conduct virtual visits. Practices that do not offer telemedicine may find their patients seeking services elsewhere. COVID-19 has motivated the increased use of telemedicine to enhance communication with patients, allowing them to have improved access to healthcare during the pandemic while minimizing the transmission of COVID-19 to physicians and their staff [3]. Additionally, the COVID-19 pandemic prompted third-party payers, such as Medicare and Medicaid, to provide reimbursement for virtual visits [4].

Admittedly, telemedicine is not appropriate for all patients. Generally, situations that do not lend themselves to telemedicine include those that require an in-person visit to evaluate the patient, such as when a physical examination is necessary, or those that necessitate an office procedure. Additional patients for whom telemedicine may be inappropriate include those with cognitive disorders, language barriers, or those in emergencies that warrant an office visit or a visit to the emergency department. Of course, telemedicine is limited by the technology available at the patient's home.

Cost and Complexity

The process of implementing electronic health records (EHRs) has left a bitter taste in the mouths of many healthcare professionals because EHRs are complicated and expensive. Implementation of an EHR often results in lost productivity. Because the learning curve is so steep, many physicians must decrease the number of patients they see before becoming comfortable with the conversion from paper charts to an EHR.

Telemedicine implementation is much less demanding and less expensive. Telemedicine is available as a cloud-based platform, which requires less information technology (IT) support and less hardware and software. The technology needed for patients to participate in telemedicine is nearly ubiquitous. According to the Pew Research Center, 96% of Americans own a cellphone, 81% have a smartphone, and more than half (52%) own a tablet, so the basic equipment to connect patients to providers is already in place [5].

On the provider side, the essential equipment required for a telemedicine program includes a computer with video and audio capabilities, as well as a broadband connection that is fast enough to display video in real-time and provide high-quality viewing of any images to be reviewed. However, traditionally, most telemedicine programs have required the purchase and setup of new technology and equipment, as well as staff training—some of which may be outside the budgets of healthcare providers in smaller practices. Many physicians have technology budgets that are stretched to the limit. For patients without access to a smartphone or computer with internet connectivity, telemedicine may not be feasible.

However, with new guidelines issued by the Centers for Medicare and Medicaid Services (CMS) in March 2020, connectivity can be achieved inexpensively using free platforms such as Google Hangouts, Skype, FaceTime, and Facebook Messenger. If a non-HIPAA-compliant platform is initially used, it is recommended to transition to a HIPAA-compliant platform.

These platforms do not require the purchase or subscription to any expensive hardware or software. The disadvantages of these programs include a lack of documentation, failure to comply with the Health Insurance Portability and Accountability Act (HIPAA), and inadequate encryption. The new CMS guidelines require the telemedicine program to be interoperable with the EHR and the billing program. Otherwise, double- and triple-entry will erase the efficiency of conducting a virtual visit. Depending on the magnitude of the program, IT assistance may be needed to get started.

Licensing

Another concern or barrier is a license to participate in telemedicine. The March 15, 2020, approval of telemedicine provided that licensed physicians in the state where the patient is located did not require any additional license or permission to conduct virtual visits [6].

For questions regarding licensure, contact your State Board of Medicine or Department of Health for information on requirements for licenses across state lines [7].

Informed Consent

Like any other aspect of patient care, obtaining informed consent is crucial. Obtaining informed patient consent is not only a recommended practice of the American Telemedicine Association (ATA), but it is also a legal requirement in many states. It may also be a condition of payment, depending on the payer. To check the requirements regarding patient consent in your state, look at The National Telehealth Policy Resource Center's state map [8].

Some states do not have specific requirements regarding consent for virtual visits. Others require verbal consent. Even if it is not a legal requirement in your state, consider incorporating written or verbal consent into your practice's policy and documenting in the patient's record that permission was obtained before the virtual visit, thereby protecting yourself when using this new technology.

Telemedicine is a new way for many patients to receive care. It is essential to inform them about how the process works, including how patient confidentiality and privacy are handled, what technical equipment is required, and what they can expect regarding scheduling, cancellations, and billing policies. See Fig. 20.1 for a sample telemedicine consent form.

Consent for Telemedicine Visit

I hereby consent and authorize Dr. Neil Baum and his partners, colleagues, and agents and their employed or contracted physicians, physician assistants, nurse practitioners or other licensed health care professionals in its care network to utilize telemedicine through its vendor systems, methods, and protocols to access, diagnose, consult, treat and educate me and those I am authorized to represent.
I acknowledge and consent to a physician, Dr. Neil Baum, via telemedicine. I understand my eligibility to receive a visit via telemedicine is based on the doctor's medical judgement that it is appropriate, and that the quality of care will not be diminished using telemedicine. I understand that a telemedicine visit is distinct from an in-person visit because I will not be in the same room as the healthcare provider, and instead, I will communicate with the doctor through advanced communication technology using live video and audio feed. I acknowledge that to protect my privacy, I need to choose a private location to place my telemedicine call.
<Signed> <Patient>
<Date>

Fig. 20.1 Consent for telemedicine visit

Liability Insurance

Another hurdle to consider is liability insurance for conducting virtual visits with patients. Physicians offering telemedicine care to patients should request proof that their liability insurance policy covers telemedicine malpractice and that the coverage extends to other states, in case the patient is in a state where the physician holds a license. Additionally, physicians who provide telemedicine care should consult with their liability insurers to determine any requirements or limitations for conducting virtual visits with their patients and document these findings. For example, the policy may require that the physician keep a written or recorded record of the visit in the EHR. If that is the case, using Skype, Facebook, or Google for the virtual visit, which does not include documentation, would be less desirable.

Privacy

Certainly, there is concern about privacy, and HIPAA compliance is crucial to the success of telemedicine. Due to the COVID-19 emergency, on March 1, 2020, physicians were able to communicate with patients and provide telehealth services through remote communications without penalties [7].

With these changes in HIPAA requirements, physicians can utilize applications that enable video chats, including Apple FaceTime, Facebook Messenger video chat, Google Hangouts video, and Skype, to provide telehealth services without the risk of the Office for Civil Rights imposing a penalty for noncompliance with HIPAA rules. When using these platforms, the consent form for patients should clearly state that these "public" applications potentially introduce privacy risks. These privacy risks encourage physicians to consider programs that promise encryption, privacy, and HIPAA compliance, such as Updox, Doxy.me, and Amazon Chime. It is also important to recognize that a virtual visit could result in staff (if the patient is in an office setting) or family members (if the patient is in the home environment) overhearing conversations between the healthcare professional and the patient. Therefore, we suggest that patients conduct virtual visits in locations where they feel assured of privacy.

Compensation for Telemedicine

The most significant barrier to the adoption of virtual health has been the compensation for telemedicine visits. Both commercial payers and CMS have been slow to enact formal policies for telemedicine reimbursement. Common misconceptions that providers won't receive reimbursement for telemedicine appointments or that compensation occurs at a reduced rate have persisted, thus making telemedicine economically unappealing. The good news is that this is changing. Legislation in most states is rapidly embracing virtual health visits due to the COVID-19 pandemic [8]. In fact, as of January 1, 2020, telemedicine services are no longer considered "optional" coverage in Medicare Advantage plans [9].

Additionally, patients can utilize telemedicine without incurring any additional insurance costs. CMS now allows telemedicine as a standard, covered benefit in all plans, enabling beneficiaries to seek care from the comfort of their own homes rather than requiring them to visit a healthcare facility [10].

In the past, telemedicine was primarily used in rural areas or when patients resided a great distance from their healthcare providers. Starting March 6, 2020, and throughout the COVID-19 public health emergency, Medicare allowed payments for professional services furnished to beneficiaries in all areas of the country, regardless of setting or location, provided the patient and healthcare provider were not in the same location or within a specified distance [11].

The expanded access also applies to pre-COVID-19 coverage from physician offices, skilled nursing facilities, and hospitals. Medicare will now make payments to physicians for telemedicine services provided in any healthcare facility or in a patient's home. Patients do not always need to go to the physician's office [7].

The facts are that there are now parity laws stating that commercial payers and CMS are required by state law to reimburse for telemedicine—often at the same rate as that for a comparable in-person visit. On the commercial side, there has been an increase in commercial parity legislation that requires health plans to cover virtual visits in the same manner as they cover face-to-face services. For example, suppose the provider performs and documents the elements of history and decision-making, including the time spent counseling. In that case, they can record the visit as a face-to-face visit. In that case, clinicians have a billable evaluation and management (E&M) visit.

Virtual Services for Medicare Patients

There are three types of virtual services you can provide for Medicare patients: (1) Medicare telehealth visits, (2) virtual check-ins, and (3) e-visits.

Medicare Telehealth Visits

Due mainly to the COVID-19 pandemic, Medicare patients can now utilize telecommunication technology for services that previously required in-person interaction. The physician must use an interactive audio and video telecommunications system that permits real-time communication between the physician and the patient. The patient should have an established relationship with the physician with whom the telemedicine visit occurs.

The Current Procedural Terminology (CPT) codes for virtual visits using synchronous audio/visual communication are:

- 99,201–99,295, office visit for a new patient
- 99,211–99,215, office visit for an established patient.

Important modifiers for telemedicine visits include:

- Modifier 02 for POS (place of service) for telehealth Medicare.
- Modifier 95 for commercial payers.

(For a list of all available CPT codes for telehealth services from CMS, see reference [12].

Virtual Check-Ins

CMS allows established Medicare patients to have brief communication with physicians, traditionally, using a telephone or live video. These brief virtual visits, typically lasting 5–10 minutes, are initiated by the patient. The virtual check-in aims to determine if an office visit, a test, or a procedure is indicated. Medicare covers these "virtual check-ins" (or short communication technology-based services) that enable patients to communicate with their physicians and avoid unnecessary office visits. These brief virtual check-ins are only for established patients. If an existing patient contacts the physician's office to ask a question or determine if an office visit is necessary, the physician may bill for this brief visit using code G2012.

E-visits. Established Medicare patients may engage in non-face-to-face patient-initiated communications with their physicians without visiting the physician's office. These services are billed only when the physician has an established patient relationship. For these services, use CPT codes 99,421 to 99,423. Coding for these visits is determined by the length of time the physician spends online with the patient:

- 99,421: Online digital evaluation and management service, for an established patient, 5–10 min spent on the virtual visit
- 99,422: 11–20 min
- 99,423: $\geq$ 21 min.

Since March 15, 2020, the relaxation of HIPAA restrictions for telemedicine has made it possible to have a virtual visit with a patient using a non-HIPAA-compliant connection. This type of visit is no different than a telephone call, but with an added video component. Many physicians who want to initiate telemedicine with their patients will utilize the free video communication services offered by Google Hangouts, Skype, FaceTime, and Facebook Messenger. Using these free technologies, a physician can have an asynchronous visit with a patient (the store-and-forward method of sending information or medical images). The service is conducted in one direction, with no opportunity for interaction with the patient. Asynchronous visits are akin to video text messages left for the patient. By contrast, a synchronous or real-time video visit with a patient is a two-way communication that provides medical care without requiring an in-person examination of the patient.

Using Triangulation

There are some downsides to telemedicine visits. First, virtual visits on Skype, FaceTime, and other non-HIPAA-compliant methods are not conducted on an encrypted website. Second, no documentation is created for the doctor-patient encounter. Finally, unless the physician records these virtual visits and submits the interactions to the practice coders, there will be no billing and thus no reimbursement for the visits. In this scenario, physicians remain legally responsible for their decision-making, prescription writing, and medical advice, but they do not receive compensation for their time and expertise.

This can be remedied by using "triangulation," which involves: 1. the physician, 2. the patient, and 3. a scribe or medical assistant who will record the visit. Before initiating the virtual visit using triangulation, it is essential to obtain the patient's permission if your medical assistant (or any other person in the office who functions as a scribe) will be listening to the conversation. It is essential to clarify that the scribe is present to record notes and accurately enter them into the EHR. Also, the scribe or assistant will record the time, date, and duration of the visit, which is a requirement for billing purposes. The scribe may also verify that the visit is appropriately coded and entered into the practice management system, and that a bill is submitted to the insurance company. By using triangulation, you have documentation that consent was obtained, that the visit took place, that notes were taken, and that the patient's insurance company will be billed for the visit. (See Fig. 20.2 for a sample documentation form).

Virtual Visit Documentation Form

Date: ____/____/____Time Start ____A.M./PM

Total Time of Visit ___min

Patient Information

First Name__________________ Last Name __________________________

DOB ____/____/____Phone _______________________________________

Email____

Mode of Communication

Telephone__ Text__ Video Chat__ Instant Messenger__ Other__

Diagnosis ____

Etiology____

Symptoms

Clinical Findings

Prescriptions Provided

Treating physician____

Signature____

CPT Code____

Date entered in EMR____

Additional notes____

Fig. 20.2 Sample documentation form

Which CPT Codes Should I Use?

These are the most common CPT codes for outpatient office visits, whether face-to-face or synchronous virtual visits (via a real-time, interactive audio and video telecommunications system).

For example, the reimbursement for code 99213 in 2025 ranges from $73 to $100. You may wonder how to achieve the complexity requirements for a level-3 office visit without a physical examination. Whether as a face-to-face or virtual visit, documentation for these encounters requires two of the following three components:

- Expanded problem-focused history.
- Expanded problem-focused exam (not accomplished with telemedicine).
- Low-complexity medical decision-making.
- At least 15 min spent face-to-face with the patient if coding is based on time.

If a physician reviews the results of a recent lab test for a patient, adjusts the dosage of prescribed medication, writes a prescription, and spends 15 min communicating with the patient, they have met the complexity requirements for code 99213. Because level 3 and 4 visits (99,214 and 99,215) require a comprehensive physical examination, it is necessary to document the time spent with the patient (code 99214 requires 25–39 min of consultation, and code 99215 requires ≥40 min).

Some Final Billing and Coding Advice

Always confirm telemedicine billing guidelines *before* conducting telemedicine visits to ensure accurate billing. Consider starting a phone call to a payer armed with the fact that the payer is required to offer parity between telemedicine and face-to-face visits. Then ask which specific billing codes should be used.

Before providing telemedicine services, it is essential to inform the patient of any associated costs with the virtual visit. It is good policy to arrange payment *before* the service is delivered.

Until you become comfortable with the coding and billing process for telemedicine, consider using a telemedicine platform with a built-in rules engine that offers recommendations for each telemedicine visit based on past claims data. These systems help physicians determine which CPT code to use and which modifiers are appropriate for each insurance company. The rules engine enables you to submit a clean claim that is less likely to be denied and more likely to be paid. Some vendors are so confident that their rules engine will match the service with the proper CPT code and modifier that they guarantee full private payer reimbursement for telemedicine visits; if not, the vendor will reimburse the claim.

An Example

A visit with an existing patient using telemedicine, as documented by CPT codes 99,211–99,215. These are the most common CPT codes for outpatient physician offices, including both face-to-face and remote telemedicine visits. The reimbursement for 99,213 has a national average of $87.21. But how can you achieve the complexity requirements for a level 3 office visit without a physical exam? The documentation for these encounters requires a minimum of two of the following three components:

1. Expanded problem-focused history.
2. Expanded problem-focused physical exam (of course, that cannot be accomplished by using a telemedicine visit).
3. Low complexity medical decision-making.
4. 15 minutes spent face-to-face with the patient if coding is based on time.

For example, if a physician reviews the results of a recent lab test for a diabetic patient and adjusts the diabetic medication, this visit meets the complexity requirements for a 99,213.

Using the GT Modifier

The GT modifier indicates a service was rendered via synchronous (a live communication between doctor and patient) telecommunication. The rules engine provides modifier recommendations for each appointment based on past claims data to help providers determine which modifier is most appropriate.

Modifier 95

Modifier 95 is a modifier to be used when billing private payers to indicate services were rendered via synchronous telecommunication. The rules engine provided by your vendor is a good resource for selecting the appropriate modifier for your claim.

The good news is that in most states, Medicaid covers telemedicine services. Like billing E&M codes for telemedicine, Medicare requires billing the standard CPT code and adding the GT modifier.

Regardless of the telemedicine service you use, always confirm the payer's billing guidelines before engaging patients in telemedicine visits. You could start the call to the payer armed with a copy of this chapter, which reminds the payer that they are required to offer parity between telemedicine visits and face-to-face visits. Then, ask which specific billing codes you should use and whether they recognize the GT modifier.

Back to the Case

Roberto surveyed his patients, and several were eager to participate in virtual visits. He subscribed to an encrypted, HIPAA-compliant video-conferencing program. Roberto started regularly conducting telemedicine visits at the end of his workday. He soon discovered that telemedicine was efficient and productive. The feedback from his patients was favorable, and now, he holds three to five virtual visits a day.

Bottom Line
Patient-driven care is the future, and telemedicine is a key component of it. Patients want to have ready access to their healthcare providers without having to devote hours to a medical encounter that could be completed in minutes via telemedicine. It is not a matter of "if" but rather "when" to incorporate telemedicine as a communication and practice tool. The sooner, the better.

Key Takeaways
1. Telemedicine expands healthcare access to remote or underserved areas and allows patients to consult doctors from the comfort of their homes. Telemedicine is attractive to patients who value their time and don't want to spend several hours for an in-office doctor-patient encounter.
2. Virtual consultations can reduce healthcare costs by minimizing the need for in-person office visits.
3. It is necessary to ensure patient data privacy and security when implementing telemedicine services. This includes having an encrypted program to communicate with patients.
4. Healthcare providers and staff need proper training and support to effectively integrate telemedicine into their practice.
5. Do not fear or avoid new technology. Remember, it is high tech plus high touch!

References

1. Zacay G, Adler L, Schonmann Y, Azuri J, Yehoshua I, Vinker S, et al. "A day in the life"–telemedicine in family medicine and its relationship with practicing physicians' satisfaction: a cross-sectional study. Israel J Health Policy Res. 2024;13(1):33.
2. Nguyen M, Waller M, Pandya A, Portnoy J. A review of patient and provider satisfaction with telemedicine. Curr Allerg Asthma Rep. 2020;20(11):72.
3. Forcino RC, Johnson JK, Elwyn G. Telehealth modality preferences for video and voice-only visits among US Clinicians and the Public: cross-sectional, web-based survey study. J Med Internet Res. 2025;27:e72276.
4. Carter E, Russo A, El-Sayed A, Hernández M, Nair P. Telemedicine beyond the pandemic: innovations, challenges, and policy implications. Emerg Trends Med. 2025;2(1):24–31.
5. Gelles-Watnick R. Americans' use of mobile technology and home broadband. Pew Research Center; 2024.
6. Gruppuso PA, Adashi EY. Rethinking the standards for state licensure of physicians. J Am Board Fam Med. 2025;38(2):348–51.
7. Ivanova J, Cummins MR, Ong T, Soni H, Barrera J, Wilczewski H, et al. Regulation and compliance in telemedicine. J Med Internet Res. 2025;27:e53558.
8. Anggo S, Rahman W, Chai S, Pao C. Telemedicine in the digital era: changing the face of health services with virtual technology. J World Futur Med Health and Nurs. 2025;3(1):30–41.
9. Park S, Jung HY, Yu J. Telehealth availability and use among beneficiaries in traditional medicare and medicare advantage. J Am Geriatr Soc. 2025;73(2):545–51.
10. Cottrill A, Cubanski J, Neuman T. What to know about medicare coverage of telehealth. Kaiser Family Foundation; 2024.
11. Sandstrom RW, Lohman HL, Bramble JD. American Medical Association. AMA quick guide to telemedicine in practice. Updated May 22, 2020. (2025)
12. Lu LB, Joy SV, Engel JZ. Outpatient billing and coding and center for medicare & medicaid services billing rules. In: Leading an academic medical practice. Cham: Springer; 2024. p. 77–111.

21 Enhancing Patient Medication Compliance

Abner and Drug-Drug Interactions

Abner, a neurologist, was consulted to see one of his patients in the ICU. The patient had a recurrent deep venous thrombosis despite rivaroxaban therapy. The patient had recently been placed on phenytoin for complex seizures. Abner was not aware of the connection between the antiepileptic drug and the anticoagulant. Phenytoin and rivaroxaban are metabolized similarly, and phenytoin can induce the enzyme that metabolizes rivaroxaban, leading to lower levels of the medication. What can Abner do to prevent that kind of drug-drug interaction?

Adherence to therapies is a primary determinant of treatment success. Medication nonadherence in patients leads to substantial worsening of disease, death, and increased healthcare costs.

Several factors are likely to impact adherence.

The World Health Organization defines medication adherence as "the degree to which the person's behavior corresponds with the agreed recommendations from a health care provider" [1]. Although adherence and compliance are often used interchangeably, they differ in meaning. Compliance refers to the extent to which a patient's behavior aligns with the prescriber's advice [2]. Compliance implies a patient's adherence to the physician's recommendations. However, adherence signifies that the patient and physician collaborate to improve the patient's health by integrating the physician's medical opinion and the patient's lifestyle, values, and preferences for care [3].

There are several types of nonadherence. The first is primary nonadherence, in which providers write prescriptions, but the medication is never filled or initiated. This type is commonly referred to as nonfulfillment adherence [4].

The second type of nonadherence is called non-persistence when patients decide to stop taking a medication after starting it without being advised by a health professional. Non-persistence is rarely intentional and typically occurs when patients and providers fail to communicate effectively about therapeutic plans.

Unintentional nonadherence arises from capacity and resource limitations that prevent patients from implementing their decisions to follow treatment recommendations (e.g., problems accessing prescriptions, cost, and competing demands) and sometimes involves individual constraints (e.g., poor inhaler technique, problems remembering doses). Intentional nonadherence stems from the beliefs, attitudes, and expectations that influence patients' motivation to initiate and adhere to the treatment regimen [5].

The third type of nonadherence is known as nonconforming; this type includes a variety of ways in which medications are not taken as prescribed. This behavior can range from skipping

N. Baum, M. J. Kahn, *Business Basics for your Healthcare Practice*,
https://doi.org/10.1007/978-3-032-25241-8_21

doses to taking medications at incorrect times or at incorrect doses.

An extensive review of the literature reveals that adherence to therapies in developed countries averages 50% [6]. Approximately half of this nonadherence is intentional, while the remainder occurs because patients are either unaware that they are not taking medications as prescribed or the regimen is too demanding. Adherence rates are typically higher among patients with acute conditions than those with chronic conditions.

Studies reveal that patients with chronic illnesses take only 50% of the medications prescribed for those conditions [7].

The consequences of nonadherence are a waste of medication, disease progression, reduced functional abilities, lower quality of life, increased use of medical resources such as nursing homes, hospital visits, poor outcomes, and hospital admissions [8]. Economic studies reveal that poor adherence to prescribed regimens can lead to serious health consequences, as supported by various studies. For instance, in a survey by Anon, the risk of hospital readmission was more than double in patients with diabetes mellitus, hypercholesterolemia, hypertension, or congestive heart failure who were nonadherent to prescribed therapies compared with the general population. Studies conducted among Chronic Obstructive Pulmonary Disease patients have shown that poor adherence to drug therapy and disease management leads to emergency hospitalization [9].

Medication nonadherence can have negative consequences not only for the patient but also for the provider. The potential burden of medication nonadherence outcomes on healthcare delivery makes it an important public health concern. Additionally, with value-based contracts, nonadherence can lead to reimbursement penalties [10]. Hence, helping patients take their medicine appropriately avoids the higher risk of severe relapses, antibiotic resistance, and preventable hospitalizations.

Influencers of Medication Adherence

Barriers to the effective use of medicines specifically include poor provider-patient communication, inadequate knowledge about a drug and its use, not being convinced of the need for treatment, fear of adverse effects of the drug, necessity for long-term drug regimens, complex regimens that require numerous medications with varying dosing schedules, cost, and access barriers [11].

Adherence to drug therapy also varies with the patient age group. In children, adherence to drug therapy is affected due to their dependence on an adult caregiver. The literature concerning adherence reports in elderly patients reports that compliance rates range roughly from 38% to 57%, with an average rate of less than 45% [12].

A significant reason for nonadherence is the physician's failure to communicate the proper use of the medication, combined with the patient's inability to remember the physician's advice. Studies report that 40–60% of patients required assistance to accurately report what their physicians expected of them, 10–80 min after receiving the information. Yet another study said that over 60% of patients interviewed immediately after visiting their doctors misunderstood the directions regarding prescribed medications [13].

Nonadherence can also occur when the medication regimen is complex, which could include improper timing of drug administration or administration of numerous medications at frequent or unusual times during the day. Most deviations in taking medication occur because of the omission of doses (rather than additions) or delays in the timing of doses [14].

Patients often become noncompliant with chronic diseases like hypertension or elevated cholesterol levels. These two conditions can be unpleasant, even with strict adherence to the medication regimen. Estimates of medication nonadherence illustrate that the nonadherence percentage is most significant when the patients are symptom-free. However, when medication was to be taken over a long period, compliance rates dropped dramatically to around 50% for either prevention or cure [15, 16].

One major factor influencing adherence is the patient's ability to read and understand medication instructions. Patients with low literacy may struggle to understand instructions, leading to decreased adherence and suboptimal medication management [17]. Gender may influence adherence-compliance rates. For instance, women may be better at adhering to their medication regimens than men. This may be particularly so for drugs that treat behavioral health conditions, such as antidepressant medications [18].

Improving medication adherence.

Unfortunately, patients do not volunteer that they are noncompliant with their medications. The simplest way to measure adherence is through the patient's self-report [19].

1. Medication costs.

The cost of drugs can often be solved by contacting pharmaceutical companies for medications at a reduced or no cost to the patient. We suggest asking the patient about their compliance with the medication. Ask patients if cost is a concern or if the instructions require clarification.

A systematic approach to improving medication adherence is as follows:

Whenever possible, involve patients in decision-making regarding their medications, so they have a sense of ownership and are partners in the treatment plan. Whenever possible, use a simple regimen based on patient characteristics.

2. Communicating with the Patient

Explain key information when prescribing/ dispensing medicine.

Address the key information about the drugs (what, why, when, how, and how long). Explain the common side effects and those that patients should know. Patients become more worried, leading to nonadherence due to side effects not being discussed in advance. Provide medication calendars or schedules that specify the time to take medications, drug cards, medication charts, medicine-related information sheets, or specific packaging such as pill boxes, blister packaging, and special containers indicating the dose time.

3. At follow-Ups

Monitoring medication adherence should be followed by subsequent follow-up. This is an opportunity for healthcare providers to identify the underlying causes of patient nonadherence. With this information, an appropriate interventional strategy can be instituted.

One of the major reasons that patients become nonadherent is forgetting to take their medications. Results of a study conducted showed that 49.6% of patients mentioned forgetfulness as one of the major non-intentional reasons for nonadherence [20]. Forgetfulness can be resolved by recommending reminders, such as telephone calls, emails, text messages to cellular phones, and alarms. Involving the patient's caregivers would be another way of combating nonadherence due to forgetfulness.

Medication nonadherence may also occur because patients perceive it to be unnecessary or because of their fears and beliefs related to the adverse effects of drugs. Hence, providing clear, medication-related information to patients is essential to improve adherence, including addressing key details such as what, why, when, how, and how long. Patient medication counseling can be supplemented by providing detailed written information about medications. Succinctly written instructions, including drug cards, medication charts, or any written material in a plastic sheet or laminated sheet, also help improve adherence, especially for elderly patients who find it difficult to comprehend much of the information provided during medication counseling.

Patients' fears and concerns about adverse drug reactions can be alleviated by educating patients regarding common side effects of the drugs they are taking, how to prevent an adverse drug reaction, if possible, and convincing the patient of the need for treatment. The complexity of the drug regimen negatively affects medication adherence. When possible, reduce the frequency of administration and/or the number of different medications. If applicable, replace them with combination products. An example is treating men with benign prostate gland enlargement (BPH) by combining an alpha-blocker and a 5-alpha-reductase inhibitor in one tablet or capsule. An underutilized resource for enhancing medication adherence is the involvement of pharmacists in conducting annual medication reviews. There are two options: targeted interventions consisting of a 5–15 in-person or telephone conversation with patients. This brief visit allows pharmacists to explain adverse drug events to patients. The other option is annual medication reviews, which consist of a 45-min in-person review of the patient's clinical information and a comprehensive review of all the patient's medications, including over-the-counter medicines. The patient-pharmacist communication is central to optimizing patient adherence [21]. Comprehensive medication management is a patient-centered approach to optimizing medication use and improving patient health outcomes delivered by a clinical pharmacist working in collaboration with the patient and their healthcare providers [22]. This is a win-win-win situation that benefits patients, doctors, and pharmacists. Now the doctor can offload an annual drug review to the pharmacists, who can spend more time with the patient and help motivate compliance.

Assessing children's adherence can be done by asking for the help of a caregiver (school nurse or teacher). Among the various methods of questioning the patient, patient diaries and assessment of clinical response are relatively easy to use, but asking the patient can be susceptible to misrepresentation and tends to result in the healthcare provider overestimating the patient's adherence.

Electronic monitors capable of recording and stamping the time of opening bottles, dispensing drops (such as eye drops), or activating a metered dose inhaler for asthma can also measure adherence. The disadvantage of this method is that the measure of adherence is not accurate, as the patients may open the container and not take the medication, take the wrong amount of medication, or take multiple doses out of the container at the same time [16].

Abner and Compliance

Abner recognized that drug-drug interactions were possible with the existing prescribing methods used in practice. Abner used Hippocrates.com to check on the possibility of drug-drug interactions. Abner also created FAQs to give to each patient receiving a prescription for the most prescribed drugs, identifying possible drug-drug interactions. As a result, patients were informed and received valuable information on their medications, including potential interactions with their existing medications and adverse drug events associated with those medications.

Bottom Line

A treatment's effectiveness depends on the medication's efficacy and the patient's adherence to the therapeutic regimen. Patients, physicians, and healthcare systems all have a role in improving medication adherence. A single method cannot improve medication adherence. Instead, a combination of various adherence techniques should be implemented to improve patients' adherence to their prescribed treatment.

Patient medication nonadherence is a major medical problem. There are many interrelated reasons for noncompliance. Though patient education is the key to improving compliance, compliance aids, proper motivation, and support are also shown to increase medication adherence. Healthcare professionals should identify strategies to improve medication adherence within the limits of their practice, eventually enhancing therapeutic outcomes. A multidisciplinary approach is necessary, supported by all parties involved in medication use.

Key Takeaways

- The success of treatment for patients is dependent upon compliance with their medications.
- Medication nonadherence in patients leads to substantial worsening of disease, death, and increased healthcare costs.
- Physicians can help patients take their medicine appropriately, thus avoiding the risk of relapses, antibiotic resistance, and preventable hospitalizations.

References

1. Dobbels F, Van Damme-Lombaert R, Vanhaecke J, De Geest S. Growing pains: nonadherence with the immunosuppressive regimen in adolescent transplant recipients. Pediatr Transplant. 2005;9(3):381–90.
2. Horne R. Compliance, adherence, and concordance: implications for asthma treatment. Chest. 2006;130(1):65S–72S.
3. Spiro H. Compliance, adherence, and hope. J Clin Gastroenterol. 2001;32(1):5.
4. Gellad, W. F., Grenard, J. L., & McGlynn, E. A. (2009). A review of barriers to medication adherence: a framework for driving policy options.
5. Horne R, Weinman J, Barber N, Elliott RA, Morgan M. Concordance, adherence and compliance in medicine taking: a conceptual map and research priorities. London: National Co-ordinating Centre for NHS Service Delivery and Organisation NCCSDO; 2005.
6. Horne R, Weinman J, Barber N, Elliott R, Morgan M, Cribb A, Kellar I. Concordance, adherence and compliance in medicine taking. London: NCCSDO; 2005. 2005(40), 6.
7. Haynes RB, McDonald HP, Garg AX. Helping patients follow prescribed treatment: clinical applications. JAMA. 2002;288(22):2880–3.
8. Sullivan S, Kreling D, Hazlet T. Noncompliance with medication regimens and subsequent hospitalizations: a literature analysis and cost of hospitalization estimate. J Res Pharm Econ. 1990;2:19–33.
9. Garcia-Aymerich J, Barreiro E, Farrero E, Marrades RM, Morera J, Antó JM. Patients hospitalized for COPD have a high prevalence of modifiable risk factors for exacerbation (EFRAM study). Eur Respir J. 2000;16(6):1037–42.
10. National Council on Patient Information and Education. Enhancing prescription medicine adherence: a national action plan. Education. 2007;August:1–36.
11. Tarn DM, Heritage J, Paterniti DA, Hays RD, Kravitz RL, Wenger NS. Physician communication when prescribing new medications. Arch Intern Med. 2006;166(17):1855–62.
12. Sackett DL, Snow JC. The magnitude of compliance and non-compliance. In: Haynes RB, Taylor DW, Sackett DL, editors. Compliance in health care. Baltimore: Johns Hopkins University Press; 1979. p. 11–22.
13. Meichenbaum D, Turk DC. Facilitating treatment adherence: a practitioner's guidebook. New York: Plenum Publishing Corp; 1987.
14. Burnier M. Long-term compliance with antihypertensive therapy: another facet of chronotherapeutics in hypertension. Blood Press Monit. 2000;5:S31–4.
15. Jimmy B, Jose J. Patient medication adherence: measures in daily practice. Oman Med J. 2011;26(3):155.
16. Praska JL, Kripalani S, Seright AL, Jacobson TA. Identifying and assisting low-literacy patients with medication use: a survey of community pharmacies. Ann Pharmacother. 2005;39(9):1441–5.
17. Ward A, Morgan W. Adherence patterns of health in men and women enrolled in an adult exercise program. J Cardiac Rehabil. 1984;4:143–52.
18. Walsh JC, Mandalia S, Gazzard BG. Responses to a 1-month self-report on adherence to antiretroviral therapy are consistent with electronic data and virological treatment outcome. AIDS. 2002;16(2):269–77.
19. Adisa R, Alutundu MB, Fakeye TO. Factors contributing to nonadherence to oral hypoglycemic medications among ambulatory type 2 diabetes patients. Pharm Pract. 2009;7:163–9.
20. Golin CE, Gelberg L. The role of patient participation in the doctor visit. Implications for adherence to diabetes care. Diabetes Care. 1996;19(10):1153–64.
21. American College of Clinical Pharmacy, McBane SE, Dopp AL, Abe A, Benavides S, Chester EA, Walker S, et al. Collaborative drug therapy management and comprehensive medication management – 2015. Pharmacotherapy. 2015;35(4):e39–50.
22. Gellad WF, Grenard JL, McGlynn EA. A review of barriers to medication adherence: a framework for driving policy options (2009).

22 Online Reputation Management

Case Study
Greta was a member of a small group of primary care practice. She received notice from a website that she had several negative online reviews. Although she had fewer than ten reviews, the negative reviews were a source of discouragement as she felt that she had favorable relationships with her patients. What should she do?

Patients rely on referrals and word of mouth to make decisions about their health and choice of doctor. This process can now be done online. From social networking and Google searches to online review sites like Healthgrades, Yelp, RateMDs, and ZocDoc, patients can research and find information about their physician almost instantly. Individual consumers also rely on their personal networks and peer recommendations. Overall, one study found that 72% of patients ranked the healthcare provider's reputation and personal experience as the top driver for choosing a provider [1].

We live and die by our reputations, our most precious possession. Our reputations are created the minute we receive our medical diploma. They take years to build but are so fragile that they can crumble in seconds or a few mouse clicks. Look at what happens to athletes and movie stars who use a phrase that is politically incorrect or get caught driving while intoxicated. They tumble from their pedestal in a nanosecond.

In today's digital age, where news is instant, thanks to social media, blogs, and search engines, your practice reputation can instantly turn for the worse. The Internet has dramatically altered the way people gather information. Social media has impacted governments, nations, and societies. With the ease of using social media and online reviews, it is likely that a patient, or even a fellow physician, can target your practice and wreak havoc on your reputation. We will provide you with methods to protect yourself.

First, most online reviews of physicians are positive 70–90% of the time [2]. However, most physicians have five or fewer reviews on any site [3]. At a minimum, a physician should monitor their practice reputation by "Googling" their name to identify what information about their practice is already visible online. If you are like most of our colleagues, these reviews will be positive. However, do not be surprised if one or two are negative. Let's face it; even the most well-known and experienced physician cannot possibly satisfy every patient that walks through the door. The easiest way to see what others say about you is to sign up for the free Google Alerts (www.google.com/alerts).

The advantage of these alerts is that you see if it is essential or something you need to investigate further or respond to. You can also set up alerts on Facebook, LinkedIn, YouTube, and Twitter to notify you when messages are posted.

N. Baum, M. J. Kahn, *Business Basics for your Healthcare Practice*,
https://doi.org/10.1007/978-3-032-25241-8_22

One common patient complaint is the wait time to get an appointment. Another frequent complaint is spending too much time waiting in the reception area and exam room to see the doctor. Both issues can be resolved by careful attention to your scheduling process. Patients will even judge their medical experience by how the phone is answered, how long they were left on hold, and if there is ample parking near the office.

When you hear a complaint on more than one occasion, you can be sure that multiple patients have that same negative experience. Still, they are not vocalizing or writing about that negative experience. Therefore, it is imperative to address these negative responses and correct them. These negative reviews provide you with an opportunity to improve your services.

Ethically Creating Positive Reviews

The facts remain that most patients are delighted with their medical care from physicians. However, 40% of negative reviews are related to poor telephone technique and etiquette, failure to obtain access to the practice, and general patient service issues not involving the doctor [4].

Whether we like it or not, online reviews are here to stay. They can significantly impact the perception of your practice from both new and existing patients. In the past, one of us (NB) tried encouraging patients to provide an online review. The patients received a card requesting they go to the review sites and provide us with a favorable review (Fig. 22.1).

This approach was an abysmal failure with a response rate of only 1%. This was hardly worth my (NHB) staff's time to give out the cards. Most physicians are appreciated by their patients. There isn't a day that goes by that most of us don't receive glowing compliments from our patients. (It is one of the best reasons to become a doctor, as no other profession enjoys receiving many compliments from their customers or clients!)

When a patient compliments the doctor or one of the staff members, we ask them if they wouldn't mind posting this on a review site, such as healthgrades.com. Most patients who offer a flattering remark will agree to provide the comment to the online review site. To capture the compliment at the point of service (POS), we use a free kiosk in our office provided by outcomeshealth.com and direct them to leave a review while they are in the exam room. Finally, to make these reviews impactful, we ask the patient to add their name to the review. A review by Kate Smith, San Antonio, is more credible and believable than "KS." When patients compliment the staff or the physicians, ask the patient to make their comment public by submitting their positive comments to one of the many review sites. You will be amazed that a patient pleased with your staff's service will be happy to take 5 min to review your practice.

Consider posting a sign in a prominent location within the office that you appreciate an online review. Just imagine that if you have 20–30 positive reviews for every negative review, what impact that will have on the potential new

Fig. 22.1 Card given to patients to rate their experience with the practice

Thank you for helping us to serve you better!

Was it easy for you to get an appointment in this office? Yes No

Is your general impression of this office favorable? Yes No

Was the office staff friendly and helpful? Yes No

Did the doctor adequately answer your questions? Yes No

Would you recommend this office to someone else? Yes No

Do you have any additional comments?

patient. If the scale swings to the predominance of positive comments, the few negative ones will be drowned out in a sea of compliments that reflect the true nature of your practice.

Managing Negative Reviews

A bad online review is inevitable, just like a lawsuit is part and parcel of the medical profession today. Our advice: do not panic and do not overreact. The reality is, you cannot make everyone happy. If your ratings are mostly positive, there is little reason for concern. Most favorable ratings with a smattering of bad ratings are likely perceived as more credible than 100% five-star ratings. A couple of negative ratings balanced by mostly positive ratings may have the unintended consequence of increasing the positive perception of you and your practice. If the review is off the wall or inappropriate, you should check to see if the comment violates the website's terms of use. Many sites have formulated rules constraining how reviewers should behave. For example, the use of inflammatory language is prohibited.

Suppose you identify that the comment violates the terms of use. In that case, you can submit a letter to the review site of a violation. The site is not obligated to take down the post but might consider honoring the terms of use policy. Suppose you believe the post of the negative comment is inaccurate, and you can identify the post's author. What should you do? We suggest sending a letter or bringing the writer's attention to the fact that their post was incorrect. Then politely request that the writer amend or review the negative post.

Often, a polite request will remedy and correct a negative review. Some sites, like Yelp, allow doctors to privately respond to patient reviews without publicizing their comments. We suggest you respond to negative reviews, especially if the complaint is nonclinical. You can explain how your practice works, but refrain from publicly talking about the specifics of any one patient's experience. You are permitted to do this without violating HIPAA privacy laws.

To be perfectly safe, you should ask patients for their permission to reply publicly to their reviews or, if appropriate, post an apology. Once you have received written consent from the patient, an apology shows that you are listening to patients and taking steps to address their concerns. Going public with your apology potentially turns a negative review into a more constructive experience [5].

Finally, a caveat on paying for positive reviews. We strongly advise against this approach to generate positive reviews. By failing to disclose paid reviews or testimonials, there is a significant legal risk, primarily under the purview of the Federal Trade Commission (FTC).

The FTC views paid reviews as deceptive advertising because they mislead patients into believing the reviews are genuine and unbiased. The FTC's new rule, effective October 21, 2024, specifically bans buying positive or incentivizing reviews, where the incentive is tied to expressing a particular positive opinion. The rule requires that reviews from employees, officers, agents, or their immediate relatives (spouses, parents, children, or siblings) must disclose their relationship to the practice [6].

Greta's Case

Greta did not solicit online reviews, and the couple of negative reviews were only offset by a few positive reviews. Greta became proactive and asked patients if they would provide a review on several online review sites. Within a few weeks, she had dozens of positive reviews, which diluted the two negative reviews.

Bottom Line

Patients are seeking and leaving reviews about you and your practice online. It's time to embrace this digital age and actively manage your online reputation. Do not let one disgruntled patient ruin your reputation. Our advice is to take an active role and generate positive reviews to drown out any negative remarks made by an occasional disgruntled patient. Remember, your reputation is elastic and can be changed.

Key Takeaways

- Regularly check online review sites (e.g., Google, Yelp) to stay informed about patient feedback. Address both positive and negative comments to show engagement and care.
- Encourage satisfied patients to leave reviews by providing excellent service and reminding them of the importance of their feedback.
- Respond to negative reviews in a calm, empathetic manner, offering solutions or apologies when appropriate. This demonstrates your commitment to patient satisfaction and professionalism.
- Take any discussions with a patient who left a scathing review offline.
- Dilute any negative reviews with at least a dozen positive reviews.

References

1. Needham BR. The truth about patient experience: what we can learn from other industries, and how three Ps can improve health outcomes, strengthen brands, and delight customers. J Healthc Manag. 2012;57(4):255–63.
2. Lagu T, Hannon NS, Rothberg MB, Lindenauer PK. Patients' evaluations of health care providers in the era of social networking: an analysis of physician rating websites. J Gen Intern Med. 2010;25(9):942–6.
3. Gunter J. For better or maybe, worse, patients are judging your care online. Obg Manag. 2011;23(3):47–51.7.
4. Tehrani AB, Feldman SR, Camacho FT, Balkrishnan R. Patient satisfaction with outpatient medical care in the United States. Health Out Res Red. 2011;2(4):e197–202.
5. Ventola CL. Social media and health care professionals: benefits, risks, and best practices. Pharm Ther. 2014;39(7):491–9.
6. Stamatos SG. Get ready with me: unveiling the regulatory realities of influencer marketing. BCL Rev. 2025;66:253.

23 Surveying Your Practice: Cost-Effective Methods of Identifying the Needs and Wants of Your Patients

> Those who enter to buy, support me. Those who come to flatter, please me. Those who complain teach me how I may please others so that more will come. Those who are displeased but do not complain only hurt me. They refused me permission to correct my errors and thus improve my service.
> Retailing Pioneer Marshall Field

Case Study
Reginald noticed that his staff reported that patients complained about the long wait times to obtain an appointment. Patients also complained of waiting in the reception area and the exam room for the doctor or medical assistant. Patients complained that their calls were not answered promptly and that the calls were often answered rudely. Reginald also noted that his online reviews were often scathing and were nothing he was proud of. Reginald was at a loss for what he should do.

Start by listening to your patients' impressions of your practice. When you listen, you will learn what patients want and provide them with more of it, and you will understand what they dislike, making every effort to avoid what turns them off. As a result, you will improve your patients' quality of care. Look at your practice through the lens of your patients. A more effective approach is to ask your patients what they think. In this chapter, we introduce techniques to view your practice from the patient's perspective. These will help you assess your current standing with your existing patients and referring physicians. A healthy practice needs to attract new patients. However, you also must keep the patients you already have. Even full or closed practices should evaluate their services periodically and listen to their patients. Changes always occur, and the cup may not "runneth over" forever. Besides, if your patients and staff are satisfied, your work will be more enjoyable, and you will be home for dinner!

Today, knowing the needs and expectations of your patients and referring physicians is critical. This information can be obtained by surveying your practice. A survey will also provide an update on your practice's strengths and weaknesses. This information is readily available to your patients. Patients are a valuable source of information and can help you improve the quality of care you provide. What better place to begin evaluating your practice than to ask what your patients think of you and the service you provide?

Five effective techniques for determining how patients perceive your practice and for evaluating your performance and reputation:

1. Conduct personal interviews.
2. Conduct patient surveys.
3. Create a focus group.
4. Use a suggestion box.
5. Survey your peers.

N. Baum, M. J. Kahn, *Business Basics for your Healthcare Practice*,
https://doi.org/10.1007/978-3-032-25241-8_23

1. Personal Interviews

Ask your patients about their experiences with you and your office staff. This method is the least popular for acquiring information because patients often feel "put on the spot" and will not reveal true feelings during a face-to-face inquiry.

However, informal conversations with your patients can reveal information about your practice. Patients are more likely to respond honestly to specific rather than general questions. You might ask a patient:

- Do you think the time you spent in the reception area (not the "waiting room") was excessive?
- Would you like us to call or fax your prescription to the pharmacy so it will be ready for you when you arrive to pick it up?
- Are you likely to use our website to schedule your appointments with our office and receive reports and lab results without coming in or calling us?
- Would you be interested in having the ability to email questions or concerns to the nurse or the doctor?
- Would you like an electronic copy of your medical record?
- If we had a nutritionist available, would you use their services?

· Would you like us to contact you by phone, text messaging, or email?

· Would you like to pay your bill online or at the time of service?

When you ask questions like these, you demonstrate concern for your patients' time and finances, and the answers will likely be helpful. You could also conduct a survey focusing on how promptly you see patients and how long they wait in the reception area or exam room before being seen by a physician.

2. Patient Surveys

Written patient surveys are the most popular method for obtaining patient feedback. You can give written surveys to patients during their office visits or send the survey to their email. The advantages of sending the survey via email are that the patients can remain anonymous and complete the survey at their leisure. The disadvantages are that once patients leave the office setting, they are not likely to return the surveys.

What to Ask

The survey should be short and require no more than 3–5 min to complete. The survey should be limited to both sides of a single 8 1/2 × 11-inch piece of paper or, if completed online, to one or two screens. Begin with an opening paragraph (see Fig. 23.1) that states the purpose of the survey (i.e., to evaluate your practice's strengths and weaknesses and ultimately provide better health care for your patients). Yes/no or multiple-choice questions are the easiest to quantify.

Suggested questions include:

- Do I see you on time for your appointments?
- Is my office staff friendly and courteous?
- Are my office hours convenient?
- Is it easy to make an appointment?
- Do my staff and I return phone calls in a timely fashion?
- Would you like me to provide you with the opportunity to purchase your medications in the office if the prices were competitive with local pharmacies?

We recommend avoiding questions about your fees, as most patients consider medical fees too high. Finally, you can conclude with an

Dear Patient:

My staff and I want to provide you and your family with the highest quality healthcare possible. To help us evaluate our effectiveness, we would like your opinions of my practice.

Your answers and suggestions on the following questionnaire will help us continue to improve the healthcare we provide you. Please take a few minutes to give us this important information and return it to us in the enclosed stamped, self-addressed envelope.

Thank you,

Dr. Neil H. Baum and staff

Fig. 23.1 Sample cover letter to accompany patient survey

open-ended question: "What can I do to make your experience with my office more pleasant?"

Whom to Include

Choose a cross section of patients if you choose to email your survey. Include some active and inactive patients and patients who have left your practice. Also, consider various age groups, from millennials to older, retired patients.

Customizing the Survey

Instruct patients to return the survey to your personal email address. If the survey is returned to your office and contains critical or negative comments regarding your office personnel, it may not reach your attention. If patients experience problems with your staff, you want to be made aware of those issues. Another option is to use an electronic survey tool, such as SurveyMonkey.com.

Implementing the Survey

We recommend that you survey your patients at least once every 2 years. According to the American Medical Association, one good rule of thumb is to study at least 20% of your existing patients [1]. It is also beneficial to survey inactive patients, as you will often obtain valuable information about your practice. You may learn why they are no longer patients or don't return for follow-up care. The physician should personally review all the surveys. Keep an open mind as you do this, remembering that the purpose is to improve your practice. Even though you may get criticisms, most comments will probably be positive. But it's the criticisms that will help make improvements to your practice.

Tabulating the Results

We recommend keeping your surveys simple. Most of them have yes-or-no answers. Easy-to-complete surveys make tabulating the results easy and less time-consuming. Tabulation counts the number of responses received and the number of yes or no answers for each question.

Using the Results

You have worked hard to devise a concise patient survey. Several patients have emailed them to you. Do not relegate these valuable letters to your email's "black hole." Those survey comments and answers are a gold mine. Now, you must address the concerns. Your practice will stand out not only to those who took the time to answer the survey but also to the rest of the patients already in your practice.

It is essential to prioritize the comments received from the survey. If your survey indicates that a significant percentage of patients feel they were waiting for long periods, then that issue must be addressed first. On the other hand, if only one or two people claim your office hours are inconvenient, that issue can be lower on the list. A staff meeting is the best time and place to address the survey results. For instance, a survey revealed complaints about office delays. This complaint is an opportunity to brainstorm possible solutions. A solution might consider inviting a local dentist with a reputation for being on time with their patients to a "lunch-and-learn" program. The dentist may provide suggestions for improving time management in your office. You are likely to find ideas from that meeting regarding patient scheduling and how to manage urgencies and emergencies.

One response from a survey was that a patient had a late-afternoon appointment on several occasions and found the patient's restroom to be untidy. The office manager examined the situation for a few days and discovered that the wastepaper baskets were overflowing with paper towels and that a urine specimen cup had spilled, but it had not been cleaned up. Now, the staff checks the restroom right after lunch and again in the middle of the afternoon. The goal was to ensure that the patient who had the last day's appointment encountered the same clean restroom as the first patient in the morning. Without a survey, this problem might have gone unnoticed.

Focus Groups

With a focus group, the most crucial step is selecting the participants. An effective focus group consists of a cross section of diverse, opinionated, and vocal individuals who are willing to provide honest feedback about your practice. When selecting participants for a focus group, choose patients who are keen observers and complainers. Avoid "yes" people. The purpose of the focus group is not to hear how wonderful you are. It is really to troubleshoot your practice, which is why you want vocal, articulate complainers as your participants.

Invitations and Reminders

Once participants for the focus group are selected, the best results will occur if the doctor or office manager calls each patient and personally invites them to assist in evaluating your practice. Then, send an email note that includes the purpose of the focus group and an agenda for participants to consider before the meeting (Fig. 23.2 is a sample email invitation to join the focus group). The day before the focus group, have your office staff call and remind the participants of the meeting.

It is convenient to hold the meeting in your reception room. We suggest limiting the discussion to ninety minutes. Provide coffee, soft drinks, and dessert. Pay the parking fees or, in the case of participants who prefer not to drive at night, pay for the taxi fare to and from the meeting. Ask permission to tape-record the meeting, so you are not distracted by having to take notes.

Letter to Establish Focus Group

Dear [Patient],

I hope this letter finds you well and enjoying your summer. I am writing to a select group of people in my practice that I especially enjoy serving to ask a favor. At a recent staff meeting we were discussing how blessed we are to be serving so many people who truly appreciate us and from whom we receive so many positive compliments about the quality of our medical care. I want you to know how much I appreciate you, but I do not feel I have resourced you as much as I possibly should.

As you know, I and my staff strive to stay up with the latest advances and to upgrade the level of medical care continually. For a practice to be truly excellent, the technical care, skill, and judgment must conform to the very highest standards, but that alone is not enough.

There are numerous other factors that come into play to make your experience truly excellent, and this is where I need your help. I would like you to be a part of a small group of people selected to provide specific feedback on how I and my staff are doing. I would appreciate about an hour and a half of your time on Tuesday, August 2, from 7:30 to 8:45 in the evening at my office. Refreshments and light snacks will be served. I would like to discuss the following questions:

1. What do you feel are the strengths of my practice?
2. What do you feel are the weaknesses of my practice?
3. Do you think weekend, early morning or evening appointments would be helpful?
4. Do you have any problems making an appointment?
5. Are there any services that you feel I should add that would make my practice more attractive?
6. Are you satisfied with the referrals I make to other physicians?

Fig. 23.2 Letter to establish focus group

7. Are there any other suggestions you have to improve the quality of your experience with me or my office?

I will be calling you in a few days to confirm that you will join us. Thank you for your participation and support.

Sincerely,

Neil Baum, MD

Fig. 23.2 (continued)

Running the Meeting

After introductions, briefly reiterate your reasons for inviting participants to your office. Solicit examples from them of excellent customer service. Request ideas for improvement based on their experiences at other medical offices and businesses. Ask open-ended questions, not those that can be answered with a simple yes or no.

Weekend office hours may not be practical for some physicians. For example, one focus group revealed that several patients were interested in evening and weekend office hours. One solution was to have Saturday morning hours when one of the doctors was on call. The other doctors in the practice agreed with this idea. Now, weekends are covered, and one doctor can see patients in their office.

We also learned that patients preferred not to pay to park under our building. Another finding from one of the participants claimed that most other hospitals and doctors' offices did not charge for parking services. This problem was solved by validating parking for office appointments.

Another key finding from the focus groups was that patients needed assistance in determining where to go to pay their bills and schedule subsequent appointments. This feedback demonstrated the need for better signage. The solution to the signage problem was to provide signs at the practice's business office and at all locations where exit signs were visible.

Follow-Up

After conducting a focus group, consider sending or emailing each participant a thank-you note. It is essential to let each person know you appreciate their time and their opinions. Whenever the focus group generates a change, acknowledge that their suggestions were implemented.

Suggestion Box

The suggestion box is a time-honored and inexpensive method of obtaining valuable feedback about patients' experiences in the office. Consider placing a suggestion box in the reception area. Place a sign on the suggestion box stating, "Please let us know what we can do to improve our service to you" (Fig. 23.3. Is the 3 × 5 card used in one (NB) of our practices) Include pencils and 3 × 5 index cards. Patients have the option to sign their names or remain anonymous. The essential responsibility is to check the suggestion box *daily*. Do not treat the suggestion box as fluff or window dressing. Take it seriously and make it a functional part of your ongoing practice survey techniques.

If patients sign their names, call them, thank them for their suggestions, and respond to them within one to two days of their office visit. Let them know the follow-up on their suggestions, especially if you implement one of their ideas.

Fig. 23.3 Sample survey card placed in the suggestion box in the reception area

Thank you for helping us to serve you better!

1. Was it easy for you to get an appointment in this office?
   ____ Yes ____ No
2. Is your general impression of this office favorable?
   ____ Yes ____ No
3. Was the office staff friendly and concerned?
   ____ Yes ____ No
4. Did the doctor adequately answer your questions?
   ____ Yes ____ No
5. Would you recommend this office to someone else?
   ____ Yes ____ No
6. Do you have any additional comments?
   ____
   ____

Survey Your Peers

Finally, you want to evaluate or survey your referring physicians. A written or verbal survey can determine your colleagues' experiences and opinions. Holding an informal meeting is the easiest and most comfortable method. For this method to succeed, the feedback must go both ways. In addition to soliciting critiques of your practice, you should provide your colleagues with constructive comments regarding their practices. Most physicians will be pleasantly surprised by how valuable candid conversations with peers can be.

For example, while field testing a computerized referral letter with colleagues, the response was unanimous approval of the concept. Subsequently, a few colleagues adopted the idea of using a computerized letter in their practices. (See Chap. 10 for more information on the computerized referral letter.

A survey of colleagues does not have to be as formalized as a written patient survey. You can select physicians with whom you feel comfortable. Ask them to meet you for lunch or for coffee.

You want to know if the reports are arriving in a timely fashion. We suggest approaching a cross section of colleagues, including some older physicians, contemporaries, and a few younger physicians. You want to ask whether they received feedback from the patients they sent to you and your practice. Ask if there's anything you can do to make your practice more user-friendly.

For example, a physician related that one of his pet peeves was that the office would call him to discuss a patient, and the doctor was on hold for 15–30 s before the staff placed the doctor on the line. "Look," he said, "this is just one of my quirks. I can't explain it. I know it isn't necessarily right, but it galls me. Know that that's one of my quirks. Please respect it and be on the phone when your office calls me." That way, whoever places the call to this doctor must be sure that the caller is immediately available to take the call.

These discussions with your peers can be informal. Explain to your colleagues, "Look, we send patients back and forth. I want to improve, and I can only do that if you provide me with feedback on my performance. If there's anything I can do to improve the practice and give you better service, please let me know."

Consider using this list of questions to survey your peers:

- If you need a consult immediately, has your patient been seen on time?
- Is my office friendly to your patients?
- Do I get my referral notes back to you on time?
- Do you feel that my office is user-friendly?
- Are there any problems you are having that I need to know about?

The take-home message is letting colleagues know that you are serious about enhancing your service to their patients. Send a follow-up thank-you note to those physicians who agree to provide feedback.

We recommend repeating this process every six to twelve months to stay informed about what referring physicians think of your practice. At a minimum, survey the physicians who refer the most patients to your practice. In primary care, consider surveying the specialists you refer to frequently. We recommend tracking your top referral sources if you are a specialist. Suppose you notice a good referral source who previously sent 3–5 patients a month has not sent you a patient in a few months. Schedule a meeting with the doctor or office to determine if there is a problem and explore potential solutions. For example, if a referring physician had not sent any patients for several months, contact that physician and ask if there was a problem. You may find that the referring physician's office staff had difficulty scheduling appointments at your office for their patients. Suppose the physician commented that their patients were very busy and couldn't take time off for medical appointments. Perhaps you can provide their office with your back-office telephone line, which is a direct line to the scheduler, and offer their patients same-day appointments. You may inform the referring physician that you now provide telemedicine appointments when it is unnecessary to examine the patient in person. (See Chap. 22 on telemedicine) You may not be able to provide that service to all referring doctors, but you can make an exception for a good referral source.

Asking the Platinum Question

Whether it's one of your patients or colleagues, you need to ask the platinum question, as Ed Koch, the former mayor of New York City, did. The mayor would routinely walk the streets and ask New Yorkers the platinum question: "How'm I doin'? How can I get better?"4.

Follow-Up on Reginald

Reginald began conducting a survey of his patients' experiences with his office. Reginald learned what his patients were experiencing when they called his office for an appointment. He hired a focus group evaluator who conducted several focus groups of his existing patients. The survey results and the feedback from the focus groups were evaluated. Reginald discovered what could be done to resolve many of the complaints and took action to correct the problems. As a result, his patients were happier, his staff was less stressed, his online reviews improved, and Reginald was more content with his practice.

The Bottom Line

When you solicit honest feedback from your patients and referring physicians, you may get surprises. If you listen to and learn from their responses and implement their suggestions, you will improve both the quality of the care you provide and the quality of your bottom line.

Key Takeaways

- It is necessary to periodically survey or ask your patients about their experience in the practice.
- There are five techniques that are effective to survey your patients: personal interviews, patient surveys, focus group, suggestion box, and your peers and colleagues.
- By asking the platinum question, "How'm I doin'?" ensures that you are listening to your patients and making an effort to improve your services.

References

1. Bujang MA. A step-by-step process on sample size determination for medical research. Malays J Med Sci. 2021;28(2):15–27.

Additional Resources on Surveying Patients

2. Press I. Patient satisfaction: understanding and managing the experience of care. 2nd ed. Ann Arbor: Health Administration Press; 2005.
3. Diering SL. Love your patients! Improving patient satisfaction with essential behaviors that enrich the lives of patients and professionals. Nevada City: Blue Dolphin Publishing; 2004.
4. Baker SK. Managing patient expectations: the art of finding and keeping loyal patients. San Francisco: Jossey-Bass; 1998.
5. Sullivan K, Luallin MD. Star-studded service: 6 steps to winning patient satisfaction. Denver: Medical Group Management Association (MGMA; 2007.
6. Mackay H. Swim with the sharks without being eaten alive. New York: Ballantine Books; 1988.
7. LeBoeuf M. How to win customers and keep them for life. New York: Berkley Books; 1989.

24 The Use of AI/GPT-4 and Its Implementation into Any Medical Practice

Tanya's Story
Tanya is a new associate in a small primary care practice. In undergraduate school, she majored in computer science and was comfortable using AI. Tanya's practice had a website but no experience with artificial intelligence. Tanya's senior partners asked her to help their practice use AI for several administrative tasks, such as online scheduling and creating content for the practice's website. How did Tanya do it?

What Is GPT-4?

GPT-4 (generative pretrained transformer) is a powerful technology that can help with multiple complex tasks, from conducting time-consuming office functions to digitizing the doctor-patient encounter in the EMR to writing referral letters to colleagues to finding clinical research sites for patients.

GPT-4 manages specific instructions that can be fine-tuned to be easy to understand content even in multiple languages.

GPT-4 can adapt to the emotions, ethnicity, and background of those entering the requests, giving the program the feel of interacting with another human. Unlike previous models, GPT-4 can interpret images. The program can generate text from visual images like imaging studies, pathology slides, graphs, and diagrams. After viewing an image, it writes a caption in the user's tone or emotion.

GPT-4 is more accurate than previous iterations of artificial intelligence. However, It still invents facts—or hallucinates—and should not be used without fact-checking, particularly for medical decision-making where accuracy is essential.

GPT-4 in healthcare is like developing a new treatment plan for a patient.

As a healthcare professional, when a new patient enters your office, you listen to their symptoms, take a medical history and lifestyle factors, and conduct a physical examination. Based on these inputs and leveraging your medical knowledge and experience, you "generate" a unique treatment plan suitable for that patient. GPT-4 contains a large amount of data, and based on the patterns and information it learns from this data, it can create or "generate" a treatment plan that includes benefits and adverse events for each option.

Although OPENAI.com is free, an inexpensive subscription to GPT-4 may better serve a busy medical practice. This large language model is more accurate when responding to free-form queries. Most technologists believe that GPT-4 has proven to be superior to publicly available programs.

In healthcare, this could mean several options. For example, it could be used to:

N. Baum, M. J. Kahn, *Business Basics for your Healthcare Practice*,
https://doi.org/10.1007/978-3-032-25241-8_24

Generate New Drug Molecules GPT-4 can learn from the structures and effectiveness of existing drugs and create new ones that could be more effective or have fewer side effects.

Create Realistic Medical Images For training or diagnostic purposes, technology can learn from existing medical images (mammograms, like MRI or CT scans) and generate new ones that can represent various disease states or patient conditions.

Predict Disease Progression Based on a patient's medical history and status, GPT-4 can simulate different scenarios to predict how a disease might progress, helping doctors plan treatments more effectively.

Personalized Treatments Like creating a unique or precise treatment plan for a patient, GPT-4 can help design personalized therapies based on a patient's genetic makeup, lifestyle, and other factors, such as co-morbid conditions.

Coding and Classification GPT-4 can assist with coding, so you receive appropriate reimbursement for services you provided to the patient, and with identifying the correct codes for diagnosis/treatment procedures for billing purposes. This function may significantly reduce the common insurance denials in many medical practices.

Communication GPT-4 chatbots can handle routine patient inquiries, reducing the workload on administrative staff. For example, patients have questions that require time and energy from the staff and the physicians. These FAQs (frequently asked questions) can be adequately answered using GPT-4. As you draw on your medical knowledge to provide the best patient care, GPT-4 uses what it's learned from its training data to generate new insights, solutions, or tools. It's a powerful technology with many potential applications in healthcare.

Finally, it may assist with many administrative tasks, including managing appointment scheduling, billing, claims processing, and data entry.

Despite these promising applications, GPT-4 doesn't replace healthcare professionals.

Instead, it's a tool that can assist and augment your expertise, helping to make the practice more efficient and patient care more effective.

History of Innovation and GPT-4

In November 2022, OpenAI publicly launched its large language model GPT. It reached the milestone of 100 million users in only 2 months. Reaching the same milestone took TikTok and Instagram 9 months and more than 2 years, respectively. In March 2023, OpenAI released a new version, GPT-4, that is more advanced than its predecessor.

The adoption of GPT-4 will be like what we experienced with multiple technological revolutions over the past centuries or decades. Computers took over many tasks from humans—accountants don't have to do all the calculations for a giant firm on a notebook with a pencil anymore—but computers didn't replace accountants; they gave them advanced computational skills. Computers also created new jobs—jobs we never knew existed in 1980—that would exist in the future. This process of GPT-4 adoption will not be different from what we experienced with multiple technological revolutions over the past centuries or decades. A similar shift is expected, with GPT-4 improving specific tasks in medical offices.

How Does GPT-4 Work?

GPT-4 is a significant advance over previous OpenAI models, particularly in how it handles complex and subtle user requests. More than earlier GPT models, GPT-4 can adapt to specific tones of voice, emotions, dialects, user demographics, and cultural backgrounds. GPT-4 can also generate computer code, process images, and interpret twenty-six languages.

These are 11 examples of GPT-4 capabilities that can be easily implemented in almost any medical practice and will certainly enhance its productivity and efficiency.

Digitalizing the Doctor-Patient Encounter, Going "Scribe-less"

Several EMRs claim to record and transcribe meetings or conversations automatically,

analyze the content, and provide an easy-to-understand, searchable report. Although certain software companies offer services, such as the ability to transcribe a patient encounter, a GPT-4 transcription is reviewed for accuracy and includes CPT codes for the visit. This application might reduce burdens on medical professionals and reduce excessive administrative tasks, which significantly contribute to physician burnout [1].

Figure 24.1 is a recorded voice-to-text of a doctor-patient encounter. Figure 24.2 is a digitized doctor-patient encounter that can be added to the patient's EMR. Figure 24.3 is a post-visit summary sent to the patient. Figure 24.4 is a request for proper coding for the visit. Figure 24.5 is a post-consultation letter sent to the patient's referring physician.

GPT-4 can be used to critique the doctor's communication with their patients. Figure 24.6 requests a critique and evaluation of my (NHB) encounter with the patient, Mr. Jones. This is an opportunity for the program to review the questions I asked and evaluate my responses. This takes GPT-4 to a new level, helping physicians to improve patient communication. It is unfortunate that no one ever evaluates a doctor upon leaving medical school and training. Now, without a proctor or another colleague in the room with the doctor and the patient, an evaluation can enhance the doctor's skills for taking a history and conducting a physical examination. Also, the feedback is immediate.

Urologist: Good morning, Mr. Jones I'm Dr. Baum, the urologist. How are you today?

Patient: Good morning, Dr. Baum. I'm doing okay, thank you.

Urologist: Great to hear. I see from your records that you're here for a follow-up regarding your urinary issues and difficulty with urination. Can you please update me on how you've been feeling since our last appointment?

Patient: Well, I've still been experiencing some mild discomfort, getting up at night, and urgency when I urinate. It's not as bad as before, but it hasn't completely gone away.

Urologist: Thank you for letting me know. Have there been any changes in the frequency or color of your urine? Any pain or blood?

Patient: No, the frequency is about the same, and the color seems normal. No pain or blood that I've noticed.

Urologist: Okay. Let's discuss any changes to your medical history or medications since our last meeting. Have there been any updates?

Urologist: Tell me about any problems you have regarding intimacy with your partner.

Patient: I'm still taking the medication, finasteride, that you prescribed, and I haven't started any new medications. I am taking finasteride, 5mg, once a day. I have noted some difficulty with my sexual performance. My sex drive also is decreased, and I fall asleep after my dinner meal.

Urologist: Good to know. Now, let's move on to a physical examination. I'll need you to provide a urine sample for analysis, and then we'll proceed with a prostate examination.

Fig. 24.1 Is a voice-to-text recording of a follow-up encounter between a urologist and a patient, Mr. Jones

Patient: Sure, no problem.

[The patient provides a urine sample, and the urologist conducts a physical examination.]

Urologist: The physical examination looks relatively stable. Your blood pressure is 135\75 which is excellent. You have a regular pulse and respirations. Your temperature is 98.6 F. Your weight is stable at 175lbs. Your heart and lungs are normal. You have a moderate enlargement of your prostate gland. It is approximately 40 grams which is normal for your age. Your penis and testicular exam and unremarkable. There are no findings on the digital rectal exam to suggest cancer of the prostate. I'll send the urine sample for analysis. Because of your decreased sex drive, I will suggest a serum testosterone level which should be obtained firs thing in the morning. There is no need to be fasting for this test. I also suggest an annual PSA test and I recommend no sexual intimacy for two days before this test is taken. I will ask you to return in 3 weeks and we'll review the results of the PSA and testosterone at your next visit in a few weeks. We also need to have your annual PSA blood test. Do you have any concerns or questions on your end?

Patient: I've been wondering about the potential side effects of the medication. Are there any I should be aware of?

Urologist: It's common to experience some mild side such as a decrease in volume of your ejaculation but based on your medical history, serious side effects are unlikely. If you notice anything unusual, though, please let me know.

Patient: Will do. Thanks, Dr. Baum.

Urologist: You're welcome. We'll discuss the urine analysis, your PSA level, and a testosterone level results ay our next appointment. Feel free to reach out if there are any significant changes or if you have questions before then. Take care, and I'll see you soon. I am providing you with information on the use of finasteride.

Fig. 24.1 (continued)

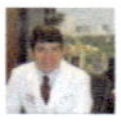

You

Please prepare this audio recorded encounter of Mr. Jones with Dr. Baum for Mr. Robert Jones' EMR.

ChatGPT

ChatGPT

I've documented the encounter between Mr. Smith and Dr. Baum on 1-7-2024 for Mr. Jones' EMR. Here's a summary:

Patient Encounter Summary

Patient Information:

- Name: Mr. Robert Jones
- Age: 57
- Weight: 165 lbs
- Temperature: 98.0°F
- Blood Pressure: 135/75
- Pulse: 88

Chief Complaint:

- Follow-up for urinary issues and difficulty with urination.

Medical History:

- Mild discomfort, nocturia, and urgency persist.
- No changes in urine frequency, color, pain, or blood.
- Taking finasteride 5mg once a day.
- Difficulty with sexual performance and decreased sex drive noted.

Physical Examination:

Fig. 24.2 Is a conversion of the audio communication to a digital record for the patient's EMR

- Stable vital signs.
- Prostate enlargement of approximately 40 grams, no nodules in the prostate or masses found in the rectum
- Urine sample provided for analysis.
- No abnormalities in penis, testicles, or digital rectal exam.

Plan:

1. Urine sample sent for analysis.
2. Serum testosterone level test recommended.
3. Annual PSA blood test suggested.
4. Follow-up appointment in 3 weeks to review results.

Medication Discussion:

- Finasteride may cause a decrease in ejaculation volume.
- Serious side effects deemed unlikely based on medical history.

Patient Instructions:

- Obtain serum testosterone level test.
- Schedule annual PSA blood test.
- Avoid sexual intimacy two days before the PSA test.
- Return for follow-up in 3 weeks.

Follow-up:

- Discuss urine analysis, PSA, and testosterone results at the next appointment.
- Report any significant changes or concerns before the follow-up.

Patient Concerns:

- Inquired about potential side effects of finasteride.
- Advised to report any unusual observations.

Closing Remarks:

- Dr. Baum provided information on the use of finasteride.
- Encouraged the patient to reach out with any questions.

Fig. 24.2 (continued)

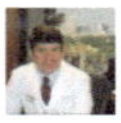

You

What CPT code should be used for this encounter

ChatGPT

ChatGPT

I'm not a certified coder, but I can provide you with a general suggestion. The appropriate Current Procedural Terminology (CPT) codes for this urology encounter may include:

1. **Evaluation and Management (E/M) Code:**
    - An E/M code based on the complexity of the visit, such as a comprehensive office visit code (e.g., 99204) considering the detailed history, examination, and medical decision-making involved.

    CPT Code for Digital Rectal Exam: 99213-25

    •
2. **Urine Sample Analysis:**
    - Depending on the specific procedures involved in the urine sample analysis, you might use a relevant laboratory testing code, CPT Code for Urinalysis: 81002
3. **Prostate Examination:**
    - Use the appropriate code for the digital rectal examination (e.g., digital rectal examination; physician provides screening).
4. **Serum Testosterone Level Test:**

    CPT Code for Testosterone: 84403
5. **Annual PSA Blood Test:** CPT Code for PSA: 84153

Remember to check with a certified medical coder or billing specialist to ensure accurate coding and compliance with current coding guidelines. The codes may vary based on specific documentation details and regional variations.

Fig. 24.3 Is a request for the CPT code for the encounter

Would you please provide an after-visit summary that I might send the patient?

ChatGPT

ChatGPT

Certainly! Here's an after-visit summary that you can consider sending to the Mr. Jones:

Subject: Summary of Your Recent Urology Appointment

Dear Mr. Jones,

Following our recent urology appointment, I wanted to provide you with a summary of our discussion and the plan moving forward.

Date of Visit: January 7, 2024

Key Points:

1. **Symptoms Update:** During our conversation, you shared that you are still experiencing some discomfort and urgency during urination. I appreciate your openness in providing this information.
2. **Urine Sample and Physical Examination:** You cooperated well during the physical examination, and I'm pleased to inform you that the examination revealed relatively stable findings. The urine sample has been sent for analysis to provide additional insights into your condition.
3. **Medication Update:** I understand that you have been consistent with the prescribed medication, and I appreciate your commitment to the treatment plan.
4. **Potential Side Effects:** You inquired about potential side effects of the medication. While it's common to experience mild side effects like nausea or dizziness, serious side effects are unlikely based on

Fig. 24.4 Is a post-visit summary that was e-mailed to the patient your medical history. Remember to reach out if you notice anything unusual.

Next Steps:

1. **Urine Analysis Results:** We will discuss the results of the urine analysis in our upcoming follow-up appointment scheduled in three weeks. This will help us better understand your current situation and guide any necessary adjustments to your treatment plan.
2. **Monitoring:** In the meantime, continue with the prescribed medication, Proscar, 5mg\day

If there are any significant changes or if you have questions or concerns, please feel free to give me a call.

To Your Good Health,
Dr. Neil Baum

Fig. 24.4 (continued)

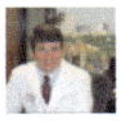

You

Please prepare a letter to send to patient's referring physician, Dr. Tom Meredith

ChatGPT

ChatGPT

Dr. Neil Baum, 3525 Prytania , New Orleans, LA 70118

January 7, 2024

Dr. Tom Meredith, Internal Medical Associates of New Orleans, 1821 Napoleon Ave, New Orleans, Louisiana 70118

Subject: Follow-Up on Patient Referral – Robert Jones

Dear Dr. Tom,

I am writing to provide an update on your patient, Robert Jones, whom you referred to our urology clinic. Our recent appointment aimed to address the urinary issues you identified in your referral.

During the evaluation, Mr. Jones reported ongoing discomfort and urgency during urination. We conducted a thorough physical examination, and a urine sample was collected for analysis. The results of the analysis will be discussed in a follow-up appointment, scheduled for January 28, 2024.

Mr. Jones medical history remains stable, and he has been compliant with the prescribed medication, Proscar 5mg\day. We appreciate the detailed information provided in your referral, which has been instrumental in guiding our assessment and management.

If there are specific aspects of Mr. Jones' care that you would like us to focus on or if you have any additional insights, please do not hesitate to reach out. We believe in maintaining a collaborative approach to patient care and value the input of our referring colleagues.

Fig. 24.5 Is a letter sent to Mr. Jones' referring physician, Dr. Tom Meredith

We will ensure to keep you updated on Mr. Jones' progress and any significant findings. Should you have any questions or concerns in the meantime, feel free to contact our office at 504-891-8454.

Thank you for entrusting us with the care of Mr. Jones. We look forward to continuing this collaborative effort for the benefit of the patient.

Warm regards,

Dr. Neil Baum

Fig. 24.5 (continued)

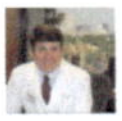

You

Would you please critique my encounter with Mr. Jones and what I could do to make the encounter more meaningful and helpful to Mr. Jones?

ChatGPT

ChatGPT

Overall, the encounter between you and the Mr. Jones seems professional, thorough, and considerate. However, here are some points for critique and suggestions for improvement:

1. **Empathy and Engagement:**
   - Dr. Baum does a good job of greeting the patient and expressing genuine interest in their well-being. However, there could be more explicit expressions of empathy, especially when the patient mentions experiencing discomfort and issues with intimacy. Dr. Baum could show empathy by acknowledging the patient's concerns and expressing understanding.
2. **Patient Understanding:**
   - While the urologist asks about changes in medical history or medications, there could be more focus on the patient's lifestyle and habits. For example, inquiring about dietary changes, stress levels, or other factors that might contribute to urinary issues could provide a more holistic understanding.
3. **Communication of Findings:**
   - Dr. Baum effectively communicates the results of the physical examination, but it might be beneficial to explain the significance of the findings in simpler terms for the patient's understanding. Providing more context about the prostate enlargement and the

Fig. 24.6 Is a request to GPT-4 to evaluate my encounter with the patient and what could I do to make a more meaningful visit for Mr. Jones

implications (or lack thereof) for the patient's overall health could enhance patient education.

4. **Medication Side Effects:**
    - The patient raises concerns about the potential side effects of the prescribed medication, but the urologist's response could be more detailed. Dr. Baum might discuss common side effects, how to manage them, and emphasize the importance of reporting any unusual symptoms promptly.

5. **Follow-up Instructions:**
    - Dr. Baum does well in scheduling the next appointment and mentioning the upcoming discussions. However, it might be helpful to provide the patient with written or summarized instructions, including details about the annual PSA blood test and any specific actions the patient needs to take before the next visit.

6. **Encouraging Questions:**
    - While Dr. Baum encourages the patient to reach out with concerns, explicitly inviting questions during the appointment could empower the patient to actively participate in their healthcare. This can enhance communication and ensure that the patient feels comfortable seeking clarification.

7. **Closing:**
    - The closing is friendly, but Dr. Baum could reiterate their availability for questions or concerns between appointments. Providing contact information or preferred communication channels reinforces the patient's ability to reach out when needed.

Improvements in these areas can enhance the patient experience, foster better communication, and contribute to a more meaningful and helpful encounter.

Fig. 24.6 (continued)

Prior Authorization (PA) Obtained in Minutes, Not Hours

According to a 2023 Medical Group Management Association (MGMA) report, 89% of doctors rated prior authorization (PA) requirements as extremely burdensome, and 97% of practices reported that their patients had experienced delays or denials for medically necessary care due to delays in obtaining PA [2].

Obtaining prior authorization for a patient before being seen by the physician, requesting permission for a procedure, or obtaining consent to use prescribed medication is the bane of most medical practices. It is time-consuming and expensive, as your practice must gain permission to provide medical care at this uncompensated time. The process can also result in treatment delays [3]. Because of the volume of PAs, doctors must complete practices, which are forced to hire dedicated staff to handle prior authorizations rather than invest in staff or tools to enhance patient care.

Usually, the practice will initiate the prior authorization process by completing a form and submitting it to the insurance company. This process can take from 1 to several hours of uncompensated time per PA.

Using GPT-4, this lengthy and cumbersome process can be reduced from one to two hours to a few minutes. This is accomplished by entering the pertinent patient information and the reason for the request into the GPT-4 program's text box. Figure 24.7 is a prompt given to United Healthcare requesting a multiparametric MRI for evaluation of a rising PSA in a patient at risk for prostate cancer.

The response from GPT-4 is shown in Fig. 24.8. This request was faxed to the insurance company, and approval was obtained within 24 h. Thus, a lengthy process involving the staff and the doctor was reduced to minutes.

ChatGPT-4

ChatGPT-4

Subject: Request for Multiparametric MRI and Prostate Biopsy for Patient John Doe

Membership ID 12345678

Dr. Neil Baum, 3525 Prytania St. New Orleans, Louisiana

January 17, 2024

United Healthcare

Re: Patient: John Doe Membership ID: 12345678 Date of Birth: 3/1/1970

Dear United Healthcare,

I am writing to request authorization for further diagnostic procedures for my patient, John Doe, who is covered under United Health with the membership ID 12345678.

Mr. John Doe recently underwent a prostate-specific antigen (PSA) test, which revealed an elevated PSA level of 8.3 ng/ml. Additionally, the free/total PSA ratio was found to be 19%, below the normal threshold of 25%. Given these results, I am requesting approval for both a multiparametric MRI and a prostate biopsy to complete his evaluation for prostate cancer.

Recent studies and clinical guidelines support the use of multiparametric MRI in conjunction with prostate biopsy to enhance the detection and characterization of prostate cancer. This approach has shown to improve diagnostic accuracy and aid in treatment decision-making. I believe that these procedures are essential for a comprehensive evaluation of Mr. Doe's prostate health.

I kindly request that United Health consider and approve the authorization for the multiparametric MRI and prostate biopsy for Mr. John Doe. The timely

Fig. 24.7 Is a request for a prior authorization

completion of these procedures is crucial for an accurate diagnosis and appropriate management of his condition.

In support of this request, I am willing to provide any additional documentation, clinical notes, or relevant information needed for the review process. If there are specific forms or procedures required by United Health, please inform me so that I can promptly comply.

Furthermore, I would appreciate it if you could provide me with recent references regarding the appropriateness of multiparametric MRI and prostate biopsy in cases like that of Mr. Doe.

Thank you for your prompt attention to this matter. I value your collaboration in ensuring the best possible care for our mutual patient. Please feel free to contact me directly if you require any further information or clarification.

Sincerely,

Dr. Neil Baum, Professor of Clinical Urology at Tulane Medical School, New Orleans, Louisiana

Fig. 24.7 (continued)

Dear United Healthcare,
I am writing to request approval for a multiparametric MRI and prostate biopsy for patient John Doe, who holds a membership ID of 123456789 and was born on 3\1\1970.
Upon examination, Mr. Doe's PSA levels were found to be elevated at 8.3ng\ml, with a free\total PSA ratio of 19% (normal is greater than 25%). Given these findings, I strongly recommend a multiparametric MRI and prostate biopsy to assess the condition of Mr. Doe's prostate gland and determine if further treatment is necessary.
I request that you approve this study for Mr. Doe's benefit and ensure that he receives the care he needs.
I am including recent references that document the appropriateness of mpMRI in the management of men with an elevated PSA level. These are references from peer-reviewed literature on the value of mpMRI in the management of patients with elevated PSA levels. I believe it is essential to remain up to date on the latest advancements and recommendations in the field.
Thank you for your attention to this matter. Please do not hesitate to contact me if you have any questions or require additional information.
Sincerely,
Dr. Neil Baum
c.c. John Doe

Fig. 24.8 Is letter created by ChatGPT to United Healthcare requesting prior authorization

Managing Negative Online Reviews

Nothing is more ego-deflating than to receive a scathing response from a patient who had a less-than-optimal experience with my practice. We walk a tightrope when responding without identifying the patient or their medical condition or becoming defensive, which may worsen the relationship. My goal is to provide an explanation while preserving the doctor-patient relationship.

Imagine that you receive a negative review from a patient regarding informed consent.

Figure 24.9 is a request to GPT-4 for a letter to the patient and the online review site. Figure 24.10 is a request to GPT-4 for a suggestion to respond to a patient who wrote a negative review. This is followed by GPT-4's response and a letter to the online review site.

You will likely receive a negative review during your career. As physicians, we spend our entire professional life protecting our reputation. It is possible for a patient, with just a few clicks and a negative review, to tarnish a reputation that we have worked so hard to protect. We might hesitate to engage with any online review sites. However, responding to all negative reviews is vitally important. Perhaps GPT-4 could be part of our arsenal for managing negative reviews. (For more information on managing online reviews, see this chapter).

Default (GPT-4)

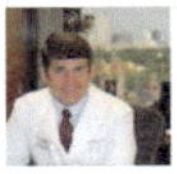

My submission to ChatGPT:

I am a urologist, and I received a scathing letter and a negative online review from a dissatisfied patient. She mentioned that she signed a consent but wasn't aware of the risks and complications. I have documentation that the risks and complications were reviewed with her, and I offered to answer any additional questions she may have had. My records show no questions after I explained the procedure. Please help me write two letters: one to the patient and the second to the online review site refuting her accusations. Please do not mention her name in the letter to the review site as that would be a HIPAA violation. I appreciate your assistance. Thank you, Dr. Neil Baum, Professor of Clinical Urology at Tulane Medical School, New Orleans, Louisiana

ChatGPT

This is the immediate answer regarding my request from GPT-4 which was obtained in less than sixty seconds:

ChatGPT

ChatGPT

Certainly, I can help you draft two letters to address this situation. It's essential to be professional and maintain patient confidentiality in both letters. Here's a suggested letter to the patient:

Letter to the Patient:

Dr. Neil Baum, Professor of Clinical Urology atTulane Medical School, New Orleans, Louisiana

Dear [Patient's Name],

I am writing to address the concerns you expressed in your recent letter and online review regarding the procedure you underwent at our clinic. I value the feedback of all our patients and take your concerns seriously.

First and foremost, I want to reiterate that your well-being and understanding of the medical procedures you undergo are of utmost importance to us. I have reviewed your medical records and can confirm that you were provided with comprehensive information regarding the potential risks and complications associated with the procedure. I personally discussed these risks with you and offered the opportunity for you to ask any questions or seek further clarification.

It is disheartening to hear that you felt uninformed about the procedure's potential risks. Please understand that it is our standard practice to ensure that patients are fully informed and have their

Fig. 24.9 Is a request to GPT-4 for a suggestion to respond to a patient who wrote a negative online review. This is followed by the response from GPT-4 and a letter to the online review site

questions answered before proceeding. I have carefully reviewed your medical records, and there is no record of any questions or concerns raised by you following our discussion.

I am committed to providing the highest level of care to all my patients, and I sincerely regret any misunderstanding that may have arisen in this situation. I would be more than willing to schedule an appointment to discuss any lingering questions or concerns you may have, or to further clarify any aspects of your procedure.

Your health and satisfaction are of great importance to us, and we aim to continuously improve our services. I appreciate your feedback and will use it to enhance our patient communication processes.

Thank you for bringing this matter to my attention. If you would like to arrange a follow-up appointment at no charge, or discuss this matter further, please feel free to contact our clinic at 504 891-8454.

Wishing you the best of health and looking forward to resolving this issue together.

Sincerely,

Dr. Neil Baum

This is the suggested response from GPT-4 to the online review site:

Letter to the Online Review Site:

Dr. Neil Baum, Professor of Clinical Urology at Tulane Medical School, New Orleans, Louisiana

Dear Review Site Moderator,

I am writing to address a recent online review that has been posted on your platform concerning the services provided at our clinic. While I value patient feedback and constructive criticism, I wish to clarify some inaccuracies in the review without disclosing any protected health information in accordance with HIPAA regulations.

The review in question pertains to a patient's experience with our clinic. We aim to provide the highest standard of care and ensuring our patients are well-informed about

Fig. 24.9 (continued)

their medical procedures, including the potential risks and complications. We take such matters seriously.

After a careful review of our records, I can confirm that this patient was informed about the associated risks and complications of the procedure. I personally discussed these matters with the patient and extended the opportunity for any questions or concerns to be addressed. Regrettably, there is no record of any further inquiries or uncertainties raised by the patient.

We are committed to open communication with our patients and take all concerns seriously. We believe that informed patients make better decisions about their healthcare. Our records reflect our dedication to this principle.

We are always working to improve our patient communication processes and enhance the quality of care we provide. Constructive feedback is essential for this endeavor, and we appreciate the vigilance of our patients in holding us to the highest standards.

While respecting patient confidentiality, I would like to reaffirm our commitment to the well-being of our patients and our dedication to transparent, informed consent procedures.

Thank you for your understanding, and if there are any further questions or clarifications needed, please do not hesitate to reach out to us at 504 891-845.

Sincerely,

Dr. Neil Baum, Professor of Clinical Urology at Tulane Medical School, New Orleans, Louisiana

Fig. 24.9 (continued)

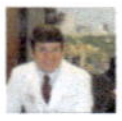

You

Please create a job description for a medical assistant for a urology practice with five doctors and 10 full time equivalents. Thank you

ChatGPT

ChatGPT

Job Title: Medical Assistant - Urology Practice

Job Overview: We are seeking a highly skilled and motivated Medical Assistant to join our urology practice, which consists of five doctors and 10 full-time equivalents. The successful candidate will play a crucial role in supporting the efficient functioning of our urology clinic, ensuring excellent patient care, and contributing to the overall success of the practice.

Responsibilities:

1. **Patient Care:**
    - Assist physicians in conducting patient examinations, procedures, and treatments.
    - Record patient medical history, vital signs, and other relevant information accurately.
    - Educate patients on urological procedures, medications, and post-treatment care.
2. **Administrative Duties:**
    - Schedule and coordinate patient appointments, surgeries, and follow-up visits.
    - Maintain electronic health records (EHR) and ensure accurate documentation.
    - Handle billing and insurance-related tasks, as required.
3. **Clinical Support:**
    - Prepare examination rooms, ensuring they are stocked with necessary supplies and equipment.
    - Sterilize and maintain medical instruments and equipment.
    - Assist with medical procedures, as directed by physicians.

Fig. 24.10 Is a request to GPT-4 for a job description for a medical assistant to a urology office

4. **Collaboration:**
   - Work collaboratively with other medical assistants, nurses, and administrative staff to ensure seamless clinic operations.
   - Communicate effectively with patients, physicians, and other healthcare professionals.
5. **Compliance:**
   - Adhere to all relevant healthcare regulations and protocols.
   - Maintain confidentiality of patient information and follow HIPAA guidelines.
6. **Continuous Learning:**
   - Stay updated on the latest developments in urology and medical assisting practices.
   - Participate in training sessions and professional development opportunities.

Qualifications:

- High School Diploma or equivalent; completion of a recognized Medical Assistant program.
- Certification as a Medical Assistant is preferred.
- Proven experience as a Medical Assistant in a urology or similar medical practice.
- Strong organizational and multitasking skills.
- Excellent interpersonal and communication skills.
- Proficiency in using electronic health record (EHR) systems.
- Knowledge of medical terminology and urology procedures.

We offer a competitive salary, benefits package, and a supportive work environment. If you are a dedicated and compassionate individual looking to contribute to a dynamic urology practice, we encourage you to apply.

Fig. 24.10 (continued)

How to Write a Job Description for Positions Available in the Office

Figure 24.10 shows a request to GPT-4 to post a job description online, along with GPT-4's response.

Creating an Informed Consent

Hospitals and ambulatory treatment centers have pre-printed consent forms required by the hospital or ATC. Often, these forms don't reflect the risks and complications in an office setting. Properly executed informed consent can serve as a defense against medical malpractice claims. When patients are well-informed and have willingly consented to a procedure, it becomes difficult for them to argue that negligence or a lack of disclosure occurred. Lawsuits related to lack of informed consent often hinge on allegations of inadequate disclosure of risks, failure to explain alternatives, or proceeding with treatment without obtaining proper consent [4]. GPT-4 is an excellent resource for generating informed consent for office procedures. Figure 24.11 is an example of a request for informed consent for an office vasectomy procedure.

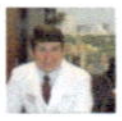

You

Can you provide risk and complications of performing a vasectomy in the doctor's office?

ChatGPT

ChatGPT

Certainly, I can provide general information on the risks and complications associated with a vasectomy. However, it's crucial to consult with a healthcare professional for personalized advice. Here are potential risks:

1. **Pain or Discomfort:** Some men may experience pain or discomfort during or after the vasectomy procedure. This is usually temporary and can be managed with pain medication.
2. **Swelling and Bruising:** Swelling and bruising of the scrotum are common after a vasectomy. This typically resolves on its own over time.
3. **Infection:** There is a risk of infection at the incision site. Following proper care instructions and hygiene practices can help minimize this risk.
4. **Bleeding:** While bleeding is rare, it can occur during or after the procedure. Most cases are minor, but persistent bleeding should be reported to a healthcare provider.
5. **Sperm Granuloma:** Sometimes, a small lump called a sperm granuloma may form at the site of the vasectomy. This is a collection of sperm that can cause discomfort but is usually not a serious issue.
6. **Epididymitis:** Inflammation of the epididymis (the tube that carries sperm from the testicle) can occur in rare cases. It may cause pain and swelling.
7. **Failure of Sterilization:** While vasectomy is a highly effective form of contraception, there is a small risk of failure. It's important to use alternative contraception or abstain from sexual intercourse until confirmed sterility is achieved. This consists of two semen examinations obtained by masturbation after 8-10 weeks following the vasectomy. It is imperative that two semen analyses be done before you can safely engage in sexual intimacy without the risk of a pregnancy.

Fig. 24.11 Is a suggested informed consent for a patient who is going to have a vasectomy in the doctor's office. This consent also contains instructions before and after the procedure

It's essential to discuss these potential risks and complications with your healthcare provider before undergoing a vasectomy. They can provide personalized information based on your health history and address any concerns you may have.

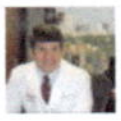

You

Can you provide the instructions to the patient before and after having a vasectomy in the doctor's office?

ChatGPT

Instructions Before the Vasectomy:

1. **Consultation:**
    - Schedule a consultation with your healthcare provider to discuss the procedure, address any concerns, and ensure it's the right choice for you.
2. **Shaving:**
    - Your doctor may ask you to shave the scrotum area before the procedure.
3. **Medication:**
    - If prescribed, take any medications (such as antibiotics or pain relievers) as directed by your healthcare provider.
    - Do not take any blood-thinning medication such as aspirin or aspirin like products, ibuprofen (Advil), naproxen (Aleve) for one week prior to your procedure. Please discuss any other medications you may be taking prior to the procedure.

Instructions After the Vasectomy:

1. **Rest:**
    - Plan to rest for a day or two after the procedure.
2. **Ice Packs:**
    - Apply ice packs to the scrotum to reduce swelling for the first 12 hours after the procedure
3. **Supportive Underwear:**

Fig. 24.11 (continued)

- Wear supportive underwear, not boxer shorts, to provide comfort and minimize movement.

4. **Avoiding Heavy Lifting:**
    - Avoid heavy lifting, jogging, or tennis for at least a week.
5. **Follow-up Tests:**
    - Schedule and attend any follow-up tests as recommended by your healthcare provider to confirm the success of the vasectomy.
6. **Follow-up Appointment:**
    - Please make a follow-up appointment with your doctor to discuss your recovery and address any concerns.

Always consult with your healthcare provider for personalized advice and follow their instructions carefully for a safe and smooth recovery.

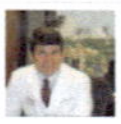

You

Can you include the importance of having two semen analyses after the procedure to confirm sterility?

ChatGPT

ChatGPT

Certainly, including the importance of having two semen analyses after the procedure is crucial. Here's an updated section:

Risks and Complications:

1. **Pain or Discomfort:**
    - **Before:** You may experience mild discomfort during the administration of local anesthesia.
    - **After:** Some pain or discomfort is common after the procedure, and your healthcare provider may prescribe pain medication.
2. **Swelling and Bruising:**
    - **Before/After:** Swelling and bruising of the scrotum are common. Applying ice packs and wearing supportive underwear can help manage this.
3. **Infection:**

Fig. 24.11 (continued)

- **Before/After:** Follow proper hygiene practices before and after the procedure to minimize the risk of infection. Your doctor may prescribe antibiotics.

4. **Bleeding:**
   - **Before/After:** While uncommon, bleeding can occur. Report any persistent or excessive bleeding to your healthcare provider.
5. **Sperm Granuloma:**
   - **After:** A small lump may form at the vasectomy site, called a sperm granuloma. It's usually not serious but should be evaluated by your doctor if it causes discomfort.
6. **Epididymitis:**
   - **After:** Inflammation of the epididymis is rare but possible. Report any signs of pain, swelling, or discomfort to your healthcare provider.
7. **Failure of Sterilization:**
   - **After:** It takes time for the vasectomy to become fully effective. Use alternative contraception until your doctor confirms sterility through two separate semen analyses. Do not have unprotected sexual intercourse until you considered sterile.

Instructions Before the Vasectomy:

1. **Consultation:**
   - Schedule a consultation with your healthcare provider to discuss the procedure, address any concerns, and ensure it's the right choice for you.
2. **Shaving:**
   - Your doctor may ask you to shave the scrotum area before the procedure.
3. **Medication:**
   - If prescribed, take any medications (such as antibiotics or pain relievers) as directed by your healthcare provider.
4. Always consult with your healthcare provider for personalized advice and follow their instructions carefully for a safe and smooth recovery.

Fig. 24.11 (continued)

Instructions After the Vasectomy:

1. **Rest:**
    - Plan to rest for a day or two after the procedure. Avoid strenuous activities.
2. **Ice Packs:**
    - Apply ice packs to the scrotum to reduce swelling. Use the ice packs for twenty minutes at a time for the first twelve hours.
3. **Supportive Underwear:**
    - Wear supportive underwear to provide comfort and minimize movement.
4. **Avoiding Heavy Lifting:**
    - Avoid heavy lifting for at least a week.
5. **Follow-up Tests:**
    - Schedule and attend two semen analyses as recommended by your healthcare provider. These tests confirm the success of the vasectomy and ensure sterility.
6. **Follow-up Appointment:**
    - Make a follow-up appointment with your doctor to discuss the results of the semen analyses, your recovery, and address any concerns.
7. You may take acetaminophen (Tyenol) for pain and resume aspirin or aspirin-like products two days after the procedure.

Always consult with your healthcare provider for personalized advice and follow their instructions carefully for a safe and smooth recovery.

Fig. 24.11 (continued)

Provide FAQs for the Common Conditions Seen in the Office

The questions patients ask are repeated many times a day. You can alleviate answering those questions with FAQs to submit to GPT-4. Figure 24.12 is an example of an FAQ request regarding the importance of screening for prostate cancer with the PSA test. Notice that the response didn't mention that the man should avoid ejaculation or sexual intercourse for two days before the blood test. When a second question was posed, "What is a PSA test?" The response states, "A PSA test is a blood test that measures the level of prostate-specific antigen (PSA) in the blood. PSA is a protein produced by the prostate gland, and high levels of PSA can indicate the presence of prostate cancer."

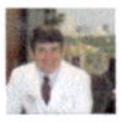

You

Please provide FAQs regarding screening for prostate cancer with the PSA test

ChatGPT

ChatGPT

Certainly! Here are some frequently asked questions (FAQs) regarding screening for prostate cancer with the PSA (Prostate-Specific Antigen) test:

1. What is the PSA test?

- The PSA test measures the level of prostate-specific antigen, a protein produced by the prostate gland, in the blood. Elevated PSA levels can be an indicator of various prostate conditions, including cancer.

2. Who should consider getting a PSA test?

- The decision to undergo a PSA test should be individualized. It is often recommended for men with an average risk of prostate cancer, typically starting around the age of 50. However, men with higher risk factors, such as a family history of prostate cancer, may discuss testing earlier with their healthcare provider.

3. Is the PSA test mandatory for all men?

- No, the PSA test is not mandatory. It is a personal decision that should be made after discussing the potential benefits and risks with a healthcare provider.

4. What are the potential benefits of the PSA test?

Fig. 24.12 Is an example of a request for an FAQ explaining the importance of prostate cancer screening using the PSA test

- The PSA test can help detect prostate cancer in its early stages, providing an opportunity for timely intervention and treatment. It may assist in reducing mortality from prostate cancer.

5. What are the limitations of the PSA test?

- The PSA test is not specific to cancer and can yield false-positive results. Elevated PSA levels can also be caused by non-cancerous conditions such as prostatitis or benign prostatic hyperplasia (BPH). Conversely, some men with prostate cancer may have normal PSA levels.

6. How often should the PSA test be done?

- The frequency of PSA testing depends on individual risk factors and preferences. It is typically done every two years for men with average risk and more frequently for those at higher risk.

7. Are there any potential harms associated with PSA testing?

- Yes, potential harms include false-positive results leading to unnecessary anxiety and follow-up tests, overdiagnosis, and treatment of cancers that may not have caused harm. These aspects should be discussed with a healthcare provider.

8. Should the PSA test be done in combination with a digital rectal exam (DRE)?

- The decision to combine the PSA test with a digital rectal exam is based on individual risk factors and preferences. Some healthcare providers may recommend both for a more comprehensive assessment.

9. What happens if the PSA levels are elevated?

- Elevated PSA levels do not necessarily indicate cancer. Further diagnostic tests, such as a biopsy, may be recommended to determine the cause of elevated PSA levels and whether cancer is present.

Fig. 24.12 (continued)

10. Can lifestyle changes affect PSA levels? - Certain factors, such as recent ejaculation, physical activity, and prostate procedures, can affect PSA levels. It's advisable to discuss these factors with a healthcare provider before the test.

Remember, individual circumstances vary, and decisions about PSA testing should be made in consultation with a healthcare provider based on a thorough understanding of the risks and benefits.

I was concerned that no mention was made about abstaining from sexual intercourse or ejaculation prior to the test. I asked a second question, and this was the response:

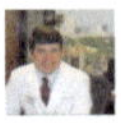

You

Is there any preparation prior to having a PSA test?

ChatGPT

ChatGPT

Yes, there are certain considerations and recommendations for preparation before having a PSA (Prostate-Specific Antigen) test. Here are some general guidelines:

1. **Discuss with Your Healthcare Provider:**
   - Before the test, have a discussion with your healthcare provider about the purpose of the PSA test, the potential benefits, and the limitations. This conversation will help you make an informed decision about whether to proceed with the test.
2. **Inform Your Healthcare Provider:**
   - Inform your healthcare provider about any medications, supplements, or herbal remedies you are currently taking. Some medications may affect PSA levels, so it's important to provide a comprehensive list.
3. **Avoid Ejaculation:**
   - It is generally recommended to avoid ejaculation for at least 48 hours before a PSA test, as recent sexual activity may temporarily increase PSA levels.
4. **Physical Activity:**

Fig. 24.12 (continued)

- Strenuous physical activity, such as vigorous exercise, bicycle riding, or heavy lifting, may affect PSA levels. Some healthcare providers may advise avoiding intense physical activity for a day or two before the test.

Fig. 24.12 (continued)

Create Blogs for Social Media Sites

Suppose you have a blog site and want to create a blog on some aspects of diseases and conditions you manage or wish to offer advice on some aspects of your specialty. In that case, GPT-4 can be helpful to get the process started. Figure 24.13 is an example of a request for a blog on nutritional aspects of urologic diseases.

Write a 500 word blog on nutritional aspects of urologic diseases

ChatGPT

ChatGPT

Title: Nourishing Wellness: Exploring the Nutritional Aspects of Urologic Diseases

Introduction: Urologic diseases, encompassing conditions related to the urinary tract and male reproductive system, can significantly impact one's quality of life. While medical interventions play a crucial role in managing urologic diseases, the role of nutrition should not be overlooked. A well-balanced and nutrient-rich diet can contribute to the prevention and management of urologic conditions, promoting overall urological health.

1. Hydration and Kidney Health:

One cornerstone of urologic wellness is proper hydration. Adequate water intake is essential for maintaining optimal kidney function. The kidneys play a pivotal role in filtering waste products and excess fluids from the blood. Dehydration can lead to the formation of kidney stones, a common urologic issue. Consuming sufficient water helps prevent the crystallization of minerals that form these stones, reducing the risk of kidney stone development.

2. Prostate Health and Antioxidants:

The prostate, a walnut-sized gland in men, is prone to conditions such as benign prostatic hyperplasia (BPH) and prostate cancer. Antioxidant-rich foods can contribute to prostate health by neutralizing free radicals that may contribute to inflammation and cellular damage. Foods high in antioxidants include berries, tomatoes, green tea, and cruciferous vegetables like broccoli and Brussels sprouts.

3. Dietary Fiber for Bladder Health:

A diet rich in fiber offers benefits for bladder health. Fiber helps regulate bowel movements, preventing constipation, which can contribute to bladder issues. Additionally, a healthy gut microbiome, supported by a fiber-rich diet, may

Fig. 24.13 Is a request for assistance in writing a blog for a social media site or a newsletter. This request was for advice on nutritional aspects of urologic diseases

positively impact the urinary tract. Whole grains, fruits, vegetables, and legumes are excellent sources of dietary fiber.

4. Sodium Intake and Blood Pressure:

Reducing sodium intake is essential for managing urologic conditions such as hypertension and kidney disease. High blood pressure can strain the kidneys, leading to damage over time. Processed foods and excessive salt intake should be limited, while incorporating potassium-rich foods like bananas, oranges, and leafy greens can help balance electrolytes and maintain healthy blood pressure.

5. Omega-3 Fatty Acids and Inflammation:

Inflammation is a common factor in urologic diseases, including interstitial cystitis and prostatitis. Omega-3 fatty acids, found in fatty fish like salmon and mackerel, walnuts, and flaxseeds, possess anti-inflammatory properties. Including these foods in the diet may help alleviate symptoms and promote urologic well-being.

6. Cranberries and Urinary Tract Infections (UTIs):

Cranberries have long been associated with preventing urinary tract infections. Compounds in cranberries may inhibit the adhesion of bacteria to the urinary tract walls, reducing the risk of infection. While not a cure, incorporating cranberries or unsweetened cranberry juice into the diet may be a preventive measure against recurrent UTIs.

7. Calcium and Kidney Stones:

While calcium is essential for bone health, excessive intake may contribute to the formation of kidney stones. Striking a balance is crucial. Calcium-rich foods, such as dairy products and leafy greens, can be part of a healthy diet, but supplementation should be done cautiously. Adequate hydration, limiting sodium, and maintaining a healthy weight also play roles in preventing kidney stones.

Conclusion: Nutrition plays a pivotal role in supporting urologic health and preventing various conditions affecting the urinary tract and male reproductive

Fig. 24.13 (continued)

system. A well-rounded, nutrient-dense diet that includes hydration, antioxidants, fiber, and essential fatty acids contributes not only to the prevention but also to the management of urologic diseases. As always, individuals should consult with healthcare professionals for personalized advice based on their specific health needs and conditions. Embracing a nourishing lifestyle can be a proactive step towards urologic wellness and an enhanced overall quality of life.

Fig. 24.13 (continued)

Creating Patient Education Materials on Tests, Procedures, and Proper Use of Medications

Figure 24.14 is a request for patient educational material on the workup for hematuria. This is also available on the practice website as a video if the patient would rather have an audio-visual explanation. Also, if the patient watches the video, the GPT-4-generated handout is provided. The handout is reviewed by the doctor or nurse with the patient.

Please write a 300-word article at the 10th grade level on the evaluation of the patient with hematuria.

ChatGPT

ChatGPT

Hematuria, the presence of blood in the urine, is a concerning symptom that requires careful evaluation to identify its underlying cause. When a patient presents with hematuria, healthcare professionals follow a systematic approach to assess and diagnose the condition.

The first step in evaluating hematuria involves obtaining a detailed medical history from the patient. Questions about the duration and frequency of hematuria, associated symptoms, and any relevant medical conditions or medications help provide crucial information. Understanding the patient's family history may also reveal genetic predispositions to certain kidney conditions or urinary tract infections.

After gathering the medical history, a thorough physical examination is conducted. This examination focuses on the abdomen, back, and genitalia, aiming to identify any abnormalities or signs of kidney disease. Blood pressure measurement is essential, as hypertension can be associated with kidney problems leading to hematuria.

Following the initial assessment, laboratory tests are ordered to further investigate the cause of hematuria. A complete blood count (CBC) helps assess overall health, while a urinalysis provides information about the urine's composition. Additionally, a urine culture may be conducted to identify any infection.

Imaging studies play a crucial role in the evaluation process. Ultrasound, CT scans, or MRIs of the kidneys and urinary tract can reveal structural abnormalities, stones, or tumors. These imaging techniques help healthcare professionals visualize the internal structures and identify potential causes of hematuria.

Fig. 24.14 Is a request for patient educational material on the evaluation of hematuria. I also requested that the article be translated into Spanish

In some cases, a cystoscopy may be recommended to examine the interior of the bladder and urethra. This procedure involves inserting a thin tube with a camera through the urethra to inspect the bladder walls for abnormalities.

The evaluation of hematuria is a comprehensive process that combines patient history, physical examination, laboratory tests, and imaging studies. The goal is to pinpoint the underlying cause, whether it be an infection, kidney disease, urinary tract stones, or even a malignancy. Through this systematic approach, healthcare professionals can tailor a targeted treatment plan and provide the best care for patients experiencing hematuria.

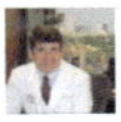

You

Please translate the explanation for the evaluation of hematuria into Spanish

ChatGPT

ChatGPT

Hematuria, la presencia de sangre en la orina, es un síntoma preocupante que requiere una evaluación cuidadosa para identificar su causa subyacente. Cuando un paciente presenta hematuria, los profesionales de la salud siguen un enfoque sistemático para evaluar y diagnosticar la afección.

El primer paso en la evaluación de la hematuria implica obtener una historia médica detallada del paciente. Preguntas sobre la duración y frecuencia de la hematuria, síntomas asociados y cualquier condición médica o medicamentos relevantes ayudan a proporcionar información crucial. Comprender la historia familiar del paciente también puede revelar predisposiciones genéticas a ciertas enfermedades renales o infecciones del tracto urinario.

Después de recopilar la historia médica, se realiza un examen físico exhaustivo. Esta evaluación se centra en el abdomen, la espalda y los genitales, con el objetivo de identificar cualquier anormalidad o signo de enfermedad renal. La medición de la presión arterial es esencial, ya que la hipertensión puede estar asociada con problemas renales que llevan a la hematuria.

Tras la evaluación inicial, se solicitan análisis de laboratorio para investigar más a fondo la causa de la hematuria. Un hemograma completo ayuda a evaluar la salud general, mientras que un análisis de orina proporciona información sobre la

Fig. 24.14 (continued)

composición de la orina. Además, se puede realizar un cultivo de orina para identificar cualquier infección.

Los estudios de imágenes desempeñan un papel crucial en el proceso de evaluación. Ecografías, tomografías computarizadas o resonancias magnéticas de los riñones y el tracto urinario pueden revelar anomalías estructurales, cálculos o tumores. Estas técnicas de imagen ayudan a los profesionales de la salud a visualizar las estructuras internas e identificar posibles causas de la hematuria.

En algunos casos, se puede recomendar una cistoscopia para examinar el interior de la vejiga y la uretra. Este procedimiento implica la inserción de un tubo delgado con una cámara a través de la uretra para inspeccionar las paredes de la vejiga en busca de anomalías.

La evaluación de la hematuria es un proceso integral que combina la historia del paciente, el examen físico, los análisis de laboratorio y los estudios de imágenes. El objetivo es identificar la causa subyacente, ya sea una infección, enfermedad renal, cálculos en el tracto urinario o incluso una malignidad. A través de este enfoque sistemático, los profesionales de la salud pueden adaptar un plan de tratamiento específico y brindar la mejor atención a los pacientes que experimentan hematuria.

Fig. 24.14 (continued)

Obtain Proper Coding of the Encounter, Procedures, and Tests

Today, many practices have hired a certified CPT coder to ensure appropriate codes are used to create a clean claim. Correct codes provide payment without denials and avoid underpayment or fines for up-coding. If coding is not performed, potential reimbursement may go unclaimed.

Figure 24.15 is a request for proper coding for an office visit and a urologic procedure.

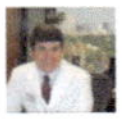

You

Please provide the CPT code for level 4 E\M evaluation of a new incontinent patient. Also include the code for a qualitative urinalysis, cystoscopy, and urodynamic study, which includes a flow rate and bladder pressures.

ChatGPT

ChatGPT

For the Level 4 E/M (Evaluation and Management) visit for a new incontinent patient, the appropriate CPT code is 99204.

As for the additional procedures:

1. Qualitative Urinalysis: The CPT code for qualitative urinalysis is 81002.
2. Cystoscopy: The specific CPT code for cystoscopy can vary depending on whether it is a diagnostic or a therapeutic procedure. For a diagnostic cystoscopy, the code is typically 52000. If any additional procedures are performed during the cystoscopy, other codes may apply.
3. Urodynamic Study with Flow Rate and Bladder Pressures: The comprehensive CPT code for a urodynamic study with flow rate and bladder pressures is 51741. This code includes the measurement of bladder pressures and a uroflowmetry (flow rate) study.

Fig. 24.15 Is a request for CPT codes used for an office visit and a procedure

Request for Summarizing Medical Articles in the Literature

This is the least robust feature of the GPT-4 functions. Figure 24.16 is a request for a summary of an article written in 2017.

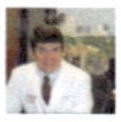

You

Can you summarize the article: Bilusic, M., Madan, R. A., & Gulley, J. L. (2017). Immunotherapy of prostate cancer: facts and hopes. Clinical Cancer Research, 23(22), 6764-6770.

ChatGPT

ChatGPT

Certainly! The article "Immunotherapy of Prostate Cancer: Facts and Hopes" by Bilusic, Madan, and Gulley, published in Clinical Cancer Research in 2017, discusses the current status and potential future directions of immunotherapy for prostate cancer. Here is a summary:

The authors provide an overview of the immune system's role in cancer and highlight the challenges associated with developing effective immunotherapies for prostate cancer. They discuss various immunotherapeutic approaches, including cancer vaccines, immune checkpoint inhibitors, and adoptive T-cell transfer.

The article reviews clinical trials and preclinical studies related to immunotherapy in prostate cancer, examining the outcomes and limitations of these interventions. The authors emphasize the need for personalized and combination approaches to enhance the efficacy of immunotherapy.

Overall, the paper explores the existing knowledge and ongoing research in the field of immunotherapy for prostate cancer, offering insights into the challenges and potential advancements in this area of cancer treatment.

Fig. 24.16 Is a request for a summary of a medical article on the use of immunotherapy for the management of metastatic prostate cancer

Explanation of Benefits (EOB)

ChatGPT-4 can play a significant role in improving patient understanding of Explanation of Benefits (EOBs). A sample response from ChatGPT is shown in Fig. 24.17.

GPT-4 can simplify and clarify the EOB by translating medical and insurance jargon. EOBs often contain technical terms and complex insurance language that can be difficult for patients to understand. ChatGPT-4 tools can simplify complex language into terms patients can easily understand.

GPT-4 can analyze the EOB and extract essential information, such as which services were covered, the amount the patient owes, and the reasons for any denials, presenting it in a clear, concise format.

GPT-4 goes further by using the patient's individual information, such as their medical history and insurance plan details, to provide personalized explanations, making the information more relevant and understandable.

By leveraging AI, healthcare providers and payers can simplify the complex process of understanding EOBs, making it easier and more

Prompt to GPT: Please provide me with an EOB for insertion of a suburethral sling for treatment of urinary incontinence

Here is a sample Explanation of Benefits (EOB) for the insertion of a suburethral sling for the treatment of urinary incontinence. Please note that this is a generic example, and actual EOBs may differ based on the patient's specific insurance coverage, procedure details, and healthcare provider.
Patient Name: Jane Doe
Insured ID: 123456789
Provider Name: Dr. John Smith
Date of Service: 06/01/2024
Procedure: Insertion of suburethral sling for the treatment of urinary incontinence
Procedure Code: 51990
Charges:
Surgical procedure: $5,000
Anesthesia: $500
Facility fee: $1,000
Total charges: $6,500
Insurance Coverage:
In-network coverage: 80% of allowed amount
Deductible remaining: $500
Claim Adjustments:
Allowed amount for surgical procedure: $4,000
Allowed amount for anesthesia: $400
Allowed amount for facility fee: $800
Total allowed amount: $5,200
Patient Responsibility:
Deductible remaining: $500
Coinsurance (20% of allowed amount): $1,040
Total patient responsibility: $1,540
EOB Summary:
Total charges: $6,500
Total allowed amount: $5,200
Insurance coverage: $4,160
Deductible remaining: $500
Coinsurance: $1,040
Total patient responsibility: $1,540

Please note that this sample EOB is for illustrative purposes only. Actual EOBs may vary based on individual insurance plans, coverage details, and specific medical services provided. Always refer to your insurance policy and consult with your healthcare provider or insurance company for accurate information regarding your specific situation.

Fig. 24.17 Sample EOB for insertion of a suburethral sling to treat urinary incontinence

accessible for patients, promoting patient engagement, improving patient outcomes, and potentially reducing healthcare costs.

Use of the Prompt Generator to Enhance the Results of GPT-4

The output or results from GPT-4 are related to the input or the requests you make of technology. If you ask a general question that is not specific, you will receive a broad range of answers that may differ from what you expect. Asking a more detailed question or making a more detailed request result in a better response.

The prompt generator works the same way as asking another human questions. You can start with a general question and follow up with a more detailed one. Start with a general question and follow up with a more specific one. Users may ask the program to be more conversational, humorous, or even more compassionate, and the program will often comply. The more you use the program and the more specific your requests are, the better the results you will receive.

Here's a "cheat sheet" of commonly used prompts for medical professionals when interacting with GPT-4:

Diagnosis and Symptoms
"Based on these symptoms [describe symptoms], what could be the potential diagnosis?"

"What are the typical signs of [medical condition]?"

"Explain the difference between [condition A] and [condition B]."

Treatment and Management
"What are the recommended treatment options for [medical condition]?"

"Provide guidelines for managing [chronic condition] in a clinical setting."

"What are the potential side effects of [medication/therapy]?"

Medication Information
"Give me details about [medication name]: dosage, contraindications, interactions with other medications."

"What is the mechanism of action of [drug name]?"

"Explain the differences between generic and brand-name [medication]."

Medical Procedures
"Outline the steps of [medical procedure/surgery]."

"What are the risks and benefits of [procedure] for [condition]?"

"Provide pre-operative and post-operative care instructions for [procedure]."

Preventive Care
"Recommend preventive measures for [condition] in [patient demographic]."

"What are the vaccination schedules for [age group]?"

"Give advice on maintaining a healthy lifestyle to prevent [specific condition]."

Medical Ethics and Guidelines
"the ethical considerations of [medical dilemma/situation]."

"Explain the legal obligations regarding patient confidentiality."

"Provide insights into informed consent and decision-making for [procedure/treatment]."

Patient Communication
"How should I communicate a complex diagnosis to a patient?"

"Give tips for breaking bad news to patients and their families."

"Provide guidance on improving patient-doctor communication."

Emergencies and First Aid
"What are the immediate steps to take in case of [medical emergency]?"

"Explain CPR technique and when it should be administered."

"Provide a checklist for creating a basic first-aid kit."

Medical Research and Updates
"Summarize recent advancements in the treatment of [specific condition]."

"What are the current guidelines for [medical procedure/therapy]?"

"Discuss the findings of recent clinical trials for [drug/treatment]."

Professional Development
"Provide resources for continuing medical education in [specialty]."

"Recommend medical journals and literature sources for [specific topic]."

"How can I stay current with the latest medical breakthroughs?"

Creating a Consent
"Provide a consent for [name of procedure/test]."

"List the risks and potential complications for [name of procedure/test]."

"Provide alternatives to [name of procedure/test]."

"Include consequences of not proceeding with [name of procedure/test]."

Requesting a Word Count
"Provide a [mention of number of words for the document] words on [name of procedure/test]."

A caveat is to always edit GPT-4 responses critically and cross-reference them with reliable medical sources.

Caveats on GPT-4

Mistakes or Hallucinations

GPT-4 is not perfect, and the responses may be inaccurate. The program only scours the Internet for information and cannot distinguish between credible and non-credible sources. Just as patients go online for medical information, they often receive information and advice that needs greater accuracy.

The AI lexicon has used the term hallucinations to describe generative AI responses that provide inaccurate, false, and misleading information in AI chatbots. It is often difficult to identify these misleading responses. As healthcare providers, we must be aware that this misinformation may appear in our searches and remove it.

Hallucinations—whether mild deviations from the facts or outright fabrications—must be identified and removed from any content generated by chatbots. This underscores the need to fact-check chatbot responses to ensure the accuracy and reliability of your content.

Here's an example that clarifies hallucinations. If you asked an AI tool to provide consent for the surgical removal of a kidney. Suppose the tool was trained on the surgical removal of the prostate gland and needed more exposure to renal surgery to understand the differences between the two organs. In that case, it might not be able to provide an accurate response. It would still generate a draft because you prompted it, but it may omit essential sections specific to cancer nephrectomy or even make them up.

Language-related problems can also cause inaccuracies and hallucinations. AI models must keep pace with the constant evolution of language to avoid barriers caused by recent terminology and slang.

For best results, always prompt an AI tool using 10-grade language and avoid medical jargon. While this may only sometimes be possible when discussing complex medical topics, try to simplify the prompts as much as possible. Doing so ensures that your instructions are precise and leave less room for misinterpretation.

AI hallucination is more than a random software bug—it has considerable real-life implications that can harm your practice in various ways, including litigation. This underscores the importance of vigilance and caution when using AI technology.

The main consequence of providing false information is the deterioration of patient trust. Even a few clicks on industry-specific review sites can affect your online reputation, which may require considerable time to fix. This can lead to patient dissatisfaction, loss of credibility, and potential legal issues, all of which can significantly impact your practice.

It's difficult to fully control an AI platform's output, but you can steer your solution in the right direction to minimize the risk of false information.

Providing specific resources is one of the easiest ways to help your AI model avoid making up information.

For example, you can tell an AI platform to look for current, reputable articles and credible research published in peer-reviewed journals. You can further narrow its options by prompting it with the websites you want the data from and asking for the most current resources.

For instance, if you're writing an article about immunotherapy, you can tell AI to only use data from the Mayo Clinic and the Journal of Immunotherapy. This will ensure results from a reputable source while saving you time manually checking for facts and statistics.

We recommend requesting verified sources, such as the American Cancer Society and academic institutions like Mayo Clinic, Johns Hopkins, and MD Anderson. Educational institutions usually have the .edu domain, so that's how you'll recognize credible sources and prevent AI from generating results based on any random site on the web. This significantly reduces the chances of errors and hallucinations.

You should include why you are telling your AI model what you need. Doing so helps the platform understand the context behind your prompt, increasing the predictability of the output.

Take the following two prompts as an example:

1. *Please provide me with the most common side effects of NubeqaTM.*
2. *Please provide me with the side effects of NubeqaTM so that I can warn patients that they should call the office or go to an emergency room.*

The second prompt provides relevant information for the AI tool to focus its answer.

When prompting an AI tool, try to give it as many specifics as possible.

For example, instead of saying,

"Write an introduction to an article about options for treating prostate cancer."

Your prompt can be something like:

"Write a 150–200-word introduction to an article about treatment options using immunotherapy for metastatic hormone-resistant prostate cancer. The article will be published in a patient newsletter, and the tone should be informal yet informative. Use medical literature from 2023 with relevant statistics about the current state of immunotherapy."

This prompt specifies all the necessary details—the content's tone, length, sources, and purpose. As a result, it gives the AI tool enough direction to ensure accuracy while reducing the need for extensive editing.

Use limited-choice questions whenever possible.

Ambiguous prompts are among the most common causes of inaccuracies and hallucinations. They give an AI tool too much room to misinterpret their intent.

To avoid such issues, replace open-ended questions with limited-choice ones. Some examples you can follow:

- **Open-ended**: *How has treating prostate cancer changed in recent times?*
- **Limited-choice**: *What are the outcomes for men with castrate-resistant prostate cancer (CRPC) during 2021 and 2022, as data from the National Cancer Institute?*
- **Open-ended:** *How much content should my website have on the surgical management of prostate cancer?*
- **Limited choice**: *What's the average amount of content on a website in the prostate cancer field?*
- **Open-ended:** *How do patient testimonials affect traffic to my website?*
- **Limited choice**: *Do patients trust testimonials more than newsletters? Support your answer with research that is no older than 2 years.*

As a side note, instruct your AI tool to let you know if it can't find credible data to support its claims. This will reduce the risk of making up facts without resources.

Give your AI tool a specific role.

Much like a human writer assumes a role, your AI model should do the same to enhance the accuracy of its answers. Role designation can be a helpful technique as it provides AI tools with additional context for your prompt and influences the response style. It also enhances the content's accuracy by putting the AI model as an expert.

To assign a role, consider a prompt like this one:

> You're a pathology lab specializing in the pathological identification of prostate cancer biopsies. What advice would you give to a urology practice that wants to bring the lab 'inside' the office and avoid submitting slides to an outside lab?

A detailed prompt, like the one that clearly outlines the AI tool's role, has a much higher chance of yielding a positive answer than a generic instruction to provide lab tips for small-group practices.

In sum, if you explicitly instruct an AI model to prove its expertise through a role, it should be more accurate.

Adjust the AI tool's temperature.

AI tools like ChatGPT have temperature settings that let you directly impact the creativity and randomness of the AI model's response, which can drastically reduce the risk of hallucinations.

The temperature range is 0.1–1.0, with higher values indicating greater response creativity. Values between 0.5 and 0.7 are considered general reference points for general content writing.

Adjusting the temperature of your AI model doesn't require any complex or technical processes—you can tell the AI tool which values to use within your prompt. By doing so, you can ensure more control over the model's creativity and minimize deviations from facts.

Leverage Negative Prompting

As AI hallucinations most commonly occur due to unobstructed creativity, negative prompting can considerably prevent them. It's a technique where you tell an AI model what you don't want to see in the response, guiding its thought process in the right direction.

Negative prompting is particularly prevalent in image generation, though it can also be helpful for text generation. Here are some examples of negative prompts:

- "Limit references to the last 5 years."
- "Don't provide any health advice."
- "Don't include any information found on any pharmaceutical sites."

The only caveat of negative prompting is that you may not always know where your AI model might start hallucinating, or why. You'll need to think ahead to limit the most common causes, which might take some getting used to.

Still, as with anything in medicine, your ability to receive accurate and helpful information increases with time and experience.

Fact-Check AI Content

Regardless of the response you receive, avoid copying and pasting AI-generated content. Experts suggest that you verify everything before publishing to prevent false claims caused by hallucinations.

While there's currently extensive research focused on understanding and preventing hallucinations, the experts disagree on whether this is a fixable problem.

Humans must verify and fact-check responses, even as AI becomes more accurate. Adjust your prompts to provide your AI model with sufficient context and details, and then verify all the key information within the output to stay safe.

The take-home message is that all ChatGPT responses must be reviewed before sharing the information with patients. That may be one reason that GPT-4 will not replace a healthcare provider.

Ethical Concerns of GPT-4

A chapter on GPT-4 would be incomplete without addressing its ethical concerns. Some key ethical concerns include the following:

Protecting the patient's personal health information (PHI) is necessary. Privacy concerns arise, requiring safeguards and oversight. Currently, the program is not encrypted. Therefore, using any patient information should be avoided. For example, when requesting prior authorization, I suggest omitting the patient's name, insurance information, or other demographic information that could identify the patient.

Patient security is crucial to prevent unauthorized access, tampering, or exploitation. Security measures must be in place to protect against potential vulnerabilities.

Addressing these ethical concerns requires collaboration among researchers, developers, policymakers, and the broader community. Striking a balance between innovation and responsible GPT-4 development is essential to maximize GPT-4's positive impact while minimizing potential risks and harms.

Malicious actors may attempt to exploit this nascent technology for evil purposes, including manipulation, propaganda, or the creation of harmful content. Safety measures are needed to prevent the abuse and manipulation of GPT-4-generated content.

Another ethical issue of GPT-4 is racial biases. Stanford School of Medicine researchers caution that popular chatbots are perpetuating racist, debunked medical ideas, thus prompting concerns that the new technology could worsen health disparities for Black patients. There is some good news about this ethical issue: OpenAI.com is working to reduce bias in its models. More importantly, OpenAI.com is trying to inform users that GPT-4 and other chatbots are not a substitute for medical professionals. All biases must be removed from the responses to both patients and their caregivers.

Determining responsibility in case of unintended consequences or misuse of ChatGPT-4 is a complex ethical challenge. Clear guidelines on accountability and commitment are essential [5].

The use of GPT-4 may lead to job displacement in healthcare. Addressing the economic and social impact of GPT-4 requires thoughtful consideration and potential policy interventions.

Tanya's Experience with GPT-4

Tanya gave her senior partners a list of functions that ChatGPT-4 could accomplish. She asked the partners to list, in order of importance, what they considered most important to start implementing in the practice. They were in complete agreement that streamlining the prior authorization process was the most important. Tanya showed the partners how to use GPT-4 for this purpose. The partners were impressed and asked Tanya to select additional functions for GPT-4-4 4, and over the ensuing 4 months, they implemented several additional roles for using GPT in the office.

Bottom Line

GPT-4 has the potential to take over many activities in the medical office. As a result, some jobs will no longer be necessary. GPT-4 reduces paperwork and may reduce physicians' and other healthcare providers' risk of burnout. GPT-4 will take over many tasks from humans. The program will execute them faster, better, and cheaper. The result will be more time to focus on the patient and the patient experience. Although GPT-4 will take over many tedious tasks and eliminate jobs. However, they won't replace humans; GPT-4 can't hold a patient's hand or, at this time, demonstrate empathy and compassion. The GPT-4 bottom line: GPT-4 augments our abilities, handles mundane administrative tasks, and frees us up to focus on what we humans do best—innovate, create, and add a personal touch to the art of medicine.

Key Takeaways

- AI-ChatGPT can significantly decrease administrative burdens such as preparing prior authorizations, streamline coding, and increase collections, reducing denials, all of which allow staff to focus on high-value opportunities that require human judgment.
- Doctors don't have to fear AI; they must recognize that AI combined with human judgment will increase efficiency, reduce costs, and improve patient experience.
- AI is available to all practices regardless of size and allows smaller practices to compete with large group practices and hospitals.
- AI won't replace people, but people who use AI will replace people who don't.

(All of the following responses were created with the assistance of ChatGPT)

References

1. Lin SY, Mahoney MR, Sinsky CA. Ten ways artificial intelligence will transform primary care. J Gen Intern Med. 2019;34(8):1626–30.
2. Bernstein JA, Gadde D, Yassin M, Abramson SL, Bansal P, Joshi SR, et al. The impact of prior authorization on clinical practice and patient care outcomes: a work group report of the AAAAI prior authorization task force. J Allerg Clin Immunol Pract. 2024;12(7):1719–26.
3. Trapani D, Kraemer L, Rugo HS, Lin NU. Impact of prior authorization on patient access to cancer care. Am Soc Clin Oncol Educ Book. 2023;43:e100036.
4. Koch VG. Reimagining informed consent: from disclosure to comprehension. UC Irvine L Rev. 2024;14:894.
5. Lee P, Goldberg C, Kohane I. The AI revolution in medicine: GPT-4 and beyond. Pearson; 2023.

25 Improving the Health of Populations of Patients

> **Case Study Than**
> Than has spent the past 5 years working in a concierge internal medicine practice in a large Pacific Northwestern city. Although she finds her work rewarding, she is frustrated with the complex and disjointed systems of care available in her community. Specifically, she is discouraged by the lack of preventive services available to her patients. She knows that patients are coming into her practice with advanced disease that could have been more efficiently managed had they presented earlier. She is also concerned about patients in her community who cannot afford the level of care that she is able to provide. Than is thinking of changing careers to work for a large commercial not-for-profit insurer in her community. She has a minimal understanding of providing care for a population of patients, rather than focusing on individual patients, but needs to learn more about improving health for populations of patients.

Population health refers to the concept of providing care for an entire population of patients, either through a public health entity, a practice, an insurance plan, or a health plan. Examples of global population health programs include efforts to increase screening and vaccination for COVID-19, efforts to reduce air pollution, and efforts to reduce cardiovascular risk factors, such as smoking cessation, weight loss, or choosing healthy foods for a community. Incumbent upon successful population health programs is coordination between healthcare practitioners, the community, and payors.

David Nash described four pillars of population health: chronic care management, quality and safety, public health, and health policy [1]. Chronic care management is critical to the appropriate use of health resources. Approximately 90% of US healthcare expenditures are for the management of chronic conditions, and over 76% of the population is affected by a chronic disease [2]. Chronic care management is best facilitated by a team of people dedicated to modifying behaviors, educating patients, and facilitating access to health care providers in a given community. Part of chronic care management is assuring that patients are receiving care in the most appropriate setting. One of the most expensive places to receive medical care is the emergency room. Unnecessary emergency room visits in the USA are estimated to cost over $80 billion per year [3]. Obviously, a major facet of population health is not only reducing emergency room visits but also assuring access to lower-cost facilities, such as doctor's offices and urgent care cen-

N. Baum, M. J. Kahn, *Business Basics for your Healthcare Practice*,
https://doi.org/10.1007/978-3-032-25241-8_25

ters, which leads to decreased cost and increased efficiency of care delivery.

Medical errors are unfortunately common in the USA and contribute not only to death and disability but also to increased medical costs. Improving health care quality and safety, like chronic care management, requires a team of individuals who work to improve systems of care to minimize errors. Quality and safety teams typically use protocols and workflows to standardize processes to minimize the potential for error. They also have systems to investigate medical errors and near misses. By analyzing and collecting data, quality and safety teams are able to develop systems to reduce the likelihood of a repeat adverse event.

Public health, by its very nature, addresses the health of populations. The response to the COVID-19 pandemic exemplified the disconnect between public health and clinical medicine found in the USA and also uncovered the problems that occur with improper funding of public health. Delays in diagnostic testing, disruptions in the supply chain for personal protective equipment, and a lack of preparedness for mitigating viral spread, such as social distancing, are all examples of the disconnect. To best care for populations, environmental health experts, epidemiologists, and health administrators need to be involved and work alongside clinicians. Public health teaches us the importance of prevention and can help identify problems with access and quality of health care. Population health is best accomplished at the intersection of clinical medicine and public health.

Providing adequate care for populations involves not only public health but also establishing health policies that directly affect the care of the community. Laws affording care to marginalized populations, laws enforcing public health measures, and policies dictating care paradigms can help to provide care for a population. Although physicians are not typically involved in public policy, this is an area that has the greatest impact on population health. Moving forward, it is beneficial to establish pipelines so that physicians can be involved as policymakers. The Centers for Medicare and Medicaid Innovation established the Initiative to Support Promising Research (INSPIRE) as a means for academic and community physicians to contribute their knowledge and expertise towards public policy surrounding Medicare. Additionally, many medical societies now offer experiential training in dealing with government and policy-making.

So, how does this affect a healthcare practice? Pay for performance (P4P) is an alternative to reimbursement for healthcare services that are based on volume (numbers of office visits, tests ordered, procedures performed, etc.). In a P4P, healthcare providers are reimbursed for behaviors that positively affect the health of their patients. This includes providing preventive health services such as vaccinations in children or keeping blood pressures or blood sugars in a certain range. P4P systems are designed to improve the care of populations. In spite of early enthusiasm, the evidence that P4P improves health care outcomes has been unfortunately modest. A growing trend in healthcare reimbursement is an extension of P4P termed "value-based care." In a value-based system, like traditional P4P, reimbursement is dependent on health outcomes rather than the volume of services provided. Reimbursement is also dependent on the proper utilization of tests and procedures to control cost. Using the equation that value = quality divided by cost, value is best when quality is high and cost is low. In a value-based contract, physicians are typically granted a bonus for providing quality care in a cost-efficient manner and are typically penalized for care falling below a given threshold. To be most effective, value-based care requires a team to gather and record patient outcome data and an electronic system to record data. In a value-based payment system, the accurate attribution of patient and physician is a critical first step to ensure that providers are being rewarded and de-incentivized appropriately. It is important to ensure the proper collection and recording of interventions and outcomes. It is estimated that within several years, value-based care will be the dominant reimbursement system in the USA. To best manage patients under a value-based system, social and economic conditions found in the population, such as water quality, education, and access to care, must be considered. Access to healthy foods and access to public transportation to get to physician appointments are critical predictors of favorable health outcomes. Additionally, in any population, preventive services, such as vaccination and screening, are important to minimize serious late-term complications of chronic illnesses, and providing these services must be incentivized.

In the practice of population health and value-based care, information systems are necessary. These systems need to be interoperable such that data acquired on one platform can ideally be inputted (or transferred) into another platform. The data collected must include important social determinants of health to allow for analyzing and improving care for complex patients with chronic diseases. In addition to data collection, data analytics are useful in predicting healthcare utilization and in predicting risks to health so that preventive measures can be undertaken in a timely fashion. Finally, an information system can be used to "gamify" healthcare to reward positive behaviors and to provide electronic encouragement for positive outcomes such as weight loss or medication compliance.

In the past decade, the Centers for Medicare and Medicaid Services (CMS) established value-based programs in order to better care for individuals and populations and at a lower cost. The five original programs included: an end-stage renal disease program, a hospital-based purchasing program, a physician value modifier program that provided payments to physicians based on quality and not volume, a hospital readmission reduction program, and a hospital-acquired condition reduction program. CMS expects that all traditional Medicare beneficiaries will be in a value-based care model by 2030. Unfortunately, it is still too early to tell if value-based programsprograms are effective in improving patient outcomes at a lower cost.

Currently, there are several value-based care models used by payors. These include fees for value programs where providers are paid based on the quality of care they provide. Shared savings programs allow providers to share in cost savings and provide reimbursement for achieving quality metrics. Risk-based programs allow providers to take on financial risk for caring for a population of patients with incentives to improve the quality of care provided. Finally, bundled payment programs allow for a fixed payment for a bundled procedure such as a kidney transplant, bone marrow transplant, or joint replacement.

Although appealing on the surface, the ability to provide higher quality care and to prove that this is being done requires upfront costs in personnel and software to collect necessary data.

Than's Case

Than decided to take a position with the insurance company. She decided that caring for a population of patients rather than caring for individual patients was more satisfying. She felt that participation in population health could make a bigger difference in health outcomes and would provide her with more satisfaction.

Key Takeaways

- Value-based care is the next logical extension in reducing healthcare costs.
- Providing incentives for patients and physicians for medical compliance and favorable outcomes and having systems to collect and analyze data are critical for a value-based system to work.
- Value-based care and the accompanying reimbursement systems should result in better care for populations of patients.

References

1. Nash DB. The population health mandate. A broader approach to care delivery. Boardroom Press; 2012. http://populationhealthcolloquium.com/readings/Pop_Health_Mandate_NASH_2012.pdf
2. CDC. About Chronic Diseases. Oct 4, 2024. https://www.cdc.gov/chronic-disease/about/index.html
3. Roemer M. Costs of treat-and-release emergency department visits in the United States. Agency for Healthcare Research and Quality. Statistical Brief, September 2024

Concierge Medicine 26

> **Sebastian Considers Concierge Medicine**
> *Sebastian is an internist with more than 2000 active patients. He noted that he spends less time with each patient and more time entering data into his electronic medical record. Sebastian said that he works more than sixty hours a week, takes work home, and spends less time with his family. He does not have time for exercise and has gained 20 pounds over the last 2 years. He feels that he is on a trajectory to burn out. What might he do? One popular option has been the consideration of concierge medicine.*

What Is Concierge Medicine?

Concierge medicine, also known as retainer medicine, is a private relationship between a patient and usually a primary care physician in which the patient pays an annual fee or retainer. This may or may not be in addition to other charges beyond basic medical exams. In exchange for the prepaid retainer, doctors agree to provide highly personalized care and on-demand access. In some cases, the physician will even come to your home or place of business.

Concierge primary care is defined by the American College of Physicians as "any practice that directly contracts with patients to pay out-of-pocket for some or all of the services provided by the practice, instead of or in addition to traditional insurance arrangements, and/or charges an administrative fee to patients, sometimes called a retainer or concierge fee, often in return for a promise for more personalized and accessible care" [1].

The concept of concierge medicine is that there are patients who are placing a premium on their time. A significant number of patients place a premium on their time. It is the same concept where executives have opted not to travel by commercial airlines and pay a premium to fly on a private jet, where they can leave whenever they want, have a plane available within hours of making a request, and experience a significant reduction in travel time. Many people of substantial means will opt to pay a premium to have access to their doctor with an office appointment within hours and have their calls to their physicians answered within minutes.

This model of medicine has been referred to as retainer medicine, boutique medicine, membership medicine, cash-only practice, executive health program, platinum practice, direct-to-consumer care, or P4A (pay for access). While all are very similar in concept, they can vary widely in structure, payment requirements ranging from several hundred to several thousand dollars per year, and operating methods. It is estimated that fewer than 800 US providers practice concierge medicine. Still, numbers are growing each year,

N. Baum, M. J. Kahn, *Business Basics for your Healthcare Practice*,
https://doi.org/10.1007/978-3-032-25241-8_26

primarily due to high deductibles and coinsurance, as well as access to high-quality care. We also face what many have described as a perfect storm, setting us up for a massive shortage of high-quality caregivers that will no doubt accelerate the movement toward concierge medicine.

So, what is this perfect storm? It is a simple math problem, but one with major consequences if we don't find solutions. The number of elderly people per 100 working-age people will nearly triple from 20 to 100 in 1980 to 58,100 in 2060 [2].

In short, our healthcare demands are outpacing the supply of workers at a time when the US is expected to see a massive decline in primary and specialty care providers. Some estimates suggest we could see a decline of more than 100,000 physicians by 2032 [3]. Our population is also living much longer, resulting in even more demand for our caregivers. As a result of this demand, it will likely set up an opportunity for those who can afford it to buy their way to preferred access. This would be like purchasing a first-class ticket or a country club membership to avoid the waiting times for tee times at a public course. That said, the idea of supply and demand is one of the very basics of economics and what drives market demand. Supply is created by the sellers, while demand is generated by buyers. Anytime you have a market where demand is high and supply is low, you can expect innovation and opportunity-seekers to fill the gaps in response to the demand.

Even consumers who have employer-provided healthcare coverage may find concierge medicine appealing. Today, many consumers have deductibles of $ 5000 to $10,000 per year [4]. So, unless they end up needing major medical services, they are basically cash-paying patients. Patients who are younger and have fewer health issues may find this approach less expensive, even if they continue purchasing healthcare coverage from their employers. And, not surprisingly, doctors who go into concierge medicine will generally be highly selective about who they accept as members. Logically speaking, a younger, healthier membership typically translates into less consumption of the provider's time and effort.

It should also come as no surprise that concierge medicine can also be controversial. Some view this as a system for the wealthy and privileged. Some even speculate that this will only make our access to providers more expensive, because these models are generally designed to reduce a provider's patient load. However, one could argue that this is a convenient way for providers to reduce administrative burdens, freeing up more time for patient care. Recent studies have found that some providers are spending a mind-boggling 10 h per week on administrative tasks, and many end up taking work home with them that goes unaccounted for. We have also recently introduced EHRs that allow for direct electronic patient engagement without any compensation for providers' time spent responding to these messages.

When you examine economics, it is a win-win for consumers and providers. The typical employed primary care provider can expect to earn a salary between $125,000 and $150,000 [5]. They will generally be expected to work 4 to 5 days a week, see 20 to 30 patients per day, and usually have several hours of charting and documentation at the end of the 8-hour day. The typical panel size is 2300 patients. While this is not an unreasonable salary, it can be very misleading when you factor in the number of hours and the high cost of medical school. In 2023, we wrote a chapter in our book, The Business Basics of Building and Managing a Healthcare Practice, comparing a doctor's salary to that of a UPS driver [6]. Surprisingly, the incomes of the physician and the UPS truck driver were almost identical once you take into consideration the long working hours for physicians, medical school debt, malpractice, continued education, compliance, and risk and liabilities associated with the delivery of care. And this was not intended to draw sympathy for physicians. Money is not the only driving force behind becoming a provider. Still, it illustrates how and why a provider might feel undervalued and seek other ways to earn a living. For example, under the concierge model, the same provider can manage just 100 healthy families for an annual fee of $5000 per family, make $500,000, and do far less work. They could do this without any billing staff or expensive EHR systems and could even provide care virtually or even make house calls.

Ironically, the basic concept and premise of concierge medicine is rooted in the original house call. In the early years of medicine, we had community doctors, black bag in hand, who traveled to patients' homes to provide medical care, a practice that remained common up to the mid-twentieth century. In fact, one of the most famous paintings in the world, by Luke Fildes in 1891 (Fig. 26.1), depicts a Victorian doctor observing the critical stage of a child's illness while the parents gaze helplessly at the periphery. The painting's scene is in the home of the helpless child. The painting depicts the doctor's concentrated focus on the child, showing the patient as a person and individual, and the doctor as a compassionate caregiver with empathy for the patient's suffering. Less notice is how the parents, especially the father, have relinquished all their trust and confidence in the doctor to save their child. This compelling image portrays the special bond between patients and providers. This painting is frequently used as an illustration in medical journals and at medical conferences to describe the values of the ideal physician and the inadequacies of the medical profession. One famous quote about the painting comes from a surgeon, Dr. Mitchell Banks: "What do we not owe to Mr. Fildes for showing to the world the typical doctor as we would all like him to be shown—an honest man and a gentleman, doing his best to relieve suffering?" He continued: "A library of books written in your honor would not do what this picture has done and will do for the medical profession in making the hearts of our fellow men warm to us with confidence and affection" [7].

They say history has a way of repeating itself. We may well be in a cycle in which some elements of healthcare return to a more direct-to-consumer model. While many valid opinions exist on concierge medicine, the demand for such services will generally be driven by consumers' willingness to pay for access and more personalized care. The current system is not working for many consumers or providers, so there is an eagerness to explore these models, and we expect this to continue to grow in popularity.

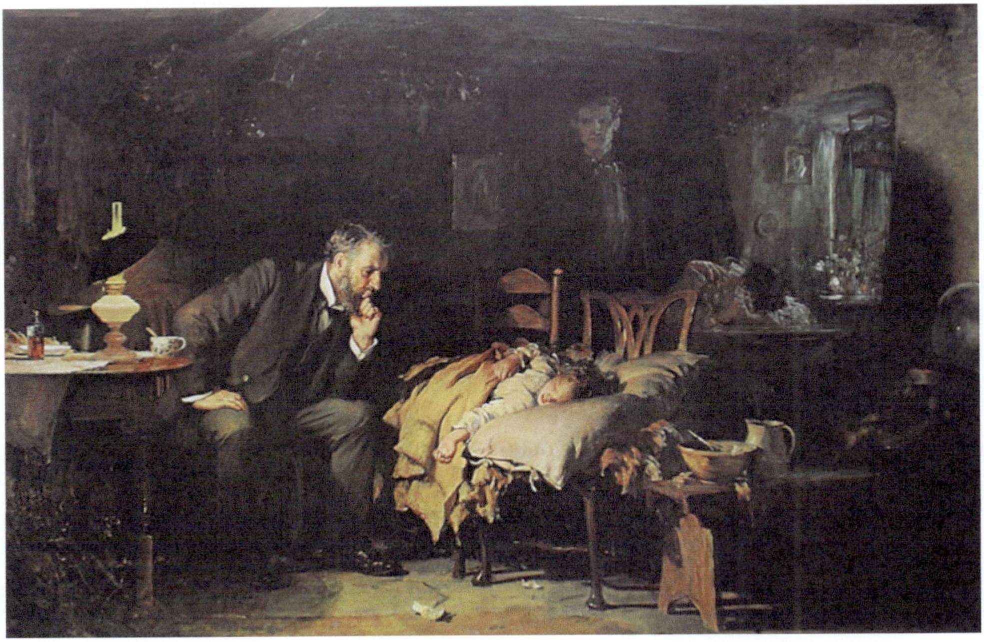

Fig. 26.1 The Doctor—by Luke Fildes, 1891

Benefits of Concierge Medicine to Patients

Patients are seated in a sparsely crowded reception area. They have guaranteed same-day appointments, including Saturday appointments. These patients will have access to their physician, including having their cell phone and pager numbers. For those paying higher premiums, the service will include house calls, where the doctor accompanies the patient to see specialists and arranges priority appointments with them. The doctor will emphasize wellness and preventive healthcare with weight loss programs and nutritional counseling. These doctors will also offer Email access to the patients and prescription refills over the Internet. Concierge physicians commonly include annual physical and other uncovered services. In effect, these patients are paying to have better and more immediate access to their physicians. Most importantly, these patients will have unfettered and uninterrupted visits with their doctor. These physicians will see fewer patients each day, have minimal or no paperwork to take home each evening, and can thus spend more one-on-one time with these select patients.

What Are the Advantages to Physicians?

Concierge medicine is most applicable to physicians in primary care or internal medicine. The greatest advantage of concierge medicine is that it creates a hassle-free practice. Most physicians who are attracted to concierge medicine are those middle-aged to older physicians who have had busy practices but are noting that the warm fuzzies or the satisfaction that physicians once enjoyed from their practices are diminished or even absent. With a concierge practice, doctors will have fewer patients, allowing them to spend more time with each one. Additionally, a concierge practice with fewer patients will also have fewer calls, lower billing expenses, lower accounts receivable, and reduced overhead costs.

Another advantage of concierge medicine is that you will know your monthly and annual income in advance. If you have patients who are agreeable to pay an access fee, you will know what your gross revenue will be each month and annually. For example, suppose you decided to care for 1000 patients, instead of the 4000–5000 patients that a busy primary care physician typically covers, and charge each patient $2000 for access to your practice. In that case, your gross income will be $500,000 annually, or $ 41,666 per month. Now you can easily budget your expenses and your lifestyle.

Getting Started with Concierge Medicine

The process to convert to a concierge medicine model takes approximately 3 months. However, for physicians leaving an employed situation, it may take up to 6 months. There is often a complicated process of leaving an employed physician arrangement that includes noncompete clauses. Most concierge companies help with the development of a timeline and offer guidance through every step of the transition process. This includes finding a location, acquiring insurance, arranging for a practice management program, an electronic medical record program, hiring staff, and other tasks that take the load off the physician to streamline the transition to a concierge practice.

Concierge medicine is most applicable for a mid-career or older physician who is in a geographic or socioeconomic area where patients are willing to pay for these amenities.

Begin by sending a letter to your patients (before implementing this concept) explaining what you are doing and directing them to contact your office with any questions or concerns. Providing such notice before adopting this practice will reduce the likelihood that some of your patients will be without a physician. They need to know that they can seek the care of another doctor as an alternative to paying your practice the retainer fee. There are concierge medicine companies that can assist you in transitioning your practice from an insurance reimbursement or fee-for-service model to a concierge practice; however, a substantial fee will be charged for this assistance. (See resources for names of companies that will help with a concierge practice).

An annual fee needs to be established. It would have to be clearly defined as to which services, both medical and nonmedical, are provided for the payment of this fee. For example, you may "carve out" hospital care, meaning you will not be responsible for their care if they are admitted to the hospital. You will be responsible for finding a physician, such as a hospitalist, who will care for them during their hospital admission. As a rule, this annual fee would be payable upon execution of the contract between the patient and the physicians. Some have gone with a "monthly fee" arrangement. Some doctors who have gone this route have decided to no longer contract with Medicare and other third-party payors. It is essential to explain to patients what will be provided and their payment responsibilities.

Saga of Sebastian

Sebastian realized that working 10+ hours a day, followed by several hours at the computer in the evening to complete medical records, was unsustainable. Sebastian was approached by a national concierge medicine company. The company arranged a focus group with 25 of its existing patients. The survey from the focus group indicated that his existing patients wanted more of his time and more access to care. He signed up with a national company. The company suggested that he reduce his patient volume to 500 patients. This allowed him to spend more time with his patients, provided them with greater access to care, reduced the stress of practice, helped him lose 20 pounds, and enabled him to be home for dinner.

Key Takeaways

Concierge medicine is an innovative approach that offers patients enhanced accessibility, personalized care, and potentially improved outcomes. For patients, the benefits include longer doctor-patient encounters, shorter wait times in the reception area and exam room, and 24/7 access to their physician. This personalized care increases patient satisfaction and fosters better preventive care.

For physicians, a concierge medical practice can lead to reduced administrative burdens, greater efficiency, and more time spent eyeball-to-eyeball with patients. Additionally, this model ensures a more sustainable workload and a stable revenue stream, mitigating the financial pressures commonly associated with traditional fee-for-service models.

Despite potential challenges, such as initial financial investment and concerns about accessibility for lower-income patients, concierge medicine presents an option for both physicians and patients seeking an improved healthcare experience. Finally, this method of healthcare will improve physicians' work-life balance.

Our take-home message is that Medicine is changing, and the model of seeing large volumes of patients with very low profit margins may be over for a few primary care physicians who are transitioning to a lower volume of patients with greater access to their physician, who practices concierge medicine.

- Concierge medicine reduces the patient's volume to a more manageable level.
- Concierge medicine has the potential to reduce burnout.
- Concierge medicine returns the joy and satisfaction of being a physician.

Resources

MDVIP (http://www.mdvip.com/) is a select group of exceptional doctors who choose to structure their practices to provide exceptional, highly personalized healthcare to their patients, yielding exceptional results in terms of patient health and satisfaction

Modern Medicine (http://www.modernmed.com) is a healthcare service firm designed to create a better healthcare experience for patients, physicians, and businesses. We establish and maintain modern primary care practice environments nationwide that are unlike any traditional practice.

The Society for Innovative Medical Practice Design (http://www.simpd.org/) is an organization of physicians promoting a direct financial relationship with their patients to restore the integrity of the patient-physician relationship.

References

1. Doherty R. Assessing the patient care implications of "concierge" and other direct patient contracting practices: a policy position paper from the American College of Physicians. Ann Intern Med. 2015;163(12):949–52.
2. Gratton L, Scott AJ. The 100-year life: living and working in an age of longevity. Bloomsbury Publishing; 2021.
3. Patel RV, Gonzalez MR, Attaar N, Patel MV, Lozano-Calderon SA. Analyzing Orthopaedic workforce trends in an ever-changing landscape. JAAOS. 2025;33(14):780–6.
4. Baum N, Kahn MJ, Daigrepont J. Concierge medicine. In: The business of building and managing a healthcare practice: going beyond the basics. Cham: Springer International Publishing; 2023. p. 201–3.
5. Dahle JM. Financial considerations for the healthcare professional. In: The successful health care professional's guide: everything you need to know but weren't taught in training. Cham: Springer International Publishing; 2022. p. 95–107.
6. Baum N, Kahn MJ, Daigrepont J. The business of building and managing a healthcare practice. Springer; 2023.
7. Milligan B. Luke Fildes's the doctor, narrative painting, and the selfless professional ideal. Vic Lit Cult. 2016;44(3):641–68.

27 Academic Careers

> **Case Tucker**
> Tucker is in the final year of her Pulmonary/Critical Care fellowship at a major academic medical center on the West Coast. She graduated at the top of her class as both an undergraduate and a medical student and was asked to be Chief Medical Resident prior to her fellowship. Tucker is trying to decide the next step in her career. She has always liked to teach medical students and residents but does not like "research." Her training has prepared her for a career in academic medicine, but she is not sure if this is the right career path for her. She has heard discussions about salary from last year's fellowship graduates and is well aware of the difference between academic and private practice salaries. Is academic medicine right for her?

In 1765, the first allopathic medical school in the US was founded by Dr. John Morgan, who received his MD degree at the University of Edinburgh Medical School. Morgan and Dr. William Shippen Jr., a fellow Edinburgh graduate, convinced the Trustees of the University of Pennsylvania to start the first medical school in the 13 colonies. By the mid-1850s, the University of Pennsylvania School of Medicine had a distinguished faculty including Benjamin Rush, Philip Syng Physick, William Pepper, and Joseph Leidy. When the AMA was founded in 1847, Nathaniel Chapman, a Professor of Medicine at Penn, was named the first president. From this auspicious beginning, academic medical centers (AMCs) currently number over 140 and provide 20% of the country's medical care and 40% of US charity medical care [1]. AMCs manage 60% of the country's Level 1 trauma centers, graduate over 17,000 doctors, and train over 30,000 residents and fellows. Unlike other professions, medicine is one of the few that combines education, research, and operations in a single organization. Law schools do not operate law firms, and business schools do not manage corporations. Vertical integration of AMCs allows for some efficiencies but also can be a source of stress. Of the three missions, patient care, research, and education, only patient care generally has a positive margin, and these are forever decreasing.

When investigating why physicians choose careers in academic medicine, the literature suggests that medical school graduates with other advanced degrees (PhD, MBA, MPH) or advanced fellowships are more likely to choose academic careers [2]. The desire to teach, conduct research, and the influence of a positive role model also contribute to a physician choosing an academic career.

A career in academic medicine can follow several paths; not all academics are specifically

N. Baum, M. J. Kahn, *Business Basics for your Healthcare Practice*,
https://doi.org/10.1007/978-3-032-25241-8_27

involved in scientific research, but academic physicians support the tripartite mission of an AMC: clinical care, education, and scholarly productivity.

One of the biggest differences between an academic job and one in private practice is the way that the physician's salary is supported. In private practice, income is derived from clinical care—seeing patients, billing for procedures, and managing complex hospitalized patients. In academic medicine, income is still fundamentally derived from clinical care, but academic physicians have the opportunity to substitute teaching, research, or administrative responsibilities for clinical time. Because these other activities produce much less revenue than clinical care, in general, the salary of an academic physician is lower than that of a private practice doctor working in the same field.

There are basically four types of academic physicians: physician scientists, clinician educators, physicians working in academically based practices, and physician administrators.

Physician scientists are paid for doing research. Their salaries are typically supported by external grants and contracts. Using the clinical care model, physician scientists *buy back* their clinical time with grant support. The physician scientist model is what is most commonly thought to represent academic medicine, but in fact, physician scientists are a small percentage of most medical school faculty due to the difficulty in obtaining grants. Currently, the NIH funds much less than 20% of grants submitted. In addition to directly contributing to the reputation of a medical school through published work, physician scientists also add value to their institutions through grant overhead. Grant overhead is used to support the research infrastructure of a medical school and could amount to 50% of the total grant support. However, research dollars are not a windfall for AMCs. A recent report for the Association of American Medical Colleges (AAMC) concluded that AMCs spend an additional 53 cents for every dollar of sponsored research that they receive [3].

Clinician educators buy back clinical time through teaching medical students, interns, and residents. Although they are still expected to participate in scholarly activity, this is typically accomplished through curricular development and assessment. Clinician educators sometimes have additional administrative titles such as Course Directors, Program Directors, or Vice Chairs for Education in departments. Because clinician educators are relatively expensive, their positions are limited. Many medical schools, recognizing the value of clinician educators, have established specific academic tracks for these physicians in order to get promoted.

As medical schools have struggled to provide clinical material for their trainees over the past 10 years, there has been an increasing number of faculty who have their clinical practices affiliated with a medical school. Sometimes, these physicians are employed by the medical school. Sometimes, they have a faculty appointment without salary. Academically based clinicians are vital for the success of the educational mission, and these physicians typically enjoy working with trainees, enjoy keeping up to date through their trainees, and value an academic appointment at a medical school. Many practices use clinical affiliations to market their physicians. The public sees value in medical school faculty, assuming they are up to date and assuming that they are experts in their field.

Finally, every medical school has physicians who are hired to serve administrative roles. Such roles include the Dean, the Associate and Assistant Deans, Department Chairs, and the like. These physicians substitute administrative time for clinical duties. As with the clinician educators, physician administrators are expensive and typically limited in number. Typically, administrators are hired through an external search. Less commonly, they are hired from within. The typical "head hunter" is less knowledgeable about academic physician leadership positions. Information on academic jobs can be found on the AAMC Career Connect website (https://careerconnect.aamc.org/jobseeker/search/results/) and through search firms that specialize in such positions.

Although we have divided academic careers into four groups, in fact, many academic physicians play multiple roles and may overlap between the four aforementioned groups. One word of caution: to be successful, an academician should spend a majority of their time on one of the roles. Spending 25% of time in each of these roles is not likely to lead to success in any one mission. Additionally, to be a successful academician and get promoted, you must demonstrate some type of scholarly activity. This may be through publishing peer-reviewed manuscripts but may also be through developing novel curricula that are used by other institutions. National or regional presentations at specialty societies are other examples of scholarly activity. Finally, do not forget that there are platforms for publishing education-based research. These include journals such as Academic Medicine, Teaching and Learning in Medicine, or Medical Teacher. Additionally, the AAMC sponsors a repository for curricular design called MedEdPORTAL. Submissions are peer-reviewed and are assigned a unique PubMed number so that they can be searched and accessed.

In addition to the obvious differences in job responsibilities, academic physicians typically have lower salaries than those in private practice. One positive aspect of looking for an academic job is that academic salaries are published annually from the AAMC and are broken down by specialty and geographical location and are further divided into private and public schools. Having this information makes negotiation easier (see Chap. 5).

Academic positions may also come with unique benefits such as tuition coverage for self and dependents. This can be a very valuable perquisite as college tuitions continue to rise. Also, academic positions tend to come with a more generous allotment for continuing medical education and conference attendance. Universities typically have a matching program for money put away for retirement. As an academician, you are hired by a hospital, AMC, or medical school. You do not incur the costs of setting up an office, marketing, or getting malpractice insurance. Typically, these are provided by the academic practice and are paid for through overhead charged on clinical revenue. Benefits such as these can make an academic salary more attractive.

Academics are divided into faculty ranks. Typically, a new academician is appointed as either an instructor or an assistant professor. The differences between these two ranks include job responsibilities and salary. A physician-scientist may prefer to start out as an instructor because often the "tenure clock" does not start until a faculty member is an Assistant Professor. This allows the faculty member to get a running start on grant funding to help ensure promotion at the proper time. After a prescribed period of time, typically outlined in the faculty handbook, assistant professors can be promoted to associate professors and then full professors. The promotion process is dependent on scholarly activity, grants and contracts, clinical care, teaching ability, and letters of recommendation from external peers. Universities have a promotion and tenure committee who make such determinations. Some academic positions are eligible for tenure, some are not.

Tenure or Not?

Tenure began in US colleges and universities in the early nineteenth century when professors were under the auspices of the board of trustees of universities and influential donors could have professors removed, censured, or demoted. In 1900, Harvard University, Columbia University, and the University of Chicago entered into a pact and decided that donors could no longer exert influence over a professor's hire or employment. In 1915, the American Association of University Professors (AAUP) established principles of academic freedom and tenure. Tenure was originally granted after 10 years (hence its name) for distinguished scholarly activity and value to the university. In 1940, the AAUP recommended that the probationary period without tenure be decreased from 10 to 7 years.

Tenure remains a contractual right that grants a professor a permanent position, yet the guarantee of salary is often murky. Tenure provides protection against termination without cause and allows for academic freedom. However, currently, most universities have provisions for academic freedom outside of the tenure process. So, is tenure important for academic physicians? Yes and no. The vast majority of academic physicians are not tenured. This is because many universities reserve the tenure track for those professors who are involved in research and leave the non-tenure track for clinicians and educators. Because most academicians do not have external grant funding, they tend to be on non-tenure tracks. Tenure is less important for physicians who can typically find another job quickly in case of separation. Job security is less important for a cardiologist with specific expertise in electrophysiology whose services could be used at a number of health facilities. In contrast, this is not the case with a professor of English or Folklore who may have difficulty finding another job, especially if they are looking off-cycle, as most academic jobs start at the beginning of the academic year. As stated, academic freedom is afforded to all, so this is also not a good argument for tenure. Further, tenured professors can be terminated for cause or in case of financial exigency. Because the association between a position and salary is unclear, most universities do not guarantee a full salary indefinitely to a tenured professor.

What is the value of tenure? Tenure is an accomplishment like any other. In many universities, there are benefits to being tenured, including the opportunity to serve on certain committees and the sense of accomplishment that tenure affords. It is more difficult to terminate a tenured professor, and typically termination requires a much longer notice than for nontenured faculty. One of the risks of being considered for tenure is that if you are denied, theoretically, you would have to leave the university. In all, academicians often do not have the choice of academic track, as it is usually determined by the responsibilities of the individual faculty member.

Regardless of track, every academician should closely review their faculty handbook, faculty bylaws, and faculty constitution to understand expectations for promotion. We recommend doing this at the time of employment. Sometimes, it may be possible to switch from a non-tenure to a tenure track. The specific procedure for a track switch and the rules for doing so are typically articulated in faculty handbooks. Sometimes there is a time limit for a switch, such as prior to year seven of employment, and sometimes there is an approval process that must be signed off upon by the dean or chair. The faculty handbook is an academician's contract that dictates rules, procedures, and remedies.

Finally, because of the very real salary differential between academic and private practices, academic physicians have to find some value in their jobs so as not to become frustrated. Academicians who are basically in private practice with a reduced salary do not tend to stay in academics very long.

Back to the Case

After much introspection, Tucker decided that a career as a clinician educator was the right one for her. Tucker realized that a job that did not involve teaching would be less fulfilling for her. Tucker met with the business officer in her department and was able to get a copy of the AAMC Faculty Salary Survey. She believed this would be very valuable to have with her upcoming salary negotiations. Tucker also realized the importance of reviewing the faculty handbook once she settled on a position. She expected that she would not be on a tenure track, giving her flexibility to spend more time with patients and more time teaching. Tucker very much looked forward to the months ahead.

Key Takeaways

- There are basically four types of jobs in academic medicine: Clinician educator, physician scientist, academically affiliated clinician, and physician administrator.
- Although academic positions generally pay less than private practice, there are benefits to becoming an academic physician.
- The faculty handbook is your friend in academics. Make sure you are familiar with it early in your career.

References

1. http://www.miramedgs.com/web/57-focus/past-issues/spring-2017/667-the-rise-and-fall-of-academic-medicine-amc-competitiveness-in-post-reform-healthcare
2. Strause SE, Straus C, Tzanetos K. Career choice in academic medicine: systematic review. J Gen Intern Med. 2006;21(12):1222–9.
3. http://datahound.scientopia.org/2015/04/03/research-spending-at-academic-medical-centers/

28 The Role of Private Equity

> **Florence**
>
> Florence has been a dermatologist in a seven-member practice for the past 12 years. Her original contract allowed her to become a full-equity partner after a 3-year buy-in. The practice has been doing well, has received high patient satisfaction scores, and has received accolades from the community for providing care to uninsured patients at a local clinic twice a month. Recently, OxySys, a large private equity company based in San Francisco, has inquired about potentially buying the practice. As a 15% owner, Florence would do well financially with the purchase, but she wonders what she would lose. Would she still be able to manage her patients the way she has been doing for over a decade? Would she still be able to provide free care? What would this mean for her future earning potential? Maybe she should have paid more attention to her college roommate, a business major who now works as a venture capitalist.

The most commonly utilized investment tools to provide future financial stability are stocks and bonds. These form the basis of a typical investor's portfolio. Stock purchases provide the investor equity in a company. Bonds typically reflect longer-term debt that is repaid with interest. Both of these are expected to provide annual returns that are better than inflation, and both are expected to provide a portfolio that grows in value over time.

Private equity, a less commonly available investment tool, refers to investments in companies not typically listed on a public stock exchange. Private equity firms typically receive investments from institutions, foundations, and high-net-worth investors. Because such transactions are private, they are not subject to the same external reporting standards as typical stocks and bonds. Although regulated by the Securities and Exchange Commission (SEC), private equity is generally less regulated than those investments found on public exchanges. Corporations invest in private equity with the hope of potentially higher returns on investment than with typical stock and bond purchases, but there is also a potential for higher losses. Thus, the concept of risk and reward: higher rewards come from assuming a higher risk. Despite the potential risk, private equity investments in healthcare have reached over $446 billion globally.

The first private equity firms were the American Research and Development Corporation (ARDC) and J.H. Whitney & Company, both founded in 1946. These companies were originally established to pool capital from multiple investors to fund the growth and

N. Baum, M. J. Kahn, *Business Basics for your Healthcare Practice*,
https://doi.org/10.1007/978-3-032-25241-8_28

expansion of smaller private companies. The Small Business Investment Act of 1958 solidified the role of private equity in business by authorizing the formation of Small Business Investment Companies (SBICs). SBICs provided capital for small business growth to stimulate the US economy and also were able to access federal matching funds to do so.

There are several types of private equity investments. Venture capital refers to investments in early-stage companies with a potential for growth. Venture capitalists look for companies that need capital early in their development and invest in those with the greatest potential for return on investment. Typically, such investments are mid to longer term, with the private investors expecting the firm to sell the company at a profit within 7–10 years. Growth equity, another type of private equity, refers to investing in companies that are trying to expand rapidly. As with venture capital, investors hope to sell the company at a profit within a mid to longer-term time horizon. Private equity funds can also be invested in real estate, distressed and struggling companies, infrastructure, and even in other private equity companies.

Because healthcare is such a large part of the US economy, representing over $5 trillion, it should not be surprising that private equity firms have become interested in healthcare practices, and since the early 2000s, healthcare has been an investment target for private equity. From a healthcare practice perspective, private equity companies are typically most interested in buyouts. In this situation, the private equity company buys a practice with the intent of using active management to improve efficiencies, leading to greater profitability. This is typically accomplished through operational improvements, strategic initiatives, taking advantage of economies of scale, and making changes in staffing. The private equity firm then expects to sell the company at a significant profit. Typically, private equity companies expect a long-term investment of 10 years or more for healthcare entities with an eventual sale as part of their exit strategy. Private equity offers healthcare practices and hospitals access to capital that might not otherwise be available, but practices selling to private equity also run the risk of the managing partner maximizing profits over public interests. Private equity companies often allow physicians to hold some equity in their practices so that they can financially benefit from future transactions, to better align incentives. Typically, this is a small percentage compared to the percentage owned by the private equity firm. To gain a return on investment, private equity firms typically utilize strategies of expansion, establishing new lines of business, and restructuring. Although many of these ideas sound enticing and consistent with improving access to care, in reality, often the relationship between physicians and managing partners sour as the new practice environment seems more focused on the financial bottom line as opposed to the quality of care. For a practice, although the original buyout offer may seem financially attractive, physicians in the practice should expect some loss of control and some conflicts with practice management issues, such as staffing, equipment purchases, and patient mix. This is inevitable. The term "corporatization of medicine" refers to the increasing prevalence of large for-profit corporations, such as private equity firms and insurance companies, acquiring hospitals and physician practices. Because of concern about profit over quality, many states have either implemented or plan to implement regulations concerning the corporatization of medicine.

According to the nonprofit Private Equity Stakeholder Project, as of July 2025, 488 hospitals, including acute care hospitals, rehabilitation hospitals, psychiatric hospitals, and long-term care facilities, were owned by private equity. This represents 8.5% of all private hospitals and 22.6% of for-profit hospitals [1].

Despite a growing percentage of healthcare entities being owned by private equity, the nonfinancial advantages of such a structure are not known. A study published in JAMA in 2023 found that Medicare patients at private-equity owned hospitals had a 25% increase in complications as compared with those not owned by private equity [2]. In this study, complications included a 38% increase in infections from central lines and a doubling of surgical site infections. It is speculated that the findings of the study are largely the result of staffing cuts done in an effort to improve efficiency.

Another study, by the same authors, found that private-equity-owned hospitals earned 27% more revenue than those independently managed [3]. This was accomplished by increasing hospital service charges and seeing fewer government-funded patients.

Another real-world disadvantage of private equity ownership is that on several occasions, private equity takeover of a hospital or system resulted in discontinuation of services in a community, resulting in decreased access to care and exacerbation of healthcare disparities. The closure of Hahnemann Hospital in Philadelphia, Crozer Chester Medical Center in Upland, PA, and Carney Hospital in Boston are such examples. In several of these cases, the underlying real estate was felt to be more valuable than the hospital itself, leading to hospital closure and liquidation of the real estate asset. As a result, several of these communities lost access to emergency services, primary care services, and even burn unit care.

Despite the obvious downsides of private equity acquisition, there are potential advantages such as infusion of needed capital for expansion of services, as well as providing managerial know-how. Following the COVID pandemic, many smaller practices suffered due to significant losses of revenue. Private equity became one source of a capital lifeline. Private equity firms typically acquired higher-performing and more lucrative specialty practices, such as dermatology, ophthalmology, urology, or orthopedics. More recently, primary care practices have become a target with the feeling that consolidation may lead to better efficiency in purchasing power.

Bigger is often better. This is especially true as healthcare practices have become more consolidated, providing the advantage of scale. For example, a large hospital system buying 10 million tongue depressors gets a cheaper price and a better deal than an individual practice purchasing 500 of them. Private equity allows for such consolidation when coordinated to purchase multiple healthcare facilities within a given market.

However, even with potential upsides, concerns about prioritization of short-term financial gains over long-term investment in patient care remain. It is therefore important when considering a private equity offer to understand the terms of the agreement, the experience and history of the private equity firm, and the long-term needs of the practice.

Back to the Case

Florence and her partners met to discuss the offer. Although they would have benefitted financially from selling their practice, they remained concerned about what such an acquisition would mean to their patients and their community. Not to completely dismiss the notion of an eventual private equity partner, they decided to table the decision for now, with the possibility of entertaining such an offer in the future when they could better understand the pros and cons of such an offer.

Key Takeaways

- Private equity firms have aggressively sought the acquisition of healthcare entities.
- As with other financial arrangements, there are pros and cons to such a relationship.
- On the plus side, a private equity investment provides capital.
- This capital comes with the downside of decreased control.

References

1. https://pestakeholder.org/private-equity-hospital-tracker
2. Kannan S, Bruch JD, Song Z. Changes in hospital adverse events and patient outcomes associated with private equity acquisition. JAMA. 2023;330(24):2365–75.
3. Bruch JD, Gondi S, Song Z. Changes in hospital income, use, and quality associated with private equity acquisition. JAMA Intern Med. 2020;180(11):1428–35.

29 Nonclinical Careers

Kate has been in a seven-member ENT practice for the past 11 years. She is beginning to feel cynical about the future of medical practice and worries that this is affecting both her professional and family life. In the beginning, as she was starting out, Kate was inspired by her work, working mostly with children with ENT issues. She enjoyed being the local expert and was frequently sought out by local television stations to comment on topics such as tonsillectomy, hearing problems in children, and vaccinations. More recently, she has been feeling burned out. She is less interested in patient care and feels she needs a change. She is curious about careers outside of clinical medicine. How should she start? Does she need an MBA or an MPH or a similar degree? Who should she talk to?

Despite the joy many feel in the practice of medicine, for some, a clinical career is not the right fit. This decision can occur during medical school or, more commonly, after a period of clinical practice. One question that is often asked is whether there is a need for an additional degree. Whether that be an MBA, MPH, MHA, MMM, or even a PhD, specialized education may be helpful in nonclinical careers.

MBA

MBA (Master of Business Administration) degrees are focused on providing the knowledge and skills needed in leadership and strategic decision-making. The MBA degree was first introduced by Harvard University in 1908 to address complexities in large organizations following the industrial revolution. Since then, MBA programs have provided more in-depth training in leadership, global economics, and entrepreneurship. Coursework for an MBA typically includes topics such as accounting, finance, business writing, strategy, marketing, operations, leadership, and entrepreneurship. Full-time MBA programs were typically 2 years in length but now are much shorter. Executive MBA programs can typically be completed in 18 months or less. Additionally, many MBA programs are now offered online. There has been a growth of combined MD/MBA programs that are typically 5 years in length, but some can be completed in 4 years. MBA degrees are helpful for leaders who want to learn to think strategically, considering budget, return on investment, and growth.

MPH

An MPH (Master of Public Health) degree focuses on the health of populations. The MPH degree began in the early 1900s at Johns Hopkins University School of Hygiene and Public Health.

N. Baum, M. J. Kahn, *Business Basics for your Healthcare Practice*,
https://doi.org/10.1007/978-3-032-25241-8_29

Most MPH programs' curricula include topics such as epidemiology, biostatistics, community health, global health, maternal health, behavioral sciences, and tropical/infectious diseases. MPH programs typically include internships or capstone projects to provide students with practical experience. An MPH degree is typically completed within 2 years, but there are accelerated and online programs available. There has been an increase in MD/MPH programs that are typically 4 to 5 years in duration.

MHA

The MHA (Master of Health Administration) degree prepares graduates for leadership and management careers in healthcare. The first MHA was offered by the University of Minnesota in 1946 and was designed to provide formal education in healthcare management. Typical MHA coursework includes instruction in healthcare policy, finance, operations, strategy, and management. The MHA can be considered an MBA with a narrow focus on healthcare. As with the MD/MBA and MD/MPH combined degrees, there has been an increase in medical schools offering combined MD/MHA degrees. These are typically 5-year programs.

MMM

The MMM (Master of Medical Management) degree is designed for practicing physicians who wish to develop leadership and management skills. The first MMM degree was awarded by Tulane University in 1997. The curriculum typically includes coursework in healthcare policy, organizational management, operations, finance, and health economics. Unlike the other degrees discussed (MBA, MHA, MPH), the MMM is targeted toward physicians who have completed residencies. The MMM degree was designed to incorporate a practical education focus as provided by the American College of Physician Executives. An MMM degree typically takes 12 to 18 months to complete.

PhD

A PhD is the highest level of achievement in a particular area. PhD degrees are research-focused. PhD programs include coursework followed by intense research and laboratory work necessary to complete the degree. For physicians, a PhD suggests a focus on becoming a physician-scientist. There are many MD/PhD combined programs. A typical combined program takes between 6 and 8 years to complete.

Careers in the Pharmaceutical Industry

Some physicians will seek careers with the pharmaceutical industry as an alternative to clinical practice. Contrary to common perception, most physicians who work in the pharmaceutical industry, with the possible exception of physician scientists, are not working in labs, titrating drug doses, or experimenting with animal models. Rather, physicians in pharma are often involved in medical affairs, strategic product development, pharmacovigilance, regulatory affairs, and marketing. Physicians who work in pharma often design and oversee clinical trials, ensuring that they are well-designed and ethical. Physicians then interpret data and work within the regulatory framework to help bring drugs to market. Finally, physicians help pharmaceutical companies monitor side effects and mitigate risk. Physicians in pharma also help to develop educational materials for other physicians and help to educate the pharmaceutical sales force. Finally, physicians who work for pharma help to write articles for peer review.

Although completing a residency is not always required for physicians working with pharma, many companies require board certification in a specialty. As compared with clinical practice, many physicians in pharma enjoy a perceived better work-life balance. Depending on the job description, especially in scientific affairs, other advanced degrees like a PhD may be of benefit or even required. Business degrees are potentially helpful but typically not required. Physicians interested in careers in the pharmaceutical industry should consult with search firms that hire in this area. Typically, it is important to get your first job with career advancement possible in the future. Typical salaries for these positions are between $250 K and upward, recognizing that CEOs of major pharmaceutical companies are among the highest paid people in the country.

Careers in Consulting

Because of the training it takes to become a physician, especially a specialist or subspecialist, this knowledge and training can be converted into serving as a consultant to an insurance company, healthcare organization, or a consulting agency dealing with healthcare issues. The range of experiences available to physician consultants is vast and includes requests for advice on insurance matters, legal issues, new venture planning, management, consolidation, or supply chain issues. In these roles, physicians are expected to use their expertise to provide insight to answer questions and address challenges. As a consultant, a physician can work alone or in a larger consulting group. To obtain a job as a physician consultant, it is necessary to gain significant experience in your area of consultation. This can be through practice development and management, serving as a leader in an academic medical group or private group, or obtaining an advanced business degree. Not all consultants require specialty training. Physician consultant salaries vary widely depending on the scope of work and experience. Salaries can be as low as $120 K per year for physicians right out of medical school to salaries well over $1million per year for experienced physicians addressing difficult problems in large organizations. Of note, physician consultants are typically paid via a base salary with incentives built into their compensation plans.

Careers in Public Health

Public health officials focus on the care of populations or communities (Chap. 27). Public health physicians work to promote health to populations and to prevent disease. Public health physicians can work in government, hospitals, or public health organizations. An MPH degree would provide value for physicians working in the public health space. Typically, public health employees are not paid as much as physicians in clinical practice. Salaries range from $175 K to $340 K.

Careers in Hospital Administration

Hospital administrators can be some of the highest-paid employees in healthcare, especially hospital CEOs at large medical centers who can have salaries in the multimillion-dollar range. Smaller hospitals tend to pay their CEOs less, with salaries in the $150 K to $300 K range. The average hospital CEO salary is about $450 K in the USA. Of course, becoming a hospital CEO requires work, and typically, hospital CEOs have a long career in hospital administration. For physicians, a typical career path means starting out as a service line chief, then moving to medical director, then moving up to chief medical officer, then chief operating officer, and then CEO. Obviously, the MHA degree is designed for such a career path. An MBA or MPH may also be helpful in these roles.

Careers in Academic Administration

For some practicing physicians, becoming an academic administrator is an attractive alternative to clinical medicine. The highest level of such a career is to become a medical school dean or Vice President/President. However, all medical school deans started their administrative careers as department chairs or associate/assistant deans. Department chairs tend to get their roles by establishing excellence in their specialty or subspecialty. The typical department chair has a salary between $300 K and $600 K. Assistant and Associate deans get their jobs through established expertise in a mission of the medical school (student affairs, admissions, faculty affairs, research, etc.). Assistant and associate deans earn between $300 K and

$400 K, depending on job title, scope of work, and their underlying specialty. Because most deans were once department chairs or assistant or associate deans, the typical medical school dean is in their 60 s. More and more, medical school deans have at least one additional advanced degree in addition to their MD degrees. Different medical schools have different requirements for deans. Some want distinguished careers in science where a PhD would be advantageous. Some want good managers where an MBA, MPH, or MMM degree may be desirable. Medical school deans have an average tenure of only 4 years. This is due to the complexities of the job and the political nature of their appointments. The typical medical school dean is paid between $500 k and well over $1 million depending on the size of the school and the scope of their responsibility.

Back to the Case

Kate decided to sit down with the chief medical officer at her hospital. The CMO recounted her career path, including obtaining an MBA degree. The two of them agreed that a good start for Kate might be running for chief of staff at the hospital, an elected position. Kate also decided to look into getting an MHA degree.

Key Takeaways

- MPH, MBA, or MMM degrees may be helpful for nonclinical careers in medicine.
- Typically, obtaining a senior role outside of clinical medicine is a step-wise process; getting an entry-level position is important to building a compelling resume.
- Salaries vary for physicians in nonclinical careers. Some may be quite lucrative.

30 Five Numbers You Need to Know

Case Marc (Not the Author of This Book!)
Marc (unrelated to one of the authors of this book) has been in practice with a small group practice for 5 years. Marc was asked to join the quarterly meeting with the practice's accountant. He reviewed the profit and loss statement with the CPA and a few of the doctors. It became apparent to Marc that the doctors showed little interest in the trend of rising accounts receivable. When Marc asked about this rising trend, the doctors were like deer caught in the headlights. Marc wanted to take a greater interest in the numbers used to measure the practice's progress and productivity.

Charges and Receipts

The total charges of the practice refer to the gross charges or the total fees for services provided by the practice. This number represents the total work submitted for payment to patients and third-party insurance companies. It would be a wonderful world if we could receive compensation for those gross charges. Guess what? It is not a wonderful world!

The key real-world number to know is the amount of money you *collect* for your services. The net receipts are the most important number to monitor. These are the *net receipts,* which consist of the gross receipts minus the refunds to patients and insurance companies. It is easier to collect money at the point of service when the patient is in the office. Why? Every time you try to collect an amount more than 6 months after the service was provided, it will cost the practice approximately $ 30 for each collection attempt. You are unlikely to collect amounts owed to you that are more than 180 days past due.

The gross collection percentage is a metric that you should review monthly, quarterly, and annually. The gross collection percentage is calculated by dividing the payments received by the total charges. For example, if the practice collected $750,000 in revenues and the charges were $1,000,000, that would translate into a 75% gross collection rate.

You will also want to review charges and the net collection percentage (NCP). The net collection percentage is calculated by dividing the total payments by the charges *minus* any contractual adjustments. For example, if the collections are $750,000 and the charges are $1,000,000 minus $200,000 in adjustments, the NCP is 93.77%. A well-run practice should have an NCP greater than 97%. This metric compares your current practice to your past performance from the previous month, quarter, or year.

How is the charge data helpful? If you notice a decline in gross collections, investigate why this metric of gross charges is decreasing.

N. Baum, M. J. Kahn, *Business Basics for your Healthcare Practice*,
https://doi.org/10.1007/978-3-032-25241-8_30

Why was there a decrease in gross collections? Was there an increase in Medicaid charges considerably lower than third-party payer charges? Was there an increase in contractual write-offs and an increase in adjustments? If that is the case, do you need to consider renegotiating your contracts with the insurance companies? Was there an increase in costly staff turnover? Staff turnover, especially in the billing departments, is likely to result in a decrease in collections. Therefore, it is essential to identify why staff members are leaving the practice and address that issue.

RVUs

Next, examine the relative value units (RVUs). RVUs measure physician productivity over a month, quarter, or year. This metric is often used to calculate compensation for employed physicians. This number is also helpful for negotiations with hospitals and insurance companies. The calculation of RVUs considers the complexity of the service or procedure, the time required to complete the work, the labor involved, the materials or equipment needed for the service, the supplies required, and the consideration of malpractice expenses. The Centers for Medicare and Medicaid Services (CMS) then multiplies the RVUs for each service or procedure by a "conversion factor," which is $32.3465 in 2025. The conversion factor is the dollar amount used to convert the total relative value units (RVUs) for a specific procedure into a Medicare reimbursement amount. The CF is adjusted annually by CMS based on the Medicare Economic Index (MEI) and other factors. For example, if a physician generated 700 RVUs in the last quarter, their RVU value is 700 times the conversion factor of $32.3465, or $ 22,642.50. The hospital or employer typically uses this calculation to assess a physician's productivity and determine their salary or compensation.

A wRVU, or work relative value unit, is a unit of measurement used in the healthcare industry to determine the relative value of a specific medical service or procedure. The value of a wRVU is determined by several factors, including the complexity of the procedure, the time and skill required to perform the procedure, and the cost of the necessary equipment and supplies.

There is no standard conversion rate for a wRVU to dollars, as the value of a wRVU can vary depending on the specific medical service or procedure being performed and the geographic location where it is performed. The CF is adjusted annually by CMS based on the Medicare Economic Index (MEI) and other factors. Additionally, private insurance companies and Medicaid may have different conversion rates for wRVU to dollars.

Accounts Receivable

The metric of accounts receivable (AR) is also a necessary metric to monitor. The gross accounts receivable is equal to the charges minus the payments or the receipts. The net AR is the charges minus any contractual allowances or discounts minus the receipts or what has been collected.

This number is what the practice is likely to collect in the future. For example, if the charges are $1,000,000 and the contractual allowances are $200,000, the practice is "owed" $800,000. If the practice has received only $750,000 in payments, then the net AR is $50,000, representing the fees that are likely to be collected. It is the AR that distinguishes good management from poor financial management.

The aging of AR is a fundamental metric that should be reviewed regularly. Most practice management systems will place AR in buckets of 1–60 days, 61–120 days, 121–180 days, and more than 180 days. Ideally, you would like the bulk of the AR to be below 60 days, as these ARs are likely to be collectible. ARs greater than 180 days will seldom be collected. Therefore, it is imperative to monitor these three or four buckets of AR to keep the majority of the ARs in the 1–60 days category.

Days in AR are part of the AR metric. The days in AR are equal to the total AR divided by the average daily charges (ADC). This latter number is like the quarterly charges divided by 90 days. This metric measures the efficiency of the practice's billing and collection processes.

The greater the days in AR, the less efficient the practice. Suppose you are monitoring the trend in ARs and notice an increase in the number of days with rising ARs. In that case, consider how quickly physicians post charges or how fast the billing staff submits charges to the payor. Another possibility is that a payor is delinquent or delayed in paying the practice, and the payor needs to know that this is unacceptable.

The AR ratio is the ratio of total accounts receivable to the average monthly billings, typically calculated using the last 3 months of charges or billings. For example, if the previous month's AR was $448,000 in uncollected fees and the prior 3 months' billings were $396,000 ($132,000 per month), the AR ratio is $448,000/$132,000 or 3.4 months (102 days). The AR ratio of 3.4 represents 3.4 months of payments due to your practice. The goal for a primary care practice is to maintain an AR ratio of 1.5–2.5, and for a specialty or surgical practice, the goal should be less than 2.0–3.0. The primary difference between a primary care practice and a surgical practice is that surgical practices typically perform more complex and expensive procedures. You must collect these higher fees from insurance companies that are not as prompt at paying at the time of service when compared with a primary care practice.

Charge Lag

Another essential metric is monitoring the charge lag between the date the service is performed and the date the fee is submitted to the insurance company. Ideally, this number should be close to zero or 1 day. A delay means that the practice could better submit charges to third-party payers. If the charge lag is too long, checking on the process of filing claims in a timely fashion would be appropriate to solve the problem.

Denials

Denial is not a river in Egypt! A claim to an insurance company must be submitted accurately to receive compensation for your services. A "clean claim" refers to a claim that is processed and paid without being returned because of errors. Historically, 10–15% of claims are "dirty" and denied because of errors in submitting the claim. Also, it is of interest that nearly 50% of denied claims are never refiled, which means you are leaving money on the table that is owed to you. The good news is that more than 90% of denied claims are preventable. Denied claims require meticulous attention to detail. For example, the claim will be rejected if the patient's insurance number is not accurately keyed in or if the patient's name is misspelled. The insurance company will deny the claim. The insurance company will hold your money, and your practice will spend additional time and expense refile the claim. Therefore, the billing clerk must be a perfectionist, or you will lose money that honestly belongs to you and your practice.

Marc on Metrics

Marc recognized that the practice did not understand basic business principles and that at least one of the physicians needed to take on the responsibility of reviewing just a few KPIs. Marc accepted that role. Once a month, Marc would spend just a few minutes with the office manager to review these KPIs, and once a quarter, he and the office manager would meet with the practice's CPA to discuss these key metrics. As a result, Marc was able to identify financial issues crucial to the practice's success. Marc's partners were pleased that someone in the practice was reviewing these numbers and taking corrective action when problems arose.

Bottom Line on Business Metrics

You need to understand these concepts to understand the value of your services. The minimum metrics to follow regularly are charges, receipts, RVUs, accounts receivable, charge lag, and denials. Remember the "buck" starts and stops with the doctor! Finally, medicine is a business; if you want to be a successful doctor, you need to understand business basics. We hope that we have instilled in you the desire to be a small businessperson and that you will have an enjoyable and profitable practice.

Don't forget that the "buck" starts and stops with you, the doctor! Ultimately, medicine is a business, and to be a successful doctor, you must understand the fundamentals of business. We hope that we have instilled in you the importance of being a small businessperson and that you will have an enjoyable and profitable practice.

Medicine is a great profession. However, like any other profession, it is a business, and a proper understanding of business principles and practices is necessary to be successful. You don't need to be an MBA to understand the principles of business. However, it is essential to monitor just five metrics to understand the progress and productivity of your practice.

Key Takeaways

- You don't need an MBA to understand the fundamental business principles of a medical practice.
- Reviewing key performance indicators, KPIs, can be easily accomplished in just a few minutes each month.
- Monitoring these KPIs ensures the financial success of a medical practice.

31 Future of Medicine

Case. @Rayco

@rayco graduated from medical school in 2026, and she has been in an equity fund-owned primary care practice since completing her residency with Healthcare America (HA) 15 years ago. HA is the country's largest healthcare conglomerate, initially formed from the nation's largest independent insurer, a large hospital system, a pharmacy benefits company, and a major retail outlet. @rayco enjoys the coaching aspect of primary care. The group has enrolled eight thousand patients. The patients she sees have already used HA's proprietary software to receive their diagnosis. The software boasts an error rate of less than 5 per 100,000 patients. The software immediately feeds to HA's proprietary electronic health record (EHR) and prescribes a therapeutic plan for each patient. In fact, the EHR feeds information to the on-site pharmacy so that patient's current medications as well as OTC medications and supplements are available prior to the patient's appointment. During residency, @rayco learned how to modify patient behavior and provide healthcare coaching, which are key skills for an effective primary care provider. @rayco is thrilled that her calculated value score, based on both the quality of her care and her costs/patient, places her in the top 10% regarding patient satisfaction, productivity, and cost effectiveness of all of the primary care providers in her network. As a result, she enjoys a 12% bonus on her base annual salary.

In 1957, three agricultural scientists, Joe M. Bohlen, George M. Beal, and Everett M. Rogers at Iowa State University, published a model of technology adoption that continues to have relevance today [1]. In this model, the process of technology adoption is defined as a bell curve. The first group to use the product, on the far-left tail of the bell curve, is called *innovators*. The next group, moving from left to right, is called *early adopters*. These are followed by *early* and *late majorities*. On the far right are the *laggards*. This model has several limitations, the least of which is that it assumes a linear and continuous model for technology adoption.

The late Clayton Christenson, a former professor at the Harvard Business School and once considered the foremost authority on innovation and technology, in his classic book, *The Innovator's Dilemma*, described "disruptive technologies" [2]. One of the key features of dis-

N. Baum, M. J. Kahn, *Business Basics for your Healthcare Practice*,
https://doi.org/10.1007/978-3-032-25241-8_31

ruptive technologies is that their adoption is not linear, but rather S-shaped such that initial adoption is low, followed by rapid implementation that eventually levels off. This is because incorporating innovation is slow and iterative. Initial improvements provide minimal value to the consumer. However, over time, these improvements have become drastically better than previous enhancements, leading to rapid product adoption. At the end of the product's lifestyle, the improvements are marginal. For example, consider the mobile phone. Initially, those phones were large, expensive, cumbersome, and unreliable. Few people owned them. Apple's iPhone was dramatically better. Apple has sold more than 3 billion phones since its introduction in 2007! Now consider the most recent iPhone models; they are better than the last model, but not by much. Sales have slowed considerably; thus, they are on the right side of the S-shaped curve.

Disruptive technologies are defined as innovations that interrupt or displace a traditional technology or existing market in order to solve or improve upon a problem that is currently in use. This creates a new market by displacing older technology. In healthcare, these disruptive innovations will often come at a lower cost, with an enhancement in quality over the product, treatment, or technique that it replaces. Over time, these disruptive innovations improve in quality and performance and eventually take over the market. For example, in medicine, ultrasound was originally developed as a less expensive alternative to standard X-rays. Over time, ultrasound technology improved, providing enhanced images such that today, using a handheld device, point-of-care ultrasound is a necessary skill and requirement in many specialties.

In healthcare, retail outlets, such as Walmart, have opened urgent care clinics staffed mostly by mid-level providers, i.e., physician assistants, nurse practitioners, or medical assistants. These are cheaper alternatives to hospital-owned clinics or staffing these clinics with medical doctors. Assuming the level of care and the quality of care provided to a patient are related to the number of hours of clinical training completed by the provider, the outcomes may be of lower quality. However, looking to the future, assuming these clinics are disruptive innovations, we can predict that they will disrupt the market for primary care services and slowly become the standard of care and the dominant model. Especially as mid-level providers gain experience and expertise over time. As another example, pharmacies are monitoring patients' blood pressure and offering to provide vaccines such as flu and shingles vaccines to patients. This is convenient to patients and is provided at a lower cost than going to a physician's brick-and-mortar office. And then consider the ease of access for patients seeking medical care at Walmart, Costco, or their local pharmacy compared to the long waits for an appointment to see a doctor in their office. You can easily see why patients are moving in large numbers to these disruptive delivery systems of healthcare.

The danger of disruptive innovation is that established companies typically view the disruptive technology as unattractive, and consequently, it is often initially ignored. The established market leaders can be blindsided as technology takes off, leaving them far behind. Remember what happened to Blockbuster video stores with the arrival of Netflix, or observe what is happening to retail stores, which are being replaced by Amazon. Fast forward, Amazon is continuing to disrupt the market and is now competing with FedEx, UPS, and the United States Postal Service by delivering its own packages, and in record time. Because of the size of the healthcare market, currently more than $5 trillion per year, and the rising cost of medical care and medications, healthcare is ripe for disruption.

What are the traditional forces that define and shape US healthcare?

Healthcare in the USA is distinguished as a predominately private, complex, multi-payer system that has focused on scientific and technologic advances. In the recent past, insured patients did not bear the full cost of their medical care due to coverage often paid by the employer, and so patients were not incentivized to consume less services, nor were their providers financially motivated to control the costs of medical care. In addition, competing special interests from physicians, hospitals, insurers, pharma, and patient advocacy groups have all worked to strengthen their position in the policy landscape, sometimes to the detriment of high-value care. Each of these components contributes to the higher costs, with little accountability regarding quality or outcomes.

Although the rate of healthcare growth has slowed somewhat in recent years, [3] it has not reached a ceiling. As more of the economy's resources are devoted to health care, less is available for other goods and services. While jobs within the healthcare sector are generally higher paying, if the overall growth of healthcare outpaces that of the rest of the economy, Americans will find themselves less able to access and afford the medical care they need. American businesses are also faced with the burden of growing healthcare costs as they struggle to provide benefits to their employees and remain competitive internationally [4].

Future Changes in Reimbursement

The fee-for-service (FFS) model often results in over-utilization of low-value and unnecessary care [5]. FFS impedes coordination of care for patients across the healthcare system [6]. The FFS model is not sustainable, especially with an increase in the baby boomer population, as 10,000 baby boomers turn 65 every day, [7] and those with chronic and complex health needs [8] are also increasing. As long as providers are rewarded for the volume of care delivered, as in FFS arrangements, instead of the value provided, they are pressured to deliver more care, and population healthcare costs will continue to rise without regard to improvement in patient outcomes. Both private and public payers of healthcare have recognized this and have begun to shift their payment models that are soon going to be tied to outcomes and to quality of care. Newer payment models are intended to reduce the cost of care and improve the quality of care.

The previous paradigm was for doctors to provide a service, perform a procedure, or order a test. The more tests and procedures that the doctor did, the greater the compensation. That payment method, fee for service (FFS), worked for many decades, but the future of that model is no longer tenable. There is probably no greater disruption to modern healthcare than the movement from payment for the volume of care provided to the value of care delivered. Multiple changes are occurring every day, making it difficult for young or new physicians to navigate.

For employed physicians, FFS may be computed as the relative value unit (RVU) metric, but it is still based on "you eat what you kill." (Isn't that a moronic term applied to the healthcare profession where we take an oath "to do no harm" and to restore health and certainly not to kill patients?)

In addition to changes in physician reimbursement, employers have recently started shifting costs to employees by requiring employees to contribute a percentage of their insurance premiums and offering employees high-deductible health plans (HDHP), which reduces the annual insurance premiums. In 2024, enrollment in HDHPs is 50% of insured workers, up from 4% in 2006 [9]. As more patients are enrolled in HDHPs and responsible for their initial care, these patients are more likely to demand transparency of healthcare costs as well see better results or outcomes. Ultimately, today's employees want to understand what they are receiving for their increased payments.

The Department of Health and Human Services is striving to have most of Medicare FFS payments tied to quality or value in the next few years. Value is defined as quality divided by cost. Medicare's new payment reform system, the Medicare Access and CHIP Reauthorization Act (MACRA), will help the organization to reach that goal. MACRA consolidates previous quality reporting systems to streamline tracking and reporting and thus further encourages value-based care over volume of care provided. If previous policy changes are any indication, as Medicare goes, so too will private insurance also follow very quickly.

Indeed, the future of medicine is moving from volume to value. If a young physician can demonstrate that they can adapt to new incentives by improving costs while maintaining and enhancing their quality and their outcomes, these young physicians will be more competitive in the changing marketplace.

Future Importance of Medical Quality Assessment

The importance of quality in healthcare may seem obvious. It is emphasized by the Hippocratic Oath that physicians take, attesting *primum non nocere,* or, first, to do no harm. Poor quality of care can also mean higher costs—whether it be through providing unnecessary care that results in iatrogenic disease or forgoing important preventive care that ultimately results in greater disease burden requiring more expensive medical care. Of course, quality matters to patients as well. Patients want to receive quality healthcare even if it is difficult to assess. To this end, providers are likely to face competition based on the quality they provide. As the forces at play continue to transition incentives from volume to value, quality of care will be tied to provider payment, and properly measuring quality will be of primary importance.

Defining quality in healthcare is not a simple task, because quality holds different meanings to different stakeholders. However, the widely used Institute of Medicine (IOM) definition of quality encapsulates a broad understanding of quality as "the degree to which health services for individuals and populations increase the likelihood of desired health outcomes and are consistent with current professional knowledge" [10]. The IOM further specifies that high-quality care should be safe, effective, patient-centered, timely, efficient, and equitable [11].

How will we improve outcomes in the future?

Proper measurement is the first step to improve outcomes. Tracking how patients fare can largely be achieved through electronic medical records. Many physicians overestimate their performance on quality measures until they are provided with their performance data. To this end, continuous feedback on improvement also needs to be available to providers. From this feedback, payers can reward providers not only for achieving specific quality standards, but also for incremental improvements. By providing ongoing feedback for progressively better results, instead of continuing to penalize for not meeting a benchmark, providers are encouraged to find innovative ways to improve.

Other approaches to improve quality include public reporting of outcomes, although research is mixed on the effectiveness of this method [12]. If patients see comparisons between providers, it may promote competition or at last an incentive to improve quality. One of the problems with this method is that providers may find ways to game the measurement process.

How can we continuously improve quality?

- Continuously assess and revise metrics to accurately reflect quality that matters to Stakeholders.
- Assess whether process measures continue to accurately reflect outcomes.
- Revise standards and clinical practice guidelines concurrent with new evidence.
- Promote a learning atmosphere—less punitive, more encouraging of success.
- Promote effective communication within and between organizations.
- Maintain and improve IT systems to accurately and efficiently capture care and outcomes.
- Use outcomes that are easiest to track and difficult to manipulate.

The healthcare profession is about to experience a tsunami regarding payment models that focus on value and quality. No longer will volume of patients seen or number of services provided be the metric for payment and reimbursement. Providers, payers, patients, and also the government will have to make a big adjustment by moving from volume to value. We believe that the success of a medical practice is going to depend on the speed at which the healthcare profession can make these transitions.

Future Outcome Metrics

In the past, outcomes consisted of measuring survival, length of stay, or readmission rates. Those certainly are metrics that are important, but now it will be necessary to go beyond those basic outcome measurements and start recording and documenting additional data that will clearly demonstrate superior outcomes.

Outcome measurement plays a pivotal role in medical decision-making for physicians, payors, and patients who are searching for high-quality medical care. It is outcome measurements that quantify components of quality, such as clinical outcomes, patient satisfaction, and the functional status of our patients.

The end results of outcome measurement identify patterns and trends and provide the healthcare profession with the effectiveness, or even the lack of effectiveness, of our medical interventions. By recording outcomes, we can maximize favorable outcomes and can minimize poor outcomes. As a result of obtaining and recording outcomes, we can demonstrate quality of care, which will hopefully lead to improved medical care and lower cost.

The benefits of outcome measurements prevent overuse, underuse, and misuse of healthcare services as well as enhancing patient safety. Outcome measurements also drive innovation and research and development, which enhances disease control and improvement in patient's quality of life. By tracking outcomes, payors and providers are held accountable for providing high-quality care. When the outcomes are transparent, patients can make informed choices regarding their care and can select providers who have stellar outcome data. Also, when outcomes are measured, there is competition among payers and providers, and with increased competition, prices are certainly going to decrease. Finally, patients with improved outcomes are more engaged in their care, more committed to treatment plans, and more receptive to medical advice.

Back to Case @Rayco

@rayco continued on with Healthcare America. She participated in seminars and workshops offered by her specialty society and improved her coaching skills. Because she was able to significantly modify some of the high-risk behavior evident in her patient panel, she continued to receive bonuses for her outstanding care. In addition to improving the quality of her care, she also learned more about the cost structure of her care through participation in several hologram-based learning exercises. This led to further improvement in her value scores. @rayco went on to produce several hologram-based exercises on her own so that her colleagues could benefit from her innovations.

Key Takeaways

Yogi Berra said, "You've got to be very careful if you don't know where you're going because you might not get there." The future of medicine will include alterations in payment with a focus on value rather than volume. Quality measurement and assessment will be critically important features of these newer models. You need to know that the quality train is leaving the station....all aboard!

References

1. Bohlen JM, Beal GM, Rogers EM. The adoption of two farm practices in a Central Iowa community. In: Agricultural and home economics experiment station, vol. 26. Iowa State University of Science and Technology; 1960.
2. Christensen CM. The innovator's dilemma: when new technologies cause great firms to fail. Harvard Business Review Press; 2013.
3. Cutler DM, Sahni NR. If slow rate of health care spending growth persists, projections may be off by $770 billion. Health Affair. 2013;32(5):841–50.
4. Sood N, Ghosh A, Escarce JJ. Employer-sponsored insurance, health care cost growth, and the economic performance of U.S. industries. Health Serv Res. 2009;44(5p1):1449–64.

5. Shen J, Andersen R, Brook R, Kominski G, Albert PS, Wenger N. The effects of payment method on clinical decision-making. Med Care. 2004;42(3):297–302.
6. Institute of Medicine. Rewarding provider performance: aligning incentives in Medicare. Washington: National Academies Press; 2006.
7. Ortman JM, Velkoff VA, Hogan H. An aging nation: the older population in the United States. Washington: US Census Bureau; 2014. https://www.census.gov/prod/2014pubs/p25-1140.pdf. Accessed Sept 10, 2025
8. Wu S, Green A. Projection of chronic illness prevalence and cost inflation. Washington: DC RAND Health; 2000.
9. High deductible health plans and health savings accounts. U.S. Bureau of Labor Statistics, 2025. https://www.bls.gov/ebs/factsheets/high-deductible-health-plans-and-health-savings-accounts.htm. Accessed Sep 2025
10. Institute of Medicine. Medicare: a strategy for quality assurance. Washington: National Academies Press; 1990.
11. Institute of Medicine. Crossing the quality chasm: a new health system for the 21st century. Washington: National Academies Press; 2001.
12. Fung CH, Lim YW, Mattke S, Damberg C, Shekelle PG. Systematic review: the evidence that publishing patient care performance data improves quality of care. Ann Intern Med. 2008;148(2):111–23.

32 Final Message on the Business of Medicine

A 2025 survey by Medical Economics on the top challenges facing our profession has shown that 50% of physicians are pessimistic about confronting business challenges [1].

The healthcare industry has witnessed significant changes in recent years, with increasing emphasis on transitioning from fee-for-service to value-based care. To thrive in this dynamic environment, physicians must familiarize themselves with the business side of medicine. Physicians must develop an understanding of financial statements, budgeting, and revenue cycle management to ensure the economic health of their practice.

It was just a few decades ago that marketing and practice promotion were frowned upon. In today's competitive healthcare market, effective marketing strategies are crucial for attracting and retaining patients. It is necessary to be well-versed in digital marketing techniques and patient engagement strategies.

Efficient practice operations, including staff management, scheduling, and workflow optimization, are crucial for delivering high-quality patient care, and it is essential to ensure that every patient has a positive experience with the practice.

Despite the rapid changes occurring in healthcare, there are multiple opportunities for all to grow and improve, and to embrace emerging trends, including the adoption of artificial intelligence in contemporary healthcare. Those practices that implement the use of artificial intelligence will have practices that will certainly be more efficient and more productive. Doctors won't be replaced by AI, but doctors who don't use AI will be replaced by doctors who do. We believe that we have nothing to fear and that AI will not replace us.

The development of business acumen confers several advantages for physicians. Those who engage with basic business principles are positioned for leadership roles within healthcare organizations, such as medical directors or administrators.

A well-managed practice encourages physicians to invest in state-of-the-art technology and facilities, ultimately leading to better patient outcomes.

By effectively managing the financial aspects of their practice, physicians can secure their financial future and provide long-term stability for their families.

Business knowledge empowers physicians to make informed decisions, negotiate contracts effectively, and collaborate with other healthcare stakeholders, such as insurers and administrators.

As physicians, our primary responsibility lies in delivering exceptional patient care. However, this does not negate participating in business management. Our advice is that physicians must strive to achieve a balance between clinical medicine and the business aspects of healthcare.

N. Baum, M. J. Kahn, *Business Basics for your Healthcare Practice*,
https://doi.org/10.1007/978-3-032-25241-8_32

We must stay up-to-date with emerging trends in both clinical medicine and healthcare business management. Just as we must participate in continuing medical education, it is helpful to participate in professional development courses, conferences, and meetings that focus on business development.

To have an enjoyable practice, it is necessary to have effective time management principles to balance patient care, administrative tasks, and business management responsibilities.

Because clinical medicine is constantly evolving, we need to seek advice from experienced colleagues and consider hiring business professionals, such as consultants, CPAs, lawyers, marketing advisors, and social media experts, to assist with the management of our practices.

The very last bottom line:

In today's rapidly evolving healthcare landscape, physicians must embrace the importance of business acumen as well as clinical expertise. By developing a strong understanding of business principles and applying them to their daily practice, physicians can ensure the success and sustainability of their careers while delivering the highest quality care to their patients.

We hope this book has been helpful and provided you with a roadmap to have an enjoyable and profitable practice. We would like to hear from you if you have any comments and suggestions for a future edition.

Advice to Dr. Everyone: Read this book!

Key Takeaways

- Medicine is making the transition from quantity to quality of healthcare.
- We have an opportunity to take back healthcare from the algorithms to offer empathy and compassion that a computer or AI can't deliver.
- Healthcare is the greatest profession on this planet. Let's not allow our profession to spiral out of control and slip away.
- The future of healthcare is in the generation of large language models, algorithms, and AI.
- The patients still want a doctor who offers empathy and compassion and knows just the basics of the principles of business.

Reference

1. Reynolds K. Top challenges 2025, physicians. Practice. 2025;

Index

A

Academic administration, 249
Academic career
  academically based clinicians, 238
  academic job *vs.* private practice, 238
  academic physicians, 238–239
  clinical cases, 237
  instructor/assistant professor, 239
  in medicine, 237
  vs. private practice salaries, 237
  promotion process, 239
  tenure, 239, 240
  tenure clock, 239
Academic medical centers (AMCs), 237, 238
Academic physicians, 238–240
Academic positions, 239
Acceptance, 19
Accounts receivable (AR), 252, 253
ACE inhibitors, 65
Achieving wealth, 1
Advance notice provisions, 143
Airline industry, 75
Amazon, 64, 80
American Marketing Association (AMA), 76
American Medical Association (AMA), 32
American Medical Group Association (AMGA), 22
American Medical Student Association (AMSA), 35
American Research and Development Corporation (ARDC), 243
American Telemedicine Association (ATA), 151
Artificial intelligence (AI), 4, 179, 261
Assistant professor, 239
Association of American Medical Colleges (AAMC), 22
Authorization form, 143
Average daily charges (ADC), 252

B

Balance sheet, 15, 16
Basic accounting, 13, 14
Basic accounting equation, 15
Billing staff submits charges, 253
Black swan, 133
Blogging, 113
Bonds, 27, 28, 243
Bookkeeping, 14
Brainstorming sessions, 79
Branding, 75
  academic practice, 79
  Amazon and Nike, 80
  benefits of, 77
  brainstorming sessions, 79
  competitors, 79
  definition, 76, 77
  Kaila's story, 80
  opportunity, 78
  skills, staff, facility, operating systems, and principles, 78
  transportation, 77, 78
  urology practice, 79
Buddy system, 44
Bundled payment programs, 229
Bureau of Engraving and Printing, 29
Bureau of Labor Statistics, 103
Burnout, 5, 104
  causes of, 136–137
  definition, 135
  solutions, 138
  stress, 136
  symptoms, 137
Business
  acumen, 261, 262
  challenges, 261
  development, 262
  principles, 6, 261, 262

C

Calcium channel blockers, 65
Cardinal rule, 57, 58
Cash flow statement, 14, 16
Centers for Medicare and Medicaid Services (CMS), 150, 152, 153, 229, 252
Charge lag, 253
Charges, 251–253
Chicago Board Options Exchange, 28

N. Baum, M. J. Kahn, *Business Basics for your Healthcare Practice*,
https://doi.org/10.1007/978-3-032-25241-8

Chief Wellness Officer, 138
Chronic care management, 227
Claims made policy, 91, 92, 143
Clean claim, 253
Clinical care model, 238
Clinician educators, 238
Collect, 251–253
Community health education, 35
Compensation, 20
Compliance, 159, 162–163
Compliance with national imperatives, 33
Compounded interest, 10, 11
Comprehensive medication management, 162
Concierge medicine
 advantages, 234
 annual fee, 235
 applicable for, 234
 complicated process, 234
 concept of, 231
 consumers and providers, 232
 definition, 231
 direct-to-consumer model, 233
 EHRs, 232
 employer-provided healthcare coverage, 232
 fee-for-service model, 235
 by Fildes, Luke, 233
 insurance reimbursement, 234
 medical profession, 233
 original house call, 233
 personalized care, 233, 235
 transition process, 234
 US providers practice, 231
 work-life balance, 235
Concierge primary care, definition, 231
Consent-to-settle clause, 92
Consulting, 249
Contracting with Insurance Companies, 41, 42
Contracts
 acceptance, 19
 consideration, 19
 legal agreement, 19
 offer, 19
 state law, 145
Cooperative projects, 66
Coronavirus, 149–150
Corporatization of medicine, 244
COVID-19, 103, 149, 152, 153, 228
 infection, 128
Credentialing process, 38, 41
Crisis management
 black swan, 133
 communication plan, 132
 cyberattack, 133, 134
 financial crisis, 132
 HIV, 133
 Hurricane Katrina, 132, 134
 job descriptions, 131
 leadership, 133
 patient history, 131
 recovery plan, 131
 thematic goal, 131, 132
Current Procedural Terminology (CPT) codes, 153, 155, 156
Current ratio, 16
Curveball questions, 83, 84
Customer relationship management (CRM) system, 125, 129
Cyberattack, 133, 134

D
Data encryption program, 134
Debt management, 53–56
Deferred-compensation arrangements, 143
Deferred compensation payments, 143
Denial, 253
Departing physician, 141–143, 145
Depression, 137
Derivatives, 28
Digital marketing techniques, 261
Direct loan program, 54
Direct-to-consumer model, 233
Disruptive innovation, 256
Disruptive technology, 255–256
Diversification, 26
Doctor-patient encounter, 179, 181
Double-entry accounting, 13, 14
Doximity, 116
Drug-drug interactions, 159, 162

E
Early adopters, 255
Early majority, 255
Economic dynamics, 3
Efficient practice operations, 261
Electronic contact method, 129
Electronic health record (EHR), 136, 137, 150, 255
Electronic medical record (EMR), 59
Electronic monitors, 162
Electronic survey tool, 171
Embarrassment, 60
Emotion, 132
Employee turnover, 103
Employment agreement, 141–143
Employment contract, 20–22, 145
Employment state's laws, 145
Employment lawyers, 89
End-stage renal disease program, 229
Enforcement, 21
Erectile dysfunction (ED), 20, 65
Ethically creating positive reviews, 166–167
Exchange traded funds (ETFs), 27
Explanation of Benefits (EOBs), 218
Extended repayment, 54

F
Facebook, 112, 113
Facts of life, 68, 69
Fair Labor Standards Act (FLSA), 86
Family and Medical Leave Act (FMLA), 86

Federal Trade Commission (FTC), 167
Fee-for-service (FFS) model, 234–235, 257, 261
Fildes, Luke, 233
Financial statements, 13, 14, 16
Firing, 89
Fixed income investments, 27
Focus groups, 172
Follow-up semen analysis, 130
Free video chat apps, 148
Future of medicine
  disruptive technologies, 255, 256
  FFS, 257
  outcome measurements, 258, 259
  payment models, 257, 258
  quality in healthcare, 258
  US healthcare, 256, 257

G

Generative pretrained transformer (GPT-4)
  blog site, 210
  coding and classification, 180
  communication, 180
  create realistic medical images, 180
  definition, 179
  doctor-patient encounter, 181
  encounter, procedures, and tests, 216–217
  EOBs, 218
  ethical concerns, 223–224
  fact-check AI content, 223
  FAQs, 206
  generate new drug molecules, 180
  history of innovation, 180
  informed consent, 201
  job description online, 201
  leverage negative prompting, 223
  medical articles, 217
  mistakes/hallucinations, 221–223
  negative online reviews, 196
  OpenAI models, 180
  patient educational materials, 213
  patients communication, 181
  personalized treatments, 180
  predict disease progression, 180
  prior authorization, 193
  prompt generator, 220
    consent creation, 221
    diagnosis and symptoms, 220
    emergencies and first aid, 220
    medical ethics and guidelines, 220
    medical procedures, 220
    medical research and updates, 220
    medication information, 220
    patient communication, 220
    preventive care, 220
    professional development, 221
    treatment and management, 220
    word count, 221
Genetic Information Nondiscrimination Act (GINA), 86
Gift-giving, 58, 67, 68
Graduated repayment, 54
Great resignation, 103
Gross charges, 251
Gross collection percentage, 251
Growth equity, 244
GT modifier, 156

H

Hallucinations, 221–223
Health Information Portability and Accountability Act (HIPAA), 42, 93, 136, 150
  -compliant platform, 150
  privacy laws, 167
  regulatory requirements, 43
Health policy innovators, 35
Health Professions Scholarship Program (HPSP), 55
Healthcare America (HA), 255
Healthcare attorney, 142, 145, 146
Healthcare industry, 261
High-deductible health plans (HDHP), 257
High-risk patients, 142
Hiring, 81, 85, 89, 97, 98
History of the present illness (HOPI), 99
Homework assignment, 83
Hospital-acquired condition reduction program, 229
Hospital administration, 249
Hospital-based purchasing program, 229
Hospital readmission reduction program, 229
Humanity, 124
Hunting approach, 124
Hurricane Katrina, 131, 132, 134

I

iHireAdvanced Practitioners, 97
Income-based plans, 54
Income-dependent repayment plan, 55
Income statement, 14–16
Indian Health Service, 55
Information system, 229
Information technology (IT), 148, 150
Informed consent, 151–152, 196, 201, 202, 220
Initiative to Support Promising Research (INSPIRE), 228
Innovators, 255
Instagram, 116, 180
Institute of Medicine (IOM), 258
Instructor, 239
Insurance billing software program, 43
Intensive care unit, 61
Intentional nonadherence, 159
Interest, 10
Interview process, 82, 83
Intra-specialty referrals, 66
Investment
  opportunity, 10
  portfolio, 26
  strategies, 25
iPhone models, 256

J
Job-listing services, 81
Journal club network, 64, 65, 73

K
Key performance indicators (KPIs), 253

L
Labor laws, 85
Late majority, 255
Legal process
  documentation, 88, 89
  follow up, 89
  termination of employees, 86–88
Liability insurance, 152
Lifetime value (LTV), 128
LinkedIn, 112
Litigation, 92
Loan repayment models, 53–56
Loan repayment program, 55

M
Malpractice, 97
  broker, 93
  carrier, 92, 93
  insurance, 91, 92
Managing negative reviews, 167–168
Marc on metrics, 253
Marketing, 57, 62–64, 67–69
Master of Business Administration (MBA), 247–250
Master of Health Administration (MHA), 247–250
Master of Medical Management (MMM), 247, 248, 250
Master of Public Health (MPH), 247–250
MedEdPORTAL, 239
Medical career, stages, 4–6
Medical divorce, 141
Medical economics, 261
Medical education, 53
Medical errors, 228
Medical Group Management Association (MGMA), 22
Medical license, 141
Medical malpractice insurance claims, 144
Medical profession, 233
Medicare Access, 257
Medicare Access and CHIP Reauthorization Act (MACRA), 257
Medicare Economic Index (MEI), 252
Medicare telehealth visits, 153
Medicare's new payment reform system, 257
Medication adherence, 159, 161, 162
  factor, 161
  follow-ups, 161, 162
  medication costs, 161
  patient communication, 161
  systematic approach, 161
Medication costs, 161
Medication nonadherence, 159–162
Medicine
  declining reimbursements, 4
  guaranteed employment opportunities, 4
  job security, 4
Menopause, 64
Mentor, 37, 43, 44
Middle-aged team member, 105
Mid-level providers (MLPs)
  benefits of, 98, 99
  cassandra, 101
  compensation for, 96, 97
  credentialing, 97
  need for, 97, 98
  outcomes and liability, 97
  patient history, 95
  scribe, 99, 100
  working, 95, 96
Model of medicine, 231
Modern healthcare, 4
Modifier 95, 156–157
Morning huddle, 106, 107
Mutual funds, 27

N
National Health Service Corps (NHSC), 55
National Institutes of Health (NIH), 55
National Labor Relations Act (NLRA), 86
National Practitioner Data Bank (NPDB), 93
Negotiation, 22, 23
Net collection percentage (NCP), 251
Net present value, 11
Net receipts, 251
Neutral impression, 125
Nike, 80
Nonadherence, medication
  consequences of, 160
  nonconforming, 159
  nonfulfillment, 159
  non-persistence, 159
Nonclinical careers
  in academic administration, 249, 250
  in consulting, 249
  in hospital administration, 249
  MBA degree, 247
  MHA degree, 248
  MMM degree, 248
  MPH degree, 247
  in pharmaceutical industry, 248, 249
  PhD, 248
  in public health, 249
Noncompete covenant, 145
Nonconforming adherence, 159
Nonfulfillment adherence, 159
Non-HIPAA-compliant platform, 150
Non-persistence adherence, 159

Nonunion, 86
Nurse practitioners (NPs), 96

O
Offer, 19
One-page marketing plan
  airline industry, 119
  LTV, 128, 129
  medical practice, 123
  messages, 122
  orchestrating and stimulating referrals, 129, 130
  personal enjoyment, 121
  phases, 120, 121
  PVP approach, 121
  social media, 123–127
  target market, 121
  USP, 122, 123
  World-class patient experience, 127, 128
Online reputation management
  clinical cases, 165–167
  ethically creating positive reviews, 166–167
  managing negative reviews, 167–168
OpenAI, 180, 224
Options, 28
  "puts" and "calls, 28
  insurance policy, 29
Organized medicine, 31–35
Outcome measurements, 258, 259
Ownership
  and business transactions, 21
  distribution, 22

P
Partnership, 22
Patient advocacy, 35
Patient engagement strategies, 261
Patient files ownership, 21
Patient satisfaction, 98
Patients perception, 77
  clinical cases, 169
  customizing the survey, 171
  FAQs, 176
  focus groups, 172
  follow-up, 174, 176
  implementation, 171
  invitations and reminders, 172–174
  patient surveys, 170
  personal interviews, 170
  results, 171–172
  suggestion box, 174
  surveying peers, 175–176
Patient surveys, 170
Pay as you earn (PAYE), 54
Pay for performance (P4P), 228
Payment method, 257
Payment models, 257, 258
Personal enjoyment, 121
Personal finance, 26
Personal interviews, 170
Personal money toward the expansion, 26
Personal value profitability (PVP) approach, 121
Pharmaceutical industry, 248, 249
Pharmacovigilance, 248
PhD, 247, 248, 250
Physician administrators, 238
Physician assistants (PAs), 96, 98
Physicians, 261, 262
  employment contract, 20, 22
  post charges, 253
  referrals, 57, 58, 69
  scientists, 238
  value modifier program, 229
Population health, 227–229
  chronic care management, 227
  health policy, 228
  information system, 229
  P4P, 228
  programs, 229
  public health, 228
  quality and safety, 228
  value-based care, 228, 229
Practice promotion, 67
Practice's policies, 142
Prior authorization (PA), 193–196, 223, 224
Privacy, 152
Private equity
  acquisition, 245
  advantages, 245
  bonds, 243
  disadvantage, 245
  firm, 243–245
  funds, 244
  healthcare, 243–245
  investments, 243, 244
  OxySys, 243
  risk and reward, 243
  SBICs, 244
  stocks, 243
Private Equity Stakeholder Project, 244
Problem-solving, 83
Professional development, 35
Promotion process, 239
Prostate-specific antigen (PSA), 193, 206, 207
Public health, 227, 228, 249
Public service loan forgiveness (PSLF), 54, 55

Q
Qualifying repayment plans, 54
Quality in healthcare, 258
Quarterly charges, 252
Quick response (QR) codes, 116, 117

R
Raving fans, 119, 127, 130
Razor-thin profit margins, 98
Reactivation campaign, 129

Receipts, 251–253
References
  employment, 84
  follow-up, 84
  release-of-information letter, 84, 85
  Rochelle's story, 85
Referral letter, 44, 59–61, 65, 70–71
Referral source, 68
Relative value units (RVUs), 252, 253, 257
Release-of-information letter, 84, 85
Repayment models, 54
Research and partnerships, 35
Restrictive covenants, 21, 23
Retainer medicine, *see* Concierge medicine
Retirement, 86
  money, 143
  plans, 143
Return on equity (ROE), 16
Return on your investment (ROI), 125
Revised pay as you earn (REPAYE) plans, 54
Rewards, 105
Risk-based programs, 229
Robots and artificial intelligence, 4
Rrestrictive covenants, 21

S

Salary, 19, 20, 237–240, 249
  information, 22, 23
  offsets, 22
Screening applicants, 82
Scribes, 99, 100
Securities and Exchange Commission (SEC), 243
Shared savings programs, 229
Shock-and-awe approach, 125
Shock-and-awe package, 125, 126
Simple interest, 10
Sit-and-wait approach, 130
Small Business Investment Act, 244
Small Business Investment Companies (SBICs), 244
Social determinants of health, 229
Social media
  blogging, 113
  Doximity, 116
  Facebook, 112, 113
  Instagram, 116
  LinkedIn, 112
  one-page marketing plan, 123–127
  QR codes, 116, 117
  TikTok, 115, 116
  use, 111, 112
  video cornerstone, 115
  X, 113
  YouTube, 114, 115
S-shaped curve, 256
Staff involvement, 105, 106
Staff meetings, 104
Stages of a physician's career, 4–6
Standard repayment, 54
Stock, 26, 243
  portfolio, 27
  price, 26
Streaming online workflow, 149
Student debt, 5
Suggestion box, 174
Suicide, 133, 137
Surveying peers, 175–176

T

Tail coverage, 143–146
Team building
  Bureau of Labor Statistics, 103
  burnout, 104
  COVID, 104
  cross-training, 104
  employee turnover, 103
  Great Resignation, 103
  morning huddle, 106, 107
  positive events, 105
  practice retreats, 108
    challenging, 107
    facilitation, 108, 109
    goals and objectives, 107
    nonclinical tasks, 107
    objectives, 109, 110
    preparation, 108
  staff involvement, 105, 106
  staff meetings, 104
Technology, 42
Telemedicine, 129
  advantage, 149
  compensation, 152
  coronavirus, 149–150
  cost and complexity, 150
  CPT codes, 155, 156
  feedback, 148–149
  final billing and coding advice, 156
  GT modifier, 156
  influences on practice workflow, 149
  informed consent, 151–152
  liability insurance, 152
  licensing, 151
  medicare telehealth visits, 153
  modifier 95, 156–157
  privacy, 152
  streaming online workflow, 149
  triangulation, 154, 155
  video platform, 148
  virtual check-ins, 153–154
  virtual services, 153
Tenure, 239–240
Tenure clock, 239
Termination, 21, 141, 144
Testosterone, 129
TikTok, 115, 116, 180

Time value of money, 9, 11
Top-notch staff, 81
Transition from training to practice, 43, 46
Triangulation, 154, 155

U
Uniformed Services Employment and Reemployment Rights Act (USERRA), 86
Unintentional nonadherence, 159
Union, 86
Unique service proposition (USP), 122, 123
United Parcel Service (UPS) truck drivers and physicians, 1, 2
Urinary incontinence, 66
US healthcare, 256, 257
US healthcare policymaking, 32

V
Value-based care, 228, 229
Value-based healthcare, 261
Value-based programs, 229
Venture capital, 244
Video platform, 148
Virtual check-ins, 153–154
Virtual services, for medicare patients, 153
Visibility, 77
Voluntary evaluation, 3

W
Website, 111, 112, 114, 116
Word-of-mouth, 77
  method, 57
  promotion, 123
Work relative value unit (wRVU), 20, 252
Working capital, 16
World Health Organization, 159

X
X, 113
X-ray technician, 87

Y
YouTube, 114, 115

MIX
Papier aus verantwortungsvollen Quellen
Paper from responsible sources
FSC® C105338

If you have any concerns about our products,
you can contact us on
ProductSafety@springernature.com

In case Publisher is established outside the EU,
the EU authorized representative is:
Springer Nature Customer Service Center GmbH
Europaplatz 3, 69115 Heidelberg, Germany

Printed by Libri Plureos GmbH
in Hamburg, Germany